2015

The Year Book of
NEONATAL AND PERINATAL MEDICINE®

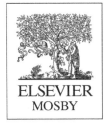

ELSEVIER
MOSBY

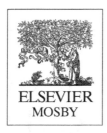

Vice President, Global Medical Reference: Mary Gatsch
Editor: Kerry Holland
Developmental Editor: Susan Showalter
Production Supervisor, Electronic Year Books: Donna M. Skelton
Electronic Article Manager: Mike Sheets
Illustrations and Permissions Coordinator: Dawn Vohsen

2015 EDITION
Copyright 2015, Elsevier, Inc. All rights reserved.

No part of this publication may be reproduced, stored in a retrieval system, or transmitted, in any form or by any means, electronic, mechanical, photocopying, recording, or otherwise, without prior written permission from the publisher.

Permission to photocopy or reproduce solely for internal or personal use is permitted for libraries or other users registered with the Copyright Clearance Center, provided that the base fee of $35.00 per chapter is paid directly to the Copyright Clearance Center, 21 Congress Street, Salem, MA 01970. This consent does not extend to other kinds of copying, such as copying for general distribution, for advertising or promotional purposes, for creating new collected works, or for resale.

Printed in the United States of America
Composition by TNQ Books and Journals Pvt Ltd, India
Printing/binding by Sheridan Books, Inc.

Editorial Office:
Elsevier
Suite 1800
1600 John F. Kennedy Blvd.
Philadelphia, PA 19106-3399

International Standard Serial Number: 8756-5005
International Standard Book Number: 978-0-323-35547-6

Editorial Board

Avroy A. Fanaroff, MD, FRCPE, FRCP&CH
Eliza Henry Barnes Chair of Neonatology, Rainbow Babies & Children's Hospital; Emeritus Professor, Department of Pediatrics and Reproductive Biology, Case Western Reserve University School of Medicine, Cleveland, Ohio

William E. Benitz, MD
Philip Sunshine Professor of Neonatology, Division of Neonatal and Developmental Medicine, Stanford University School of Medicine, Lucile Packard Children's Hospital, Palo Alto, California

Steven M. Donn, MD
Professor of Pediatrics, Division of Neonatal-Perinatal Medicine, C.S. Mott Children's Hospital, University of Michigan Health System, Ann Arbor, Michigan

Josef Neu, MD
Professor of Pediatrics, University of Florida College of Medicine, Gainesville, Florida

Lu-Ann Papile, MD
Professor of Pediatrics, Division of Neonatal-Perinatal Medicine, Indiana University School of Medicine, Riley Hospital for Children, Indianapolis, Indiana

Linda J. Van Marter, MD, MPH
Associate Professor of Pediatrics, Harvard Medical School; Vice-Chair, Department of Pediatric Newborn Medicine, Brigham and Women's Hospital, Boston, Massachusetts

Contributing Editors

David H. Adamkin, MD
Professor of Pediatrics; Director of Division of Neonatology; Director of Nutritional Research; Rounsavall Chair of Neonatal Medicine; Co-Director of Neonatal Fellowship, University of Louisville, Louisville, Kentucky

Monika Bhola, MD
Associate Professor, Department of Pediatrics, Case Western Reserve University; Director, Neonatal Follow-Up Clinic, Rainbow Babies & Children's Hospital, Cleveland, Ohio

Heather Burris, MD, MPH
Assistant Professor of Pediatrics, Division of Newborn Medicine, Boston Children's Hospital; Attending Neonatologist, Department of Neonatology, Beth Israel Deaconess Medical Center, Boston, Massachusetts

Kate Wan-Chu Chang, MA, MS
Department of Neurosurgery, University of Michigan, Ann Arbor, Michigan

Valerie Y. Chock, MD, MSEpi
Clinical Associate Professor of Pediatrics, Division of Neonatal and Developmental Medicine, Department of Pediatrics, Stanford University School of Medicine, Stanford, California

Karl C. Desch, MD
Assistant Professor, Department of Pediatrics and Communicable Diseases, Division of Neonatal-Perinatal Medicine, University of Michigan C.S. Mott Children's Hospital, Ann Arbor, Michigan

DeAnne Costello-Wilson, MD
Professor of Pediatrics, Case Western Reserve University; Director, Neonatal Follow-Up Clinic, Rainbow Babies & Children's Hospital; Director of Neonatology, UH Geauga Medical Center, Cleveland, Ohio

Jonathan M. Fanaroff, MD, JD
Associate Professor of Pediatrics, CWRU School of Medicine; Director, Rainbow Center for Pediatric Ethics; Co-Director, NICU, Rainbow Babies & Children's Hospital, Cleveland, Ohio

Jay P. Goldsmith, MD
Elsie Schaefer Professor of Pediatrics; Section Chief, Neonatology, Tulane University School of Medicine, New Orleans, Louisiana

Katherine E. Gregory, PhD, RN
Associate Director of Research, Department of Pediatric Newborn Medicine; Haley Nurse Scientist, Department of Nursing, Brigham and Women's Hospital, Boston, Massachusetts

Samir Gupta, DM, MD, FRCPCH, FRCPI
Professor of Neonatology, Durham University; Deputy Director, Research and Development; Consultant Neonatologist, University Hospital of North Tees, Stockton, United Kingdom

M. Jeffrey Maisels, MD, DSc
Chair Emeritus and Professor; Director, Academic Affairs, Department of Pediatrics, Oakland University William Beaumont School of Medicine, Beaumont Children's Hospital, Royal Oak, Michigan

Richard J. Martin, MD
Drusinsky-Fanaroff Chair in Neonatology; Professor of Pediatrics, Reproductive Biology and Physiology, Case Western Reserve University; Director, Neonatal Research Programs, Rainbow Babies & Children's Hospital, Cleveland, Ohio

Christopher McPherson, PharmD
Clinical Pharmacist, Department of Pediatric Newborn Medicine, Brigham and Women's Hospital; Instructor, Department of Pediatrics, Harvard Medical School, Boston, Massachusetts

Fernando Moya, MD
Medical Director, Betty Cameron Children's Hospital; CEO, Coastal Carolina Neonatology, PLLC, Wilmington, North Carolina

Robin K. Ohls, MD
Professor of Pediatrics; Director, Neonatal Research, University of New Mexico, Albuquerque, New Mexico

Brenda B. Poindexter, MD, MS
Professor of Pediatrics; Director of Clinical and Translational Research, Perinatal Institute, Cincinnati Children's Hospital Medical Center, Cincinnati, Ohio

Richard Polin, MD
William T. Speck Professor of Neonatology; Director, Division of Neonatology, Children's Hospital of New York; Professor of Pediatrics, Columbia University College of Physicians and Surgeons, New York, New York

Ann R. Stark, MD
Professor of Pediatrics, Vanderbilt University School of Medicine, Mildred Stahlman Division of Neonatology, Monroe Carell Jr Children's Hospital, Nashville, Tennessee

David K. Stevenson, MD
Harold K. Faber Professor of Pediatrics, Division of Neonatal & Developmental Medicine, Department of Pediatrics, Stanford University School of Medicine, Stanford, California

Eileen K. Stork, MD
Professor of Pediatrics, Case Western Reserve University; Director, Neonatal ECMO Program, Rainbow Babies & Children's Hospital, Cleveland, Ohio

Win Tin, FRCPCH
Professor of Paediatrics and Neonatal Medicine, The James Cook University Hospital, Middlesbrough, United Kingdom; Professor of Paediatrics and Neonatal Medicine, University of Durham, Durham, United Kingdom

Kristi Watterberg, MD
Professor of Pediatrics/Neonatology, University of New Mexico School of Medicine, Albuquerque, New Mexico

Thomas J. Wilson, MD
Department of Neurosurgery, University of Michigan, Ann Arbor, Michigan
Lynda J.-S. Yang, MD, PhD
Department of Neurosurgery, University of Michigan, Ann Arbor, Michigan

Table of Content

JOURNALS REPRESENTED	xi
INTRODUCTION	xiii
1. The Fetus	1
2. Epidemiology and Pregnancy Complications	7
3. Genetics and Teratology	27
4. Labor and Delivery	35
5. Infectious Disease and Immunology	55
6. Cardiovascular System	93
7. Respiratory Disorders	105
8. Central Nervous System and Special Senses	137
9. Gastrointestinal Health and Nutrition	167
10. Hematology and Bilirubin	203
11. Renal, Metabolism, and Endocrine Disorders	215
12. Miscellaneous	221
13. Pharmacology	235
14. Postnatal Growth and Development/Follow-up	245
15. Ethics	265
16. Behavior Pain	271
ARTICLE INDEX	279
AUTHOR INDEX	287

Journals Represented

Journals represented in this YEAR BOOK are listed below.
Acta Anaesthesiologica Scandinavica
Acta Ophthalmologica
Acta Paediatrica
Acta Paediatrica Journal of Paediatric
American Journal of Obstetrics and Gynecology
American Journal of Perinatology
American Journal of Roentgenology
Archives of Disease in Childhood
Archives of Disease in Childhood Fetal and Neonatal Edition
Arthritis Care & Research (Hoboken)
Australia & New Zealand Journal of Obstetrics & Gynaecology
Cell Biology International
Circulation
Clinical Infectious Diseases
Dermatology
Environmental Health Perspectives
Fertility and Sterility
Journal of Allergy and Clinical Immunology
Journal of Applied Physiology
Journal of Cellular Biochemistry
Journal of Pediatric Gastroenterology and Nutrition
Journal of Pediatric Orthopaedics
Journal of Pediatric Surgery
Journal of Pediatrics
Journal of Paediatrics and Child Health
Journal of Perinatology
Journal of the American Medical Association
Journal of the American Medical Association Ophthalmology
Journal of the American Medical Association Pediatrics
JPEN Journal of Parenteral and Enteral Nutrition
Lancet
National Vital Statistics Reports
Nature Medicine
New England Journal of Medicine
Nutrients
Obstetrics & Gynecology
Pediatric Infectious Disease Journal
Pediatric Neurology
Pediatric Research
Pediatrics
Scientific Reports
Thyroid
Transfusion
Ultrasound in Obstetrics & Gynecology

Standard Abbreviations

The following terms are abbreviated in this edition: acquired immunodeficiency syndrome (AIDS), cardiopulmonary resuscitation (CPR), central nervous system (CNS), cerebrospinal fluid (CSF), computed tomography (CT), deoxyribonucleic acid (DNA), electrocardiography (ECG), health maintenance organization (HMO), human immunodeficiency virus (HIV), intensive care unit (ICU), intramuscular (IM), intravenous (IV), magnetic resonance (MR) imaging (MRI), ribonucleic acid (RNA), and ultrasound (US).

Note

The YEAR BOOK OF NEONATAL AND PERINATAL MEDICINE® is a literature survey service providing abstracts of articles published in the professional literature. Every effort is made to assure the accuracy of the information presented in these pages. Neither the editors nor the publisher of the YEAR BOOK OF NEONATAL AND PERINATAL MEDICINE® can be responsible for errors in the original materials. The editors' comments are their own opinions. Mention of specific products within this publication does not constitute endorsement.

To facilitate the use of the YEAR BOOK OF NEONATAL AND PERINATAL MEDICINE® as a reference tool, all illustrations and tables included in this publication are now identified as they appear in the original article. This change is meant to help the reader recognize that any illustration or table appearing in the YEAR BOOK OF NEONATAL AND PERINATAL MEDICINE® may be only one of many in the original article. For this reason, figure and table numbers will often appear to be out of sequence within the YEAR BOOK OF NEONATAL AND PERINATAL MEDICINE®.

Introduction

It is with great pleasure that we have assembled the 28th rendition of the YEAR BOOK of Neonatal and Perinatal Medicine. Remarkably, the editors working independently selected a variety of topics for commentary, and we are able to include 16 different chapters. By size, the leading topics include gastroenterology and feeding, respiratory disorders, and disorders of the central nervous system, including special senses. Critical topics include a wealth of information on the human gastrointestinal biome (we are, after all, hosts for literally trillions of bacteria), important information on human colostrum and its critical role in establishing the immune defense system, the various benefits of human milk nutrition, and the evidence for and against refeeding measured gastric residuals.

Before addressing some of the other advances, I thought it would be interesting to see what was featured in the YEAR BOOK of Neonatal Perinatal Medicine 25 years ago and attempt to relate those topics to what takes place in 2015 in similar situations.

The commentaries in 1990 were selected from 6000 published studies, whereas today there are many more articles from which to select. A key article reported on the discovery of the cystic fibrosis gene, with the hope that the gene would be soon inserted into the body and the disease would be cured. As we are now aware, there are many mutations of the cystic fibrosis gene, and whereas the treatment of the disease has progressed at a rapid rate and long-term survival has improved, gene replacement therapy remains a distant prospect.

> The problem [with genetic research] is, we're just starting down this path, feeling our way in the dark. We have a small lantern in the form of a gene, but the lantern doesn't penetrate more than a couple of hundred feet. We don't know whether we're going to encounter chasms, rock walls or mountain ranges along the way. We don't even know how long the path is.
> —Francis S. Collins MD, PhD Director NIH

The 1990 YEAR BOOK also included randomized trials on surfactant (which was not yet available for general use) as well as ECMO and high frequency ventilation. In 2015, we review less invasive delivery of surfactant, await the emergence of aerosolized surfactants, and read more about minimally invasive ventilation, mainly CPAP. In 1990, there was an article on the reconstitution of the bone marrow of a child using cord blood. There have been substantial advances in stem cell research and therapy and management of the cord remains very topical. The 2015 YEAR BOOK includes a number of articles and critical comments relating to management of the cord. Milking of the cord is emerging as a viable, and some would even argue superior, alternate therapy to delayed cord clamping. The evidence from the randomized trials is presented. Indeed, there have been so many trials on management of the cord that the meta-analyses have been updated every two years.

An article of interest 25 years ago was on the use of an artificial larynx to stimulate the fetus. The article entitled "Vibro-acoustic Stimulation of the Human Fetus: Effect on Behavioral State Organization" by Visser et al (Early Human Dev 1989:19;285) reported that vibroacoustic stimulation performed to assess fetal health resulted in excessive fetal movements, a prolonged tachycardia, and disorganization of fetal state. My colleague Marshall Klaus called it a form of "fetal abuse" and recommended that it was time "to cease and desist as the risks seem greater than the benefits." This indeed has occurred and there are more sophisticated ways of assessing fetal behavior and well-being.

There was also an invited commentary by M. Jeffrey Maisels and Thomas B. Newman entitled "Jaundice in the Healthy Full Term Infant: Time for Reevaluation," which was the forerunner of the American Academy of Pediatrics Guidelines published in 1994. Their final paragraph rings so true: "If we can agree, and it seems that we should, that the laboratory investigation of most normal infants is painful for the infant, worrisome for parents, costly and rarely enlightening." The use of the transcutaneous bilirubin measurements (covered in 2015 YEAR BOOK), together with the published bilirubin nomograms and guidelines, have standardized the care of the full term newborn with jaundice.

The seeds for evidence-based practice today were already starting to flourish in 1990.

The 2015 volume includes a number of topics where more than one editor has commented on the same article, providing similar or, in some instances, different insights and perspectives. There are many randomized trials included, but it is frustrating to read the last sentence in many of these trials which call for further studies. It is time for the power analyses to be done *a priori*, and the studies to enroll sufficient patients to definitively answer the question posed.

All of the editors attempt to find articles and topics in journals, which may not be routinely available to our readers. We all strive to provide insight into clinical issues and to pose questions that when answered can close the gaps in our knowledge. We are forever grateful to our colleagues who lend their expertize to the process and enhance the quality of the book. We thank Kerry Holland, our executive editor, Barbara Cohen-Kligerman, and Susan Showalter for their continued assistance and for helping us to complete our task on time. We thank the Elsevier team for their professionalism and support in producing this book.

Avroy A. Fanaroff, MD
William E. Benitz, MD
Steven M. Donn, MD
Josef Neu, MD
Lu-Ann Papile, MD
Linda Van Marter, MD, MPH

1 The Fetus

Fetal Surgery: Principles, Indications, and Evidence
Wenstrom KD, Carr SR (Alpert Med School of Brown Univ, Providence, RI)
Obstet Gynecol 124:817-835, 2014

Since the first human fetal surgery was reported in 1965, several different fetal surgical procedures have been developed and perfected, resulting in significantly improved outcomes for many fetuses. The currently accepted list of fetal conditions for which antenatal surgery is considered include lower urinary tract obstruction, twin—twin transfusion syndrome, myelomeningocele, congenital diaphragmatic hernia, neck masses occluding the trachea, and tumors such as congenital cystic adenomatoid malformation or sacrococcygeal teratoma when associated with developing fetal hydrops. Until recently, it has been difficult to determine the true benefits of several fetal surgeries because outcomes were reported as uncontrolled case series. However, several prospective randomized trials have been attempted and others are ongoing, supporting a more evidence-based approach to antenatal intervention. Problems that have yet to be completely overcome include the inability to identify ideal fetal candidates for antenatal intervention, to determine the optimal timing of intervention, and to prevent preterm birth after fetal surgery. Confronting a fetal abnormality raises unique and complex issues for the family. For this reason, in addition to a maternal-fetal medicine specialist experienced in prenatal diagnosis, a pediatric surgeon, an experienced operating room team including a knowledgeable anesthesiologist, and a neonatologist, the family considering fetal surgery should have access to psychosocial support and a bioethicist.

▶ This is not the typical article that we usually select for the Year Book. However, it represents a wonderful historical review as well as state-of-the-art of fetal surgery ranging from intrauterine transfusions to the EXIT procedure. The striking inability to find better tocolytic agents and avoid the inevitable premature delivery after invasion of the fetal domain continues to frustrate perinatal specialists.
There is extensive discussion of all the randomized trials including the MOMS trial dealing with in utero repair of neural tube defects. Although the infants did better, there were risks to the mother because maternal-fetal surgery for repair of myelomeningocele requires an upper-segment hysterotomy, which increases maternal postsurgical risks. Belfort[1] reported repairing a fetus with a L3-S1 meningomyelocele by laparotomy and fetoscopic repair using a 2-port,

in-CO_2 approach at 23 2/7 weeks of gestation. The neonate was delivered at 30 6/7 weeks of gestation by lower segment cesarean delivery and required no further surgery, has not needed a shunt (5 months), and has normal, age-appropriate neurologic function. If and when fetoscopic repair of myelomeningocele achieves better fetal outcomes while at the same time decreasing maternal risks, it would be a better option. The section on twin-to-twin transfusion is interesting and evidence-based, as are the management of the many renal lesions. Hydronephrosis in utero presents an ongoing challenge with the search for the best markers ongoing. Most of these lesions are best handled after delivery.

It was rather revealing for the authors to note "importantly, as neonatal care of preterm newborns has improved, and with the advent of betamethasone, magnesium sulfate for neuroprotection, and surfactant, elective preterm delivery has become preferable to fetal intervention in many cases." Advances in imaging, application of the new genetics, and improved ability to follow the natural progression of many of these lesions will reinforce the concepts expressed in this article and assist with more precise timing when interventions are needed. Perhaps many of these lesions will be managed less invasively and with better long-term outcomes.

A. A. Fanaroff, MBBCh, FRCPE

Reference

1. Belfort MA, Whitehead WE, Shamshirsaz AA, Ruano R, Cass DL, Olutoya OO. Fetoscopic repair of meningomyelocele. *Obstet Gynecol*. 2015 [Epub ahead of print].

Risk of selected structural abnormalities in infants after increased nuchal translucency measurement
Baer RJ, Norton ME, Shaw GM, et al (California Dept of Public Health, Richmond; Univ of California, San Francisco; Stanford Univ School of Medicine, CA)
Am J Obstet Gynecol 211:675.e1-675.e19, 2014

Objective.—We sought to examine the association between increased first-trimester fetal nuchal translucency (NT) measurement and major noncardiac structural birth defects in euploid infants.

Study Design.—Included were 75,899 singleton infants without aneuploidy or critical congenital heart defects born in California in 2009 through 2010 with NT measured between 11-14 weeks of gestation. Logistic binomial regression was employed to estimate relative risks (RRs) and 95% confidence intervals (CIs) for occurrence of birth defects in infants with an increased NT measurement (by percentile at crown-rump length [CRL] and by ≥3.5 mm compared to those with measurements <90th percentile for CRL).

Results.—When considered by CRL adjusted percentile and by measurement ≥3.5 mm, infants with a NT ≥95th percentile were at risk of having ≥1 major structural birth defects (any defect, RR, 1.6; 95% CI, 1.3—1.9; multiple defects, RR, 2.1; 95% CI, 1.3—3.4). Infants with a NT measurement ≥95th percentile were at particularly high risk for pulmonary, gastrointestinal, genitourinary, and musculoskeletal anomalies (RR, 1.6-2.7; 95% CI, 1.1—5.4).

Conclusion.—Our findings demonstrate that risks of major pulmonary, gastrointestinal, genitourinary, and musculoskeletal structural birth defects exist for NT measurements ≥95th percentile. The ≥3-fold risks were observed for congenital hydrocephalus; agenesis, hypoplasia, and dysplasia of the lung; atresia and stenosis of the small intestine; osteodystrophies; and diaphragm anomalies.

▶ Nuchal translucency (NT) is a hypoechoic region in the posterior neck at the level of the cervical spine between the skin and soft tissues found at 10 to 14 weeks' gestation. Normal values are usually less than 2.5 mm, but these values must be related to the crown-rump length and gestational age. Increased NT measurements place the fetus at increased risk for chromosomal and structural abnormalities. How reliable are these NT measurements? Cuckle et al[1] sought to evaluate the performance of first trimester NT measurement by providers (physician-sonologists and sonographers within the Nuchal Translucency Quality Review program). They reviewed a million and a half evaluations, related to crown-rump length and concluded, "Even with extensive training, credentialing, and monitoring, there remains considerable variability between NT providers. There was a general tendency toward under-measurement of NT compared with expected values, although more experienced providers had performance closer to that expected."

Three primary theories exist to explain the presence of increased NT: altered composition of the cellular matrix, abnormalities of the heart and great arteries, and disturbed or delayed lymphatic vessels. It is possible that the mechanisms consistently implicated as leading to increased NT also hold etiologic clues for defects where there is a propensity for increased NT. This is an impressive report from California establishing beyond reasonable doubt an association between increased NT and major noncardiac malformations in euploid infants. Infants with NT measurements above the 95th percentile, adjusted for crown-rump length were at risk for a variety of anomalies involving the lung, gastrointestinal tract, diaphragm, brain (hydrocephalus), genitourinary, and musculoskeletal systems. Surprisingly, this is the first large study addressing this question. The association between increased NT and an abnormal karyotype as well as critical congenital heart disease had been established. Why did it take so long to look beyond these anomalies in fetuses with increased NT in the first trimester?

A. A. Fanaroff, MBBCh, FRCPE

Reference

1. Cuckle H, Platt L, Thornburg L, et al. Nuchal translucency quality review (NTQR) program: first one and half million results. *Ultrasound Obstet Gynecol.* 2015;45:199-204.

Accuracy of prenatal ultrasound in detecting jejunal and ileal atresia: systematic review and meta-analysis

Virgone C, D'antonio F, Khalil A, et al (Univ of London, UK; St George's Univ of London, UK; et al)
Ultrasound Obstet Gynecol 45:523-529, 2015

Objective.—The accuracy of prenatal ultrasound examination in detecting jejunal and ileal atresia has been reported in the literature to be highly variable, at 25—90%. The aim of this systematic review was to evaluate the accuracy of prenatal ultrasound in detecting non-duodenal small bowel atresia (ND-SBA).

Methods.—MEDLINE, EMBASE and The Cochrane Library, including The Cochrane Database of Systematic Reviews (CDSR), Database of Abstracts of Reviews of Effects (DARE) and The Cochrane Central Register of Controlled Trials (CENTRAL), were searched electronically. The overall detection rate of jejunal or ileal atresia using ultrasound was reported. The accuracy of using polyhydramnios and dilated loops of bowel as diagnostic signs was also explored.

Results.—Sixteen studies involving 640 fetuses were included in this review. The detection rate of ND-SBA by prenatal ultrasound was highly variable, with values ranging from 10 to 100%, with an overall prediction of 50.6% (95% CI, 38.0—63.2%). When analyzed separately, the detection rates of jejunal and ileal atresia were 66.3%, (95% CI, 33.9—91.8%) and 25.9% (95% CI, 4.0—58.0%), respectively. Both dilated loops of bowel and polyhydramnios as diagnostic signs for ND-SBA provided a low overall detection rate.

Conclusions.—The diagnostic performance of prenatal ultrasound in identifying ND-SBA is extremely variable. Large studies are needed in order to identify objective and combined criteria for the diagnosis of these anomalies.

▶ In the United States, congenital anomalies are now the leading cause of neonatal mortality, surpassing extreme prematurity and respiratory disorders. Advances in technology have markedly improved the ability to recognize congenital anomalies in the fetus. Complemented by the noninvasive fetal plasma-free DNA from maternal blood, more and more diagnoses are made earlier in gestation. Nonetheless, many lesions are still difficult to detect despite all these advances. The article abstracted here is 1 of 2 reports from the same group exploring the accuracy of prenatal ultrasound in identifying jejunal and ileal atresia. The initial publication was from John et al,[1] followed by the literature review including only 640 subjects and published by Virgone. They report that the sensitivity of ultrasound in detecting small bowel atresia beyond the duodenum has a sensitivity of 50% and a specificity of 71%. If the bowel is dilated ≥17 mm and polyhydramnios is present beyond 32 weeks' gestation, the sensitivity is increased to 67% and the specificity to 80%.[1]

Because ultrasound missed so many lesions beyond the duodenum, careful consideration needs to be given to other potential warning signs. For example, Baer et al,[2] who probed the California Genetic Screening program, reported that nuchal thickness (NT) screens above the 95th percentile were strongly associated with congenital malformations. When considered by crown-rump length—adjusted percentile and by measurement ≥3.5 mm, infants with a NT ≥95th percentile had a 2-fold risk of having ≥1 major structural birth defects. There was also a more than 3-fold risk for congenital hydrocephalus; agenesis, hypoplasia, and dysplasia of the lung; atresia and stenosis of the small intestine; osteodystrophies; and diaphragm anomalies.

Approximately 1 in 1000 infants will require abdominal surgical intervention.

A. A. Fanaroff, MBBCh, FRCPE

References

1. John R, D'Antonio F, Khalil A, Bradley S, Giuliani S. Diagnostic accuracy of prenatal ultrasound in identifying jejunal and ileal atresia. *Fetal Diagn Ther.* 2015 [Epub ahead of print].
2. Baer RJ, Norton ME, Shaw GM, et al. Risk of selected structural abnormalities in infants after increased nuchal translucency measurement. *Am J Obstet Gynecol.* 2014;211:675.e1-675.e19.

Thoracoamniotic shunts for the management of fetal lung lesions and pleural effusions: a single-institution review and predictors of survival in 75 cases
Peranteau WH, Adzick NS, Boelig MM, et al (Children's Hosp of Philadelphia, PA; Univ of Pennsylvania, Philadelphia)
J Pediatr Surg 50:301-305, 2015

Purpose.—Hydrops and pulmonary hypoplasia are associated with significant morbidity and mortality in the setting of a congenital lung lesion or pleural effusion (PE). We reviewed our experience using in utero thoracoamniotic shunts (TA) to manage fetuses with these diagnoses.

Methods.—A retrospective review of fetuses diagnosed with a congenital lung lesion or pleural effusion who underwent TA shunt placement from 1998—2013 was performed.

Results.—Ninety-seven shunts were placed in 75 fetuses. Average gestational age (± SD) at shunt placement and birth was 25 ± 3 and 34 ± 5 weeks. Shunt placement resulted in a 55 ± 21% decrease in macrocystic lung lesion volume and complete or partial drainage of the PE in 29% and 71% of fetuses. 69% of fetuses presented with hydrops, which resolved following shunt placement in 83%. Survival was 68%, which correlated with GA at birth, % reduction in lesion size, unilateral pleural effusions, and hydrops resolution. Surviving infants had prolonged NICU courses and often required either surgical resection or tube thoracostomy in the perinatal period.

Conclusion.—TA shunts provide a therapeutic option for select fetuses with large macrocystic lung lesions or PEs at risk for hydrops and/or pulmonary hypoplasia. Survival following shunting depends on GA at birth, reduction in mass size, and hydrops resolution.

▶ This article reports a single-center experience in placing in utero thoracoamniotic shunts for fetal pulmonary lesions and pleural effusions. Seventy-five cases were reported over a 15-year period at the Center for Fetal Diagnosis and Treatment at Children's Hospital of Philadelphia. Nineteen fetuses received multiple shunts, bringing the total number of procedures to 97. About half had macrocystic congenital pulmonary airway malformation (CPAM), and half had pleural effusions. For those with CPAM, the change in lung lesion volume and CPAM volume-to-head circumference ratio were used to assess shunt effectiveness.

Shunt placement resulted in a 55% reduction in the macrocystic lung lesion volume and complete (29%) or partial (71%) drainage of pleural effusions. Data were analyzed to determine which, if any, factors were associated with improved survival, and gestational age, reduction in mass size, and resolution of hydrops were so correlated.

I commend these investigators for this review. They have the largest series to date and made an effort to analyze the results of their program. As with any retrospective observational study, it is difficult to draw many conclusions, especially when dealing with a rather heterogeneous patient group with a high risk of both mortality and morbidity. It would have been nice to know whether these parameters changed over the 15 years of the study period, both from the standpoint of experience gained by the fetal surgeons as well as the improvements in neonatal intensive care.

The authors also acknowledge that despite improvements in survival, there is a considerable complication risk with shunt placement, including shunt failure, occlusion, or migration. Chest wall deformities have been described with early (18–20 week) placement, and there was a high incidence of preterm delivery.

Determination of the long-term risk to benefit ratio will only be resolved through a large, multicenter randomized trial like the Management of Myelomeningocele Study (MOMS) trial for in utero myelodysplasia repair. Are we ready?

S. M. Donn, MD

2 Epidemiology and Pregnancy Complications

A population-based, multifaceted strategy to implement antenatal corticosteroid treatment versus standard care for the reduction of neonatal mortality due to preterm birth in low-income and middle-income countries: the ACT cluster-randomised trial
Althabe F, Belizán JM, McClure EM, et al (Inst for Clinical Effectiveness and Health Policy (IECS), Buenos Aires, Argentina; RTI International, Durham, NC; et al)
Lancet 385:629-639, 2015

Background.—Antenatal corticosteroids for pregnant women at risk of preterm birth are among the most effective hospital-based interventions to reduce neonatal mortality. We aimed to assess the feasibility, effectiveness, and safety of a multifaceted intervention designed to increase the use of antenatal corticosteroids at all levels of health care in low-income and middle-income countries.

Methods.—In this 18-month, cluster-randomised trial, we randomly assigned (1:1) rural and semi-urban clusters within six countries (Argentina, Guatemala, India, Kenya, Pakistan, and Zambia) to standard care or a multifaceted intervention including components to improve identification of women at risk of preterm birth and to facilitate appropriate use of antenatal corticosteroids. The primary outcome was 28-day neonatal mortality among infants less than the 5th percentile for birthweight (a proxy for preterm birth) across the clusters. Use of antenatal corticosteroids and suspected maternal infection were additional main outcomes. This trial is registered with ClinicalTrials.gov, number NCT01084096.

Findings.—The ACT trial took place between October, 2011, and March, 2014 (start dates varied by site). 51 intervention clusters with 47 394 livebirths (2520 [5%] less than 5th percentile for birthweight) and 50 control clusters with 50 743 livebirths (2258 [4%] less than 5th percentile) completed follow-up. 1052 (45%) of 2327 women in intervention clusters who delivered less-than-5th-percentile infants received antenatal corticosteroids, compared with 215 (10%) of 2062 in control clusters ($p < 0.0001$). Among the less-than-5th-percentile infants, 28-day neonatal mortality was 225 per 1000 livebirths for the intervention group and 232 per 1000 livebirths for the control group (relative risk [RR] 0·96, 95% CI 0·87–1·06, $p = 0·65$) and suspected maternal infection was reported in 236 (10%) of 2361 women in the intervention group and 133 (6%) of 2094 in the control group (odds ratio [OR] 1·67, 1·33–2·09, $p < 0·0001$). Among the whole population, 28-day neonatal mortality was 27·4 per 1000 livebirths for the intervention group and 23·9 per 1000 livebirths for the control group (RR 1·12, 1·02–1·22, $p = 0·0127$) and suspected maternal infection was reported in 1207 (3%) of 48 219 women in the intervention group and 867 (2%) of 51 523 in the control group (OR 1·45, 1·33–1·58, $p < 0·0001$).

Interpretation.—Despite increased use of antenatal corticosteroids in low-birthweight infants in the intervention groups, neonatal mortality did not decrease in this group, and increased in the population overall. For every 1000 women exposed to this strategy, an excess of 3·5 neonatal deaths occurred, and the risk of maternal infection seems to have been increased.

▶ The study was designed to assess the health effects of a population-based multifaceted strategy to identify women at high risk of preterm birth and administer antenatal corticosteroids in low-resource settings. This is the first such attempt at such a trial. Before commencing the study, a systematic review of the mortality data with the use of antenatal steroids was undertaken. According to an extensive literature, neonatal mortality was reduced 31% in babies who received either dexamethasone or betamethasone before delivery.[1] It was thus disturbing to find that despite increasing the use of antenatal corticosteroids to 45% of women delivering infants less than the 5th percentile for birth weight (the study definition of prematurity), compared with about 10% in control clusters, there was an increased mortality among the population exposed to antenatal steroids. Antenatal corticosteroids were used in 2322 (7%) of 33 870 of higher birth weight (≥25th percentile) births in the intervention group, compared with 279 (1%) of 36 511 in the control group. Similarly among infants born at a gestational age of 37 weeks or older, 3198 (8%) of 38 594 in the intervention group and 424 (1%) of 41 385 in the control group received antenatal corticosteroids. Thus, more larger, mature infants were exposed to steroids, and although overall 28-day neonatal mortality in the preterm infants did not differ between the intervention and the control groups (relative risk [RR] 0.96, 95% confidence interval [CI] 0.86–1.08, $P = .497$), a higher mortality was seen in the intervention group for infants born at a gestational age of 37 weeks or older (RR 1.21, 95% CI 1.07–1.36, $P = .0018$). The authors are delving into the reasons for the increased mortality and have postulated that it relates to infection. This cannot be verified from their data because the information related to infections was not rigorously collected.

The message that you cannot extrapolate findings from developed countries with precise definitions of gestational age to countries with limited resources is loud and clear. Great caution must be exercised before scale-up of antenatal corticosteroids to reduce preterm deaths in low-income settings.[2,3] Whereas antenatal corticosteroids are beneficial and lifesaving for infants between 23 and 34 weeks' gestation, they may be harmful beyond these gestational ages.[4]

A. A. Fanaroff, MBBCh, FRCPE

References

1. Roberts D, Dalziel S. Antenatal corticosteroids for accelerating fetal lung maturation for women at risk of preterm birth. *Cochrane Database Syst Rev.* 2006;(3): CD004454.
2. McClure EM, de Graft-Johnson J, Jobe AH, et al. A conference report on prenatal corticosteroid use in low- and middle-income countries. *Int J Gynaecol Obstet.* 2011;115:215-219.
3. Azad K, Costello A. Extreme caution is needed before scale-up of antenatal corticosteroids to reduce preterm deaths in low-income settings. *Lancet Glob Health.* 2014;2:e191-e192.
4. Porto AM, Coutinho IC, Correia JB, Amorim MM. Effectiveness of antenatal corticosteroids in reducing respiratory disorders in late preterm infants: randomised clinical trial. *BMJ.* 2011;342:d1696.

A Universal Transvaginal Cervical Length Screening Program for Preterm Birth Prevention
Orzechowski KM, Boelig RC, Baxter JK, et al (Thomas Jefferson Univ, Philadelphia, PA)
Obstet Gynecol 124:520-525, 2014

Objective.—To evaluate a universal transvaginal ultrasonogram cervical length screening program on the incidence of a cervical length 20 mm or less and adherence to the management protocol for a cervical length less than 25 mm.

Methods.—We conducted a prospective cohort study of women with singleton gestations 18 0/7 to 23 6/7 weeks of gestation eligible for universal transvaginal ultrasonogram cervical length screening over an 18-month period. Only women receiving antenatal care at our institution were included. Women with a prior spontaneous preterm birth and without delivery data available were excluded. A transvaginal ultrasonogram cervical length of less than 25 mm was managed according to a predetermined protocol. Primary outcomes were the incidence of a cervical length 20 mm or less and adherence to the management protocol for a cervical length less than 25 mm. Secondary outcomes were the incidences of spontaneous preterm birth at less than 37, less than 34, or less than 32 weeks of gestation among women undergoing transvaginal ultrasonogram cervical length screening compared with those not screened.

Results.—One thousand five hundred sixty-nine of 2,171 (72.3%) eligible women underwent transvaginal ultrasonogram cervical length screening. Overall, 17 (1.1%, 95% confidence interval [CI] 0.66—1.74) women had a cervical length 20 mm or less before 24 weeks of gestation. Management protocol deviations occurred in nine women with a cervical length less than 25 mm (43%, 95% CI 24.3—63.5). There was no difference in the incidence of spontaneous preterm birth at less than 37 weeks of gestation (4.1 compared with 4.7%, adjusted odds ratio [OR] 0.91, 95% CI 0.57—1.45), less than 34 weeks of gestation (1.5 compared with 1.3%, adjusted OR 1.19, 95% CI 0.52—2.74), or less than 32 weeks of gestation (0.8 compared with 0.8%, adjusted OR 0.0.76, 95% CI 0.26—2.25) among women receiving transvaginal ultrasonogram cervical length screening compared with those not screened.

Conclusion.—In a universal transvaginal ultrasonogram cervical length screening program, the incidence of a cervical length 20 mm or less was 1.1% in women with singleton gestations without prior spontaneous preterm birth. Protocol deviations occurred in 43% of women with a cervical length less than 25 mm. The incidence of spontaneous preterm birth was similar among women undergoing transvaginal cervical length screening compared with those not screened.

Level of Eviedence.—II.

▶ Prematurity remains a tremendous burden for obstetricians and neonatologists. Preterm birth is the leading cause of perinatal morbidity and mortality worldwide. Although the rates of prematurity and stillbirth have declined globally, further reduction in these 2 parameters remains a major health care priority and Millennium Goal. In the United States, congenital malformations are now the leading cause of neonatal mortality; however, prematurity remains a major contributor to perinatal mortality and long-term morbidity. Short cervical length has been identified as the most accurate way to predict preterm delivery. One of the mechanisms leading to a clinically silent, short cervix in midtrimester is the untimely decline in progesterone action. There have been a number of randomized trials exploring the use of vaginal progesterone to prevent preterm delivery in women with a short cervix. Some of these trials have generated significant controversy and discussion.[1-7]

Romero[1] concluded in a review that "Vaginal progesterone can reduce the rate of preterm delivery by 45% and the rate of neonatal morbidity (admission to the neonatal intensive care unit, respiratory distress syndrome, need for mechanical ventilation, etc.). To prevent one case of spontaneous preterm birth < 33 weeks of gestation, 11 patients with a short cervix would need to be treated (based on an individual patient meta-analysis).[2,3] Vaginal progesterone reduces the rate of spontaneous preterm birth in women with a short cervix, both with and without a prior history of preterm birth. In patients with a prior history of preterm birth, vaginal progesterone is as effective as cervical cerclage to prevent preterm delivery." However, van Os et al[4] concluded that "In women with a short cervix, who are otherwise low risk, we could not show a significant benefit of progesterone in reducing adverse neonatal outcome and preterm birth." Winer et al[5] were also unable to demonstrate the benefits of progesterone. They concluded that "17 hydroxy progesterone caproate did not prolong pregnancy in women with singleton gestations, a sonographic short cervix, and other risk factors of preterm delivery (prior history, uterine malformations cervical surgery, or prenatal DES exposure)." Parry and Elovitz[6] agreed that large randomized controlled trials have demonstrated that universal maternal cervical length screening and treatment with daily vaginal progesterone in women with short cervical length reduces the risk of preterm birth, but they were concerned by the large numbers of women who need to be screened to detect those with short cervices and prevent a relatively small number of preterm births. They raised some interesting points regarding universal screening including "(1) the standards of quality and reproducibility for transvaginal ultrasound cervical length ascertainment; and (2) the implications of screening on the application of therapeutic strategies to populations not known to benefit (so-called "indication creep"). Optimal strategies to employ cervical ultrasound and progesterone treatment might be revealed by additional studies investigating cervical length cutoffs, frequency of screening, selective screening in higher-risk groups, and the use of transabdominal cervical length screening as a surrogate for transvaginal cervical length screening." Pizzi et al[7] have indeed found cervical measurement and the intervention to be cost-effective.

The data from the study abstracted her speaks for itself. Short cervix is uncommon (1.1%), and less than half the women so identified followed the treatment protocol. The debate on progesterone and a short cervix will no doubt continue.

A. A. Fanaroff, MBBCh, FRCPE

References

1. Romero R, Yeo L, Chaemsaithong P, Chaiworapongsa T, Hassan SS. Progesterone to prevent spontaneous preterm birth. *Semin Fetal Neonatal Med.* 2014;19:15-26.
2. Hassan SS, Romero R, Vidyadhari D, et al. Vaginal progesterone reduces the rate of preterm birth in women with a sonographic short cervix: a multicenter, randomized, double-blind, placebo-controlled trial. *Ultrasound Obstet Gynecol.* 2011;38:18-31.
3. McKay LA, Holford TR, Bracken MB. Re-analysis of the PREGNANT trial confirms that vaginal progesterone reduces the rate of preterm birth in women with a sonographic short cervix. *Ultrasound Obstet Gynecol.* 2014;43:596-597.
4. van Os MA, van der Ven AJ, Kleinrouweler CE, et al. Preventing preterm birth with progesterone in women with a short cervical length from a low-risk population: a multicenter double-blind placebo-controlled randomized trial. *Am J Perinatol.* 2015 [Epub ahead of print].
5. Winer N, Bretelle F, Senat MV, et al; Groupe de Recherche en Obstétrique et Gynécologie. 17 alpha-hydroxyprogesterone caproate does not prolong pregnancy or reduce the rate of preterm birth in women at high risk for preterm delivery and a short cervix: a randomized controlled trial. *Am J Obstet Gynecol.* 2015; 212:485.e1-485.e10.
6. Parry S, Elovitz MA. Pros and cons of maternal cervical length screening to identify women at risk of spontaneous preterm delivery. *Clin Obstet Gynecol.* 2014; 57:537-546.
7. Pizzi LT, Seligman NS, Baxter JK, Jutkowitz E, Berghella V. Cost and cost effectiveness of vaginal progesterone gel in reducing preterm birth: an economic analysis of the PREGNANT trial. *Pharmacoeconomics.* 2014;32:467-478.

Urinary Bisphenol A Levels during Pregnancy and Risk of Preterm Birth
Cantonwine DE, Ferguson KK, Mukherjee B, et al (Brigham and Women's Hosp, Boston, MA; Univ of Michigan School of Public Health, Ann Arbor)
Environ Health Perspect, 2015 [Epub ahead of print]

Background.—Preterm birth (PTB), a leading cause of infant mortality and morbidity, has a complex etiology with a multitude of interacting causes and risk factors. The role of environmental contaminants, particularly bisphenol A (BPA), is understudied with regards to PTB.

Objectives.—In the present study we examined the relationship between longitudinally measured BPA exposure during gestation and PTB.

Methods.—A nested case-control study was performed from women enrolled in a prospective birth cohort study at Brigham and Women's Hospital in Boston during 2006-2008. Urine samples were analyzed for BPA concentrations at a minimum of three time points during pregnancy on 130 cases of PTB and 352 randomly assigned controls. Clinical classifications of PTB were defined as "spontaneous", which was preceded by spontaneous preterm labor or preterm premature rupture of membranes, or "placental", which was preceded by preeclampsia or intrauterine growth restriction.

Results.—Geometric mean concentrations of BPA did not differ significantly between cases and controls. In adjusted models, urinary BPA averaged across pregnancy was not significantly associated with PTB. When examining clinical classifications of PTB, urinary BPA late in pregnancy was significantly associated with increased odds of delivering a spontaneous PTB. After stratification on infant's sex, averaged BPA exposure during pregnancy was associated with significantly increased odds of being delivered preterm among females, but not males.

Conclusions.—These results provide little evidence of a relationship between BPA and prematurity, though further research may be warranted given the generalizability of participant recruitment from a tertiary teaching hospital, limited sample size, and significant associations among females and within the clinical subcategories of PTB.

▶ Cantonwide and colleagues performed a nested case-control study of 130 preterm cases and 352 full-term controls to analyze associations between maternal urine bisphenol-A (BPA) concentrations and preterm birth. They used a hospital-based cohort in Massachusetts of mother-infant pairs from 2006 to 2008. They analyzed BPA at a minimum of 3 time points during pregnancy to assess a mother's average BPA exposure. This is an improvement over previous studies and important because BPA has a short half-life. Geometric mean concentrations did not differ between cases and controls. However, a secondary analysis revealed positive associations between BPA and odds of spontaneous preterm delivery specifically among female infants. The null results of the primary analysis of this study might be due to lack of power to detect an association and/or potential misclassification given that a woman's overall BPA exposure, given that the exposure might not be captured even with 3 time points of collection given the rapid urinary excretion of BPA.

H. H. Burris, MD, MPH

Climate change is associated with male:female ratios of fetal deaths and newborn infants in Japan
Fukuda M, Fukuda K, Shimizu T, et al (M&K Health Inst, Ako, Japan; Shimizu Women's Clinic, Takarazuka, Hyogo, Japan; et al)
Fertil Steril 102:1364-1370, 2014

Objective.—To evaluate whether climate change is associated with male:female ratios (sex ratios) of fetal deaths and births in Japan.
Design.—A population-based cohort study.
Setting.—Not applicable.
Patient(s).—Newborn infants and fetuses spontaneously aborted after 12 weeks of gestation.
Intervention(s).—None.
Main Outcome Measure(s).—Yearly sex ratios of fetal deaths and newborn infants and monthly fetal death rates and sex ratios of newborn infants.
Result(s).—A statistically significant positive association was found between yearly temperature differences and sex ratios of fetal deaths; a statistically significant negative association was found between temperature differences and sex ratios of newborn infants from 1968 to 2012, and between sex ratios of births and of fetal deaths. The sex ratios of fetal deaths have been increasing steadily along with temperature differences, whereas the sex ratios of newborn infants have been decreasing since the 1970s. Two climate extremes, a very hot summer in 2010 and a very cold winter in January 2011, showed not only statistically significant declines in sex ratios of newborn infants 9 months later in June 2011 and October 2011 but also statistically significant increases of fetal death rates immediately, in September 2010 and January 2011.
Conclusion(s).—The recent temperature fluctuations in Japan seem to be linked to a lower male:female sex ratio of newborn infants, partly via increased male fetal deaths. Male concepti seem to be especially vulnerable to external stress factors, including climate changes (Fig 1).

▶ A decline in male births after environmental stresses is apparently a well-known phenomenon. This article cites articles where sex ratios are related to latitude, temperature, toxins, and earthquakes to be related to sex ratio birth differences. They thus questioned whether sex ratio along with fetal death could be affected by recent large fluctuations in climate. Using several decades of data, they found that along with changes in temperature fluctuations, there was a significant positive correlation with male fetal death and subsequent birth sex ratios (Fig 1). They also evaluated 2 separate periods after a

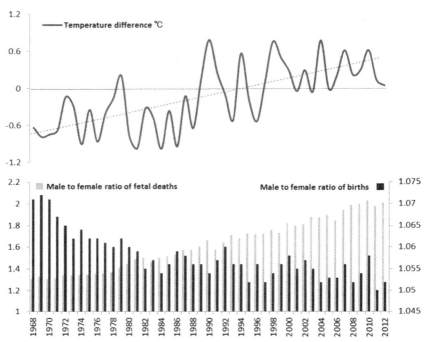

FIGURE 1.—Yearly mean temperature differences (°C); male:female ratio of spontaneous fetal deaths after 12 weeks of gestation; and male:female ratio of births from 1968 to 2012 in Japan. (Reprinted from Fertility and Sterility. Fukuda M, Fukuda K, Shimizu T, et al. Climate change is associated with male:female ratios of fetal deaths and newborn infants in Japan. *Fertil Steril*. 2014;102:1364-1370, Copyright 2014, with permission of the American Society for Reproductive Medicine.)

particularly hot summer and cold winter and found significant increases in male fetal death and decreases in male/female sex ratios 9 months later.

Although this work is preliminary, only provides an association rather than causation, and was localized to Japan, it does raise an important question about climate extremes and its effect on the human population. If the extremes in climate change as seen in Fig 1 are actually causing the change in male/female birth ratio with an increase in male fetal death, what is the mechanism? The phenomenon of temperature-dependent sex determination is well known in nonmammalian vertebrates such as reptiles and amphibians. Potential theoretical mechanisms of why this may be a persistent phenomenon in the evolution to mammalian vertebrates including humans is discussed in McLachlan and Storey.[1] They mention an interesting adaptation in humans where the testicles are found "external" to the rest of the body and appear to protect the sperm through temperature-mediated mechanisms. Sex determination is mediated by the *Sex Determining Region Y* gene, which seems to be activated at certain temperatures. Whether this or other mechanisms are the cause of temperature fluctuations increasing fetal male death, thus altering the sex ratio, remains to be determined and is of major interest both scientifically and for society as a whole.

J. Neu, MD

Reference

1. McLachlan JC, Storey H. Hot male: can sex in humans be modified by temperature? *J Theor Biol.* 2003;222:71-72.

Prescription Opioid Epidemic and Infant Outcomes
Patrick SW, Dudley J, Martin PR, et al (Vanderbilt Univ, Nashville, TN; et al)
Pediatrics 135:842-850, 2015

Background and Objectives.—Although opioid pain relievers are commonly prescribed in pregnancy, their association with neonatal outcomes is poorly described. Our objectives were to identify neonatal complications associated with antenatal opioid pain reliever exposure and to establish predictors of neonatal abstinence syndrome (NAS).

Methods.—We used prescription and administrative data linked to vital statistics for mothers and infants enrolled in the Tennessee Medicaid program between 2009 and 2011. A random sample of NAS cases was validated by medical record review. The association of antenatal exposures with NAS was evaluated by using multivariable logistic regression, controlling for maternal and infant characteristics.

Results.—Of 112 029 pregnant women, 31 354 (28%) filled ≥1 opioid prescription. Women prescribed opioid pain relievers were more likely than those not prescribed opioids ($P < .001$) to have depression (5.3% vs 2.7%), anxiety disorder (4.3% vs 1.6%) and to smoke tobacco (41.8% vs 25.8%). Infants with NAS and opioid-exposed infants were more likely than unexposed infants to be born at a low birth weight (21.2% vs 11.8% vs 9.9%; $P < .001$). In a multivariable model, higher cumulative opioid exposure for short-acting preparations ($P < .001$), opioid type ($P < .001$), number of daily cigarettes smoked ($P < .001$), and selective serotonin reuptake inhibitor use (odds ratio: 2.08 [95% confidence interval: 1.67–2.60]) were associated with greater risk of developing NAS.

Conclusions.—Prescription opioid use in pregnancy is common and strongly associated with neonatal complications. Antenatal cumulative prescription opioid exposure, opioid type, tobacco use, and selective serotonin reuptake inhibitor use increase the risk of NAS.

▶ For many years, it was presumed that infants at risk for neonatal abstinence syndrome (NAS) were born to mothers who either participated in maintenance opiod programs or used narcotic-containing street drugs. Over the past 10 years, it had become increasingly apparent that this paradigm has shifted to include women who are given prescriptions for opioid pain relievers (OPRs) during pregnancy. The statistics in this abstract included women who were receiving maintenance opioid therapy. If women who were on maintenance therapy are excluded from the analyses, the following facts emerge: 27% of pregnant women filled at least 1 opioid prescription while pregnant, and 42% of the infants with NAS were born to mothers who took OPRs during pregnancy. Of the 1089 infants with NAS, more than one-third were born to women who filled a prescription for a greater than 7-day supply, and almost a quarter were born to mothers who filled prescriptions in the last 30 days of pregnancy. The most common reasons for OPRs were musculoskeletal pain and headache or migraine.

US statistics indicate that between 2009 and 2012 the incidence of NAS has increased from 3.4 per 1000 hospital births to 5.8 per 1000 hospital births and has increased 5-fold since 2000. There has been a parallel increase in the use of OPR prescriptions. Nationally, more than 80% of infants with NAS are enrolled in state Medicaid programs. In addition to administering and partially funding Medicaid, states also regulate prescribers and pharmacists. Thus, it would seem that states are in a position to employ public health interventions to cope with this epidemic of OPR overuse.

L. A. Papile, MD

Etiologies of NICU Deaths

Jacob J, Kamitsuka M, Clark RH, et al (Ctr for Res and Education, Sunrise, FL)
Pediatrics 135:e59-e65, 2015

Background and Objectives.—Infant mortality is an indicator of overall societal health, and a significant proportion of infant deaths occur in NICUs. The objectives were to identify causes of death and to define potentially preventable factors associated with death as areas for quality improvement efforts in the NICU.

Methods.—In a prospectively defined study, the principal investigator in 46 level III NICUs agreed to review health care records of infants who died. For each infant, the principal investigator reviewed the medical record to identify the primary cause of death and to look for preventable factors associated with the infant's death. Infants born at ≥22 weeks estimated gestational age who were born alive were included. Stillborn infants were excluded.

Results.—Data were collected on 641 infants who died. At lower gestational ages, mortality was most commonly due to extreme prematurity and the complications of premature birth (respiratory distress progressing to respiratory failure, intraventricular hemorrhage, necrotizing enterocolitis, and sepsis). With increasing gestational age, the etiology of mortality shifted to hypoxic—ischemic encephalopathy and genetic or structural anomalies. Reviewers of clinical care identified 197 (31%) infants with potentially modifiable factors that may have contributed to their deaths.

Conclusions.—The factors associated with death in infants admitted for intensive care are multifactorial and diverse, and they change with gestational age. In 31% of the deaths, potentially modifiable factors were identified, and these factors suggest important targets for reducing infant mortality.

▶ This article prospectively examined the etiologies of nonstillborn infants beyond 22 weeks' gestation in 46 neonatal intensive care units (NICUs) over a 2-year period. Not surprisingly, the incidence of death directly attributed to complications of prematurity, such as respiratory distress syndrome, necrotizing enterocolitis, intraventricular hemorrhage, and sepsis were inversely proportional to gestational age. The more mature babies were succumbed to congenital anomalies and hypoxic-ischemic encephalopathy. Analysis of the 641 infants who died suggested that nearly one-third (197, 31%) had potentially modifiable factors that might have enabled survival and reflect opportunities for reducing infant mortality.

Although none of this is particularly novel, the data were collected prospectively, reducing the selection bias, determination of the cause of death was made by the principal investigator, a neonatologist, in each participating NICU. It is unclear whether there was postmortem corroboration or whether a pathologist was involved. Nevertheless, there were some important features of the study that have importance and implications for care. The authors noted that the overwhelming majority of deaths occurred in the extremely low gestational age infants, especially less than 25 weeks. Importantly, among all nonsurviving infants irrespective of gestational age, the vast majority expired within the first week of life, usually within the first 2 days. This may have been influenced by redirection of care.

Also of importance was the finding that 6 of the 89 mothers delivering extremely preterm infants had not received prenatal care, and only 56% of mothers had seen a maternal-fetal specialist.

Among the potentially modifiable factors, delivery at a center without the appropriate level of support (10%), limited or no prenatal care (8.9%), and maternal smoking or use of drugs and/or alcohol were the most common. It appears that this is the low-hanging fruit.

S. M. Donn, MD

Etiologies of NICU Deaths
Jacob J, Kamitsuka M, Clark RH, et al (Pediatrix Med Group, Sunrise, FL)
Pediatrics 135:e59-e65, 2015

Background and Objectives.—Infant mortality is an indicator of overall societal health, and a significant proportion of infant deaths occur in NICUs. The objectives were to identify causes of death and to define potentially preventable factors associated with death as areas for quality improvement efforts in the NICU.

Methods.—In a prospectively defined study, the principal investigator in 46 level III NICUs agreed to review health care records of infants who died. For each infant, the principal investigator reviewed the medical record to identify the primary cause of death and to look for preventable factors associated with the infant's death. Infants born at ≥22 weeks estimated gestational age who were born alive were included. Stillborn infants were excluded.

Results.—Data were collected on 641 infants who died. At lower gestational ages, mortality was most commonly due to extreme prematurity and the complications of premature birth (respiratory distress progressing to respiratory failure, intraventricular hemorrhage, necrotizing enterocolitis, and sepsis). With increasing gestational age, the etiology of mortality shifted to hypoxic—ischemic encephalopathy and genetic or structural anomalies. Reviewers of clinical care identified 197 (31%) infants with potentially modifiable factors that may have contributed to their deaths.

Conclusions.—The factors associated with death in infants admitted for intensive care are multifactorial and diverse, and they change with gestational age. In 31% of the deaths, potentially modifiable factors were identified, and these factors suggest important targets for reducing infant mortality (Fig 3).

▶ If we are to prevent mortality in neonatal intensive care, one of the first steps is to define targets that can be prevented. In this prospectively defined review,

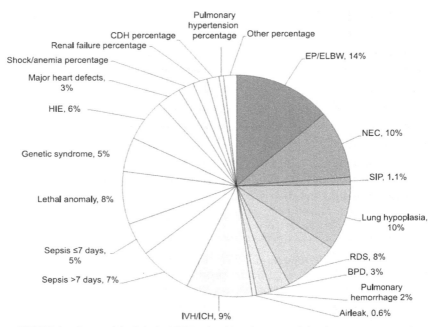

FIGURE 3.—Causes of death in the NICU ordered in subgroups and then by most common to least common. BPD, bronchopulmonary dysplasia; CDH, congenital diaphragmatic hernia; EP/ELBW, extreme prematurity or extremely low birth weight; ICH, intracranial hemorrhage; SIP, spontaneous intestinal perforation. (Reproduced with permission from Pediatrics. Jacob J, Kamitsuka M, Clark RH, et al. Etiologies of NICU deaths. *Pediatrics.* 2015;135:e59-e65, Copyright 2015, with permission from the American Academy of Pediatrics.)

health records from 46 level III NICUs were analyzed. Of 641 infants who died, 31% were identified as potentially modifiable. Generalizability of these outcomes was evaluated by reviewing data on all deaths included in the Pediatrix Data Warehouse that occurred between 2010 and 2012. These data were derived from admission to discharge in daily progress notes generated in the electronic medical records.

There are several salient results. As might be expected, a large number of deaths occurred in the most immature infants (<25 weeks' gestation) and in the first week after birth. Sepsis (most often late onset) and accuired bowel disease (necrotizing enterocolitis and spontaneous intestinal perforation) were the most common causes of death. These were followed by lung hypoplasia (related to renal anomalies and prolonged rupture of membranes), intraventricular, or intracranial hemorrhage and other causes as seen in Fig 3.

One surprise to me was the number of infants reported dying of respiratory distress syndrome (RDS; 8%) given that, at least in my personal experience, death by pure RDS in the past decade appears to be rare. One wonders whether these infants dying of "RDS" actually had other highly related respiratory causes of death, but "RDS" was simply easier to code, hence leading to some potentially misleading diagnoses. The article provides discussion about "cause of death" instructions that are provided with the death summary packets, but where 26% of the data provided by the clinicians was still "nonspecific." Nevertheless, this study provides a reasonable factual database on which efforts can be aimed for death prevention and quality improvement.

J. Neu, MD

Impact of Late Preterm and Early Term Infants on Canadian Neonatal Intensive Care Units

Bassil KL, the Canadian Neonatal Network (Mount Sinai Hosp, Toronto, Ontario, Canada)
Am J Perinatol 31:269-278, 2014

Objective.—To examine the short-term morbidities, mortality, and use of neonatal intensive care unit (NICU) resources for late preterm, early term, and term infants.

Study Design.—Infants born between 34 and 40 weeks of gestation and admitted to a Canadian NICU in 2010 were designated late preterm ($34^{0/7}$ to $36^{6/7}$ weeks), early term ($37^{0/7}$ to $38^{6/7}$ weeks), or term ($39^{0/7}$ to $40^{6/7}$ weeks). Mortality, short-term morbidities, and resource utilization were compared between the three groups using chi-square tests and analysis of variance.

Results.—Among 6,636 included infants, 44.2% ($n = 2,935$) were late preterm, 26.2% ($n = 1,737$) early term, and 29.6% ($n = 1,964$) term. Term infants were more likely to require resuscitation at birth and had lower Apgar scores than late preterm and early term infants ($p < 0.001$). Length of stay and need for respiratory support decreased with increasing gestational age; however, the proportion of hospital days that intensive care was required increased.

Conclusion.—The greatest impact of late preterm infants is on NICU bed occupancy, whereas for term infants it is on intensity of care. Early term infants experience greater rates of some complications than term, demonstrating that risk persists for these infants. These findings have important implications for NICU resource planning and practice.

▶ In 1950, the World Health Organization defined "preterm" as birth before 37 weeks of completed gestation.[1] Since then, there have been further refinements and definitions of preterm births; "late preterm" as birth at 34–36 weeks' gestation, "moderate preterm" as birth at 32–33 weeks, "very preterm" as birth < 32 weeks, and "extremely preterm" as births < 28 weeks. Historically, much of our focus has been on very preterm infants, but over the past decade, there has also been a growing interest in late preterm infants in terms of the epidemiology, developmental physiology, obstetric management, neonatal problems, and the short- and long-term outcomes. However, the information related to neonatal mortality and morbidity, resource utilization in the neonatal intensive care unit (NICU), as well as long-term outcomes of "term" infants, born beyond 37 weeks' gestation, who were admitted to neonatal nurseries is still limited.

In the article by Bassil et al, investigators in the Canadian Neonatal Network (CNN) highlighted the importance of examining neonatal outcomes and NICU resource utilization of infants born > 37 weeks' gestation. The data represent nearly all (approximately 96%) tertiary-level neonatal admissions in Canada. The study is further strengthened by the adherence to uniform definitions for data collection. The information that late preterm infants accounted for approximately 22% of all tertiary-level neonatal admissions and also that their biggest impact on resource use is on bed occupancy, rather than the need for intensive care, is important for health care providers in reorganization of perinatal services. This study is unique in the sense that the investigators have examined the impact on NICUs of "early term" and "term" infants in 2 separate groups, thereby demonstrating that the increased risk of serious respiratory morbidity and NICU resource use persist in infants born at 37 and 38 weeks' gestation. This information is important, and clinicians should seriously question the wisdom of some existing practices of "elective deliveries" at these gestational ages because of the perceived notion that the pregnancy has passed the "preterm" threshold. The result from this study is perhaps applicable to most tertiary NICUs with similar perinatal networks as in the CNN but could not be generalized to all infants delivered within these defined gestational ages because the data represent only tertiary-level neonatal admissions. The authors have clearly recognized this limitation. It is not clear why the investigators did not look at the NICU admissions after delivery at 41 weeks' gestation and beyond (ie, "late term" and "postterm") because the neonatal illness severity and need for intensive care, as well as neonatal mortality and morbidity, may differ in this group.

The arbitrary definitions of "preterm," "term," and "postterm" were invented more than 60 years ago without a clear scientific basis.[1] It is only appropriate that the "perinatal community" is now searching for more evidence and attempting to refine these definitions based on the evidence.

W. Tin, MD

Reference

1. Madar J, Richmond S, Hey E. Surfactant-deficient respiratory distress after elective delivery at "term". *Acta Paediatr.* 1999;88:1244-1248.

Measuring Gestational Age in Vital Statistics Data: Transitioning to the Obstetric Estimate
Martin JA, Osterman MJK, Kirmeyer SE, et al (Division of Vital Statistics, U.S. Department of Health and Human Services, Centers for Disease Control and Prevention, GA, USA)
Natl Vital Stat Rep 64:1-20, 2015

Objectives.—Beginning with the 2014 data year, the National Center for Health Statistics is transitioning to a new standard for estimating the gestational age of a newborn. The new measure, the obstetric estimate of gestation at delivery (OE), replaces the measure based on the date of the last normal menses (LMP). This transition is being made because of increasing evidence of the greater validity of the OE compared with the LMP-based measure. This report describes the relationship between the two measures. Agreement between the two measures is shown for 2013. Comparisons between the two measures for single gestational weeks and selected gestational age categories for 2013, and trends in the two measures for 2007–2013 by gestational category, focusing on preterm births, are shown for the United States and by race and Hispanic origin and state.

Methods.—Data are derived from U.S. birth certificates for 2007–2013 for 100% of reported resident births.

Results.—Estimates of pregnancy length were the same for the OE- and LMP-based measures for 62.1% of all births, and within 1 week for 83.4% in 2013. The mean OE-based gestational age for all 2013 births was 38.5 weeks, lower than the LMP-based average of 38.7. Births were less likely to be classified as preterm using the OE (9.62%) than with the LMP (11.39%). The 2013 OE preterm rate was lower than the LMP rate for 49 states and the District of Columbia. The OE-based percentage of full-term deliveries was higher than the LMP-based percentage; levels of late-term and postterm deliveries were lower. Preterm birth rates declined for both measures from 2007 through 2013 (8% compared with 10%). The OE-based 2013 preterm infant mortality rate was 19% higher than the LMP rate.

▶ The National Center for Health Statistics is transitioning to using the obstetric estimate (OE) of gestation at delivery instead of the date of the last menstrual period (LMP) to assign infants' gestational ages at birth. The OE is defined as the "best obstetric estimate of the infant's gestation in completed weeks based on the birth attendant's final estimate of gestation." The OE is found to have greater validity compared with LMP-based dating. In this report, Martin et al compare the 2 measures for US birth certificates from 2013. They report that pregnancy lengths were the same using the 2 measures for 62.1% of births and were within 1 week for 83.7%. Births were less likely to be classified as preterm using OE versus LMP (9.6% vs 11.4%, respectively). Furthermore, the OE-based preterm infant mortality rate was 19% higher than the LMP rate (41.5 per 1000 compared with 34.8 per 1000). Rates of preterm birth are lower across all racial/ethnic groups, but black/white disparities persist. Using LMP, preterm birth rates were 16.27% and 10.17% for black and white infants, respectively (relative risk [RR], 1.6). Using OE, preterm birth rates were 13.25% and 8.94% for black and white infants, respectively (RR, 1.5). Recognition of differences in methods of measuring preterm birth should be taken into consideration when comparing trends in gestational age and related outcomes over time.

H. H. Burris, MD, MPH

Survival and Morbidity of Preterm Children Born at 22 Through 34 weeks' Gestation in France in 2011: Results of the EPIPAGE-2 Cohort Study
Ancel P-Y, the EPIPAGE-2 Writing Group (Sorbonne Paris Cité Research Ctr, France)
JAMA Pediatr 169:230-238, 2015

Importance.—Up-to-date estimates of the health outcomes of preterm children are needed for assessing perinatal care, informing parents, making decisions about care, and providing evidence for clinical guidelines.

Objectives.—To determine survival and neonatal morbidity of infants born from 22 through 34 completed weeks' gestation in France in 2011 and compare these outcomes with a comparable cohort in 1997.

Design, Setting, and Participants.—The EPIPAGE-2 study is a national, prospective, population-based cohort study conducted in all maternity and neonatal units in France in 2011. A total of 2205 births (stillbirths and live births) and terminations of pregnancy at 22 through 26 weeks' gestation, 3257 at 27 through 31 weeks, and 1234 at 32 through 34 weeks were studied. Cohort data were collected from January 1 through December 31, 1997, and from March 28 through December 31, 2011. Analyses for 1997 were run for the entire year and then separately for April to December; the rates for survival and morbidities did not differ. Data are therefore presented for the whole year in 1997 and the 8-month and 6-month periods in 2011.

Main Outcomes and Measures.—Survival to discharge and survival without any of the following adverse outcomes: grade III or IV intraventricular hemorrhage, cystic periventricular leukomalacia, severe bronchopulmonary dysplasia, retinopathy of prematurity (stage 3 or higher), or necrotizing enterocolitis (stages 2-3).

Results.—A total of 0.7% of infants born before 24 weeks' gestation survived to discharge: 31.2% of those born at 24 weeks, 59.1% at 25 weeks, and 75.3% at 26 weeks. Survival rates were 93.6% at 27 through 31 weeks and 98.9% at 32 through 34 weeks. Infants discharged home without severe neonatal morbidity represented 0% at 23 weeks, 11.6% at 24 weeks, 30.0% at 25 weeks, 47.5% at 26 weeks, 81.3% at 27 through 31 weeks, and 96.8% at 32 through 34 weeks. Compared with 1997, the proportion of infants surviving without severe morbidity in 2011 increased by 14.4% ($P < .001$) at 25 through 29 weeks and 6% ($P < .001$) at 30 through 31 weeks but did not change appreciably for those born at less than 25 weeks. The rates of antenatal corticosteroid use, induced preterm deliveries, cesarean deliveries, and surfactant use increased significantly in all gestational-age groups, except at 22 through 23 weeks.

Conclusions and Relevance.—The substantial improvement in survival in France for newborns born at 25 through 31 weeks' gestation was accompanied by an important reduction in severe morbidity, but survival remained rare before 25 weeks. Although improvement in survival at extremely low gestational age may be possible, its effect on long-term outcomes requires further studies. The long-term results of the EPIPAGE-2 study will be informative in this regard.

▶ There is general consensus that counseling of incipient parents about expected outcomes and treatment options for extremely preterm infants should be informed by relevant empirical data. Translating that sentiment into practice is not simple, however, because outcomes have improved over time, and, especially at the margins of viability, may be heavily influenced by practice preferences that result in self-fulfilling prophecies of mortality. These recent data from France exemplify both of these challenges. For example, survival rates at 25 and 26 weeks' gestation improved from 50% and 56% in 1997 to 61% and 74% in 2011, respectively. On the other hand, survival rates for infants born before 24 weeks' gestation remained essentially zero, reflecting the usual practice in France of providing palliative but not intensive care to infants at those gestational ages, so this report cannot directly inform care of infants born (or about to be born) at 22 or 23 weeks. That approach may have influenced care choices for infants up to 27 weeks' gestation, for whom survival rates in France were lower than those recently reported from the United States, Japan, and Sweden. However, the currency of these data (from the present decade) makes them useful for more advanced pregnancies or more mature preterm babies, and they merit a more detailed examination than this space permits. Two observations may be particularly salient. First, the rates of severe neonatal morbidities (grade III-IV intraventricular hemorrhage, cystic periventricular leukomalacia, stage II-III necrotizing enterocolitis, retinopathy of prematurity stage ≥3, or severe bronchopulmonary dysplasia) remain substantial up to 28 weeks' gestation (59%, 45%, 35%, 28%, and 18% at 24, 25, 26, 27, and 28 weeks, respectively). Rates of long-term neurodevelopmental and sensory impairments are yet to be determined. These outcomes, in addition to survival alone, may require consideration in reaching decisions about obstetrical interventions or neonatal intensive care. Second, it should be recognized that the denominator changes over the trajectory of infants at each gestational age. For example, in this cohort, only 20% of pregnancies delivered at 25 weeks resulted in survival without severe neonatal morbidity, but 30% of those that resulted in live birth did so, and 50% of surviving infants did not have severe morbidity. These distinctions are important because parents may value different outcomes (death or survival with severe morbidity) quite differently. These principles are applicable to less mature infants in settings where intensive care is more frequently provided before 24 weeks' gestation as well.

W. E. Benitz, MD

Using Satellite-Based Spatiotemporal Resolved Air Temperature Exposure to Study the Association between Ambient Air Temperature and Birth Outcomes in Massachusetts

Kloog I, Melly SJ, Coull BA, et al (Ben-Gurion Univ of the Negev, Beer Sheva, Israel; Harvard T.H. Chan School of Public Health, Boston, MA)
Environ Health Perspect, 2015 [Epub ahead of print]

Background.—Studies looking at air temperature (Ta) and birth outcomes are rare.

Methods.—We evaluated birth outcomes and average daily Ta during various prenatal exposure periods in Massachusetts (USA) using both traditional Ta stations and modeled address Ta. We used linear and logistic mixed models, and accelerated failure time models, to estimate associations between Ta and the following outcomes among live births >22 weeks: term birth weight (≥37 weeks), low birth weight (LBW) (<2,500 g at term), gestational age and preterm delivery (PT) (<37 weeks). Models were adjusted for individual level socioeconomic status, traffic density, $PM_{2.5}$, random intercept for census tract and mothers health.

Results.—Predicted Ta during multiple time windows before birth was negatively associated with birth weight: average birth weight was 16.7 g lower (95% CI: −29.7, −3.7) in association with an IQR increase (8.4°C) in Ta during the last trimester. Ta over the entire pregnancy was positively associated with PT (OR = 1.02; 95% CI: 1.00, 1.05) and LBW (OR = 1.04; 95% CI: 0.96, 1.13).

Conclusions.—Ta during pregnancy was associated with lower birth weight and shorter gestational age in our study population.

▶ Although individual characteristics such as race/ethnicity, prior preterm birth, short cervix, and smoking modestly predict preterm birth, most preterm birth is not explained by such factors. Whether differences in environmental temperature in a given geographic setting play a role has not been established. Kloog and colleagues used Massachusetts birth data from birth certificates (2000-2008) to analyze associations of temperature and birth outcomes in more than 450 000 births. The authors report that per interquartile range increase (8.4°C) was negatively associated with birth weight and positively associated with preterm birth (odds ratio 1.02, 95% confidence interval: 1.00-1.05). Although these associations were modest, if replicated, implications in the setting of climate change are that increased temperatures could affect perinatal health. Economic models of climate change often take into account effects on elderly but should also consider burdens to the neonatal care systems. Furthermore, the stronger associations in urban (vs rural) areas between temperature and preterm birth found in this might explain some of the ongoing racial and socioeconomic disparities in preterm birth.

H. H. Burris, MD, MPH

Neonatal and early childhood outcomes following early vs later preterm premature rupture of membranes

Manuck TA, Varner MW (Univ of Utah Health Sciences Ctr, Salt Lake City)
Am J Obstet Gynecol 211:308.e1-308.e6, 2014

Objective.—Data regarding long-term outcomes of neonates reaching viability following early preterm premature rupture of membranes (PPROM; <25.0 weeks at rupture) are limited. We hypothesized that babies delivered after early PPROM would have increased rates of major childhood morbidity compared with those with later PPROM (≥25.0 weeks at rupture).

Study Design.—This was a secondary analysis of a multicenter randomized controlled trial of magnesium sulfate vs placebo for cerebral palsy prevention. Women with singletons and PPROM of 15-32 weeks were included. All women delivered at 24.0 weeks or longer. Those with PPROM less than 25.0 weeks (cases) were compared with women with PPROM at 25.0-31.9 weeks (controls). Composite severe neonatal morbidity (sepsis, severe intraventricular hemorrhage, periventricular leukomalacia, severe necrotizing enterocolitis, bronchopulmonary dysplasia, and/or death) and composite severe childhood morbidity at age 2 years (moderate or severe cerebral palsy and/or Bayley II Infant and Toddler Development scores greater than 2 SD below the mean) were compared.

Results.—A total of 1531 women (275 early PPROM cases) were included. Demographics were similar between the groups. Cases delivered earlier (26.6 vs 30.1 weeks, $P < .001$) and had a longer rupture-to-delivery interval (20.0 vs 10.4 days, $P < .001$). Case neonates had high rates of severe composite neonatal morbidity (75.6% vs 21.8%, $P < .001$). Children with early PPROM had higher composite severe childhood morbidity (51.6% vs 22.5%, $P < .001$). Early PPROM remained associated with composite severe childhood morbidity in multivariable models, even when controlling for delivery gestational age and other confounders.

Conclusion.—Early PPROM is associated with high rates of neonatal morbidity. Early childhood outcomes at age 2 years remain poor compared with those delivered after later PPROM.

▶ This observational study is a secondary analysis of the Eunice Shriver Kennedy National Institute of Child and Human Development Maternal Fetal Network's multicenter randomized controlled trial of magnesium sulfate for the prevention of cerebral palsy.[1] This analysis was restricted to women with singleton gestations who had a confirmed diagnosis of preterm premature rupture of the membranes (PPROM) between 15 and 32 weeks of gestation and subsequently delivered at less than 35 weeks of gestation. Thus, of the 2241 women enrolled in the main trial, only 64% were included. It should be noted that initially enrollment in the main trial did not specify a lower gestational age restriction for PPROM; however, partway through the recruitment, the protocol was amended to exclude women with PPROM at less than 22 weeks of gestational age.

On multivariable logistic regression analysis PPROM before 25 weeks of gestational age (early PPROM) was associated with neurodevelopmental disability in early childhood when compared with PPROM after 25 weeks of gestational age (later PPROM), even when controlling for gestational age at delivery. From the information presented in the article, it is difficult to ascertain whether this association is clinically relevant.

There were vast differences in birth weight and gestation age between the 2 groups, which may have had a greater impact on neonatal morbidity and early childhood outcome than the timing of PPROM. The infant cohort in the early PPROM (before 25 weeks of gestational age) had a mean birth weight of 930 ± 415 grams and a mean gestational age of 26.6 ± 2.5 weeks compared with a mean birth weight of 1481 ± 44 grams and a mean gestational age of 30.1 ± 2.2 weeks in the later PPROM (26—32 weeks of gestational age) cohort. Because medical morbidity occurs more frequently in extremely immature infants, it is also not surprising that the rate of the medical conditions included in the severe medical morbidity composite were 2- to 5-fold higher in the early PPROM group. The subsequent difference in neurodevelopmental outcome in early childhood may be a reflection of the severity of these medical complications, each of which is known to have a detrimental effect on neurodevelopmental outcome. A study design in which delivery gestational age was matched in the 2 groups would have been ideal; however, because of the marked difference in gestational age between the 2 groups and the small number of infants in the early PPROM cohort, this was not feasible.

L. A. Papile, MD

Reference

1. Rouse DJ, Hirtz DG, Thom E, et al. A randomized controlled trial of magnesium sulfate for the prevention of cerebral palsy. *N Engl J Med.* 2008;359:895-905.

3 Genetics and Teratology

Severity of Birth Defects After Propylthiouracil Exposure in Early Pregnancy

Andersen SL, Olsen J, Wu CS, et al (Aalborg Univ Hosp, Denmark; Aarhus Univ, Denmark; et al)
Thyroid 24:1533-1540, 2014

Background.—Propylthiouracil (PTU) used in the treatment of maternal hyperthyroidism in early pregnancy may be associated with a higher prevalence of birth defects in the face and neck region and in the urinary system but the severity of these complications remains to be elucidated.

Methods.—Review of hospital-registered cases of birth defects in the face and neck region and in the urinary system after PTU exposure in early pregnancy. We obtained information on maternal redeemed prescription of PTU and child diagnosis of birth defect from nationwide registers for all children born in Denmark between 1996 and 2008 ($n = 817{,}093$). The children were followed until December 31, 2010 (median age, 8.3 years) and the Cox proportional hazards model was used to estimate adjusted hazard ratio (HR) with 95% confidence interval (CI) for having a birth defect after PTU exposure versus nonexposed children ($n = 811{,}730$).

Results.—Fourteen cases of birth defects were identified in the face and neck region and in the urinary system after PTU exposure in early pregnancy; 11 children were exposed to PTU only ($n = 564$), whereas 3 children were born to mothers who switched from methimazole (MMI)/carbimazole (CMZ) to PTU in early pregnancy ($n = 159$). Among children exposed to PTU only, the adjusted HR for having a birth defect in the face and neck region was 4.92 (95% CI 2.04–11.86) and in the urinary system 2.73 (1.22–6.07). Looking into details of the 14 cases, 7 children were diagnosed with a birth defect in the face and neck region (preauricular and branchial sinus/fistula/cyst) and 7 children had a birth defect in the urinary system (single cyst of kidney and hydronephrosis). Surgical treatment was registered in 6 of the cases with a birth defect in the face and neck region and 3 of the cases with a birth defect in the urinary system. Two of the children with a birth defect in the urinary system also had other birth defects (genital organs).

Conclusions.—We report details on possible PTU-associated birth defects. They tend to be less severe than the defects observed after MMI/CMZ exposure. Yet, the majority of affected children had to undergo surgery.

▶ Methimazole (MMI) and its prodrug carbimazole (CMZ), together with propylthiouracil (PTU), are the spectrum of agents available for the treatment of hyperthyroidism. In the management of hyperthyroidism in pregnancy, the clinician is caught between a rock and a hard place, somewhat akin to the situation with maternal epilepsy, in that the maternal therapy may be effective, but there are substantial risks for birth defects in the fetus. In a Danish population-based cohort study of 817 093 children, the same investigative team reported that both MMI/CMZ and PTU exposure in early pregnancy were significantly associated with a higher prevalence of having 1 or more birth defect diagnosed before age 2 years.[1] The birth defects described after MMI/CMZ exposure were similar to previous reports and in line with the MMI/CMZ embryopathy,[2] but the finding that PTU was also associated with a higher prevalence of birth defects was new and intriguing. The study abstracted here further explores the relationship between PTU and birth defects, clearly establishing risk, in contrast to the findings from Japan where no such relationship was found.[3] They reviewed almost 7000 cases of maternal hyperthyroidism including more than 1500 mothers treated in the first trimester with PTU in which the prevalence of birth defects was similar to the controls mothers with hyperthyroidism who had not received therapy in the first trimester. The explanation for the difference with the Danish experience is that the Danes looked for and found "minor anomalies" including tags and sinuses, evidence of branchial arch disturbances that may not have been searched for in the Japanese cohort. Yoshihara[3] reported: "In utero exposure to MMI during the first trimester of pregnancy increased the rate of congenital malformations, and it significantly increased the rate of aplasia cutis congenita, omphalocele, and a symptomatic omphalomesenteric duct anomaly." Overall, Hackmon et al[4] concluded from their literature review that there was insufficient statistical power to determine accurate rates of either MMI teratogenicity or PTU hepatotoxicity in cohort studies. However, a case-control study helped identify the relative risk of MMI-induced choanal atresia. Esophageal atresia may also be added to the list of anomalies associated with MMI. A second case-control study failed to show that aplasia cutis congenita is associated with MMI. PTU has been associated with a rare but serious form of hepatic failure. Hackmon et al concluded that after first trimester exposure MMI causes a specific pattern of rare teratogenic, while PTU therapy may be followed by rare but severe hepatotoxic sequelae. "It is therefore appropriate to use PTU to treat maternal hyperthyroidism during the first trimester of pregnancy, and to switch to MMI for the remainder of the pregnancy." These appear to be reasonable conclusions bearing in mind that PTU may also cause facial and genitourinary anomalies.

A. A. Fanaroff, MBBCh, FRCPE

References

1. Andersen SL, Olsen J, Wu CS, Laurberg P. Birth defects after early pregnancy use of antithyroid drugs: a Danish nationwide study. *J Clin Endocrinol Metab*. 2013; 98:4373-4381.
2. Taylor PN, Vaidya B. Side effects of anti-thyroid drugs and their impact on the choice of treatment for thyrotoxicosis in pregnancy. *Eur Thyroid J*. 2012;1: 176-185.
3. Yoshihara A, Noh J, Yamaguchi T, et al. Treatment of graves' disease with antithyroid drugs in the first trimester of pregnancy and the prevalence of congenital malformation. J Clin Endocrinol Metab 97:2396-2403
4. Hackmon R, Blichowski M, Koren G. The safety of methimazole and propylthiouracil in pregnancy: a systematic review. *J Obstet Gynaecol Can*. 2012;34: 1077-1086.

Hypermethylation of *SHH* in the pathogenesis of congenital anorectal malformations

Huang Y, Zhang P, Zheng S, et al (Children's Hosp of Fudan Univ, Shanghai, P.R. China)
J Pediatr Surg 49:1400-1404, 2014

Objective.—This study sought to examine promoter methylation and expression of the identified *sonic hedgehog (SHH)* gene in terminal rectal tissues of children with congenital anorectal malformations (ARMs).

Methods.—Tissue samples from the terminal rectum of pediatric patients with ARMs (five cases each of high and intermediate malformation — two cases of rectovesical fistula, two cases of rectourethral prostatic fistula, one case of cloaca with > 3 cm common channel, four cases of rectourethral bulbar fistula and one case of imperforate anus without fistula, respectively, and ten cases of low malformation — five cases of perineal fistula and five cases of vestibular fistula, respectively), and patients with nongastrointestinal tract malformation (six cases, anal fistula) were collected and divided into three groups: high-intermediate ARM (ARMhi-int), low ARM (ARMlo), and control (Cont.). Real-time RT-PCR was used to detect mRNA expression levels of the verified differentially methylated gene *SHH*, and bisulfite genomic sequencing was performed to evaluate DNA methylation in the *SHH* promoter region.

Results.—The average methylation levels of the *SHH* promoter were significantly higher in ARMhi-int (0.850 ± 0.030, $P = 0.0036$) and ARMlo (0.540 ± 0.053, $P = 0.0087$) groups than in Cont. group (0.280 ± 0.032). SHH mRNA expression levels were lower in ARMhi-int (0.340 ± 0.015, $P = 0.0065$) and ARMlo (0.530 ± 0.042, $P = 0.0156$) groups than in Cont. group (0.870 ± 0.046). The average methylation levels of the *SHH* promoter were higher in ARMhi-int group than in ARMlo group (0.850 ± 0.030 vs. 0.540 ± 0.053, $P = 0.0095$), while *SHH* expression was significantly reduced in ARMhi-int group compared to ARMlo group (0.340 ± 0.15 vs. 0.530 ± 0.042, $P = 0.0252$). The methylation levels of the *SHH* promoter in ARMhi-int group were negatively correlated with *SHH* gene expression (r = −0.89, $P < 0.01$).

Conclusions.—The *SHH* gene, which plays a major role in the development of the anorectum and enteric nervous system, is hypermethylated at its promoter, and this is correlated with low levels of *SHH* gene expression. This epigenetic modification may therefore be responsible for the observed changes in *SHH* expression, which could in turn underlie the pathogenesis of congenital ARMs.

▶ During early fetal development, the distal large intestine and the urinary tract emerge from a large mass of cells that undergo differentiation in which the rectum and anus separate from the urinary tract. Failure of this normal differentiation may lead to congenital malformations anomalies termed anorectal malformations. Several proteins are coded by genes that are involved in differentiation, including the one that the authors of this article focus on, sonic hedgehog (SHH). The gene that encodes this protein apparently is not affected when these anorectal malformations occur, but rather according to this research is an epigenetic phenomenon that involves a heritable change in gene activity and expression that occurs without alteration in the DNA sequence. There are several epigenetic modifications that may cause this alteration in gene expression, one of which is DNA methylation. If a certain region of a gene, especially the promoter region, is highly methylated, transcription will be blunted, and less of the protein product will be produced.

If one searches for a genetic mutation or chromosomal anomaly underlying anorectal malformations using karyotyping, microarrays, or even exome sequencing, a defect may not be found. From this study, it is clear that messenger RNA transcription of SHH is highest in the control samples and lowest in the samples from the patients with intermediate or high (usually the more serious) anorectal malformations. This is accompanied by the highest methylation in the samples from the patients with the anorectal malformations and lowest in the control patients. This reciprocal association suggests a relationship where the increased methylation of the SHH gene may result in decreased production of SHH protein, suggesting an epigenetic cause.

One can criticize some of the methodology from this study. For example, it is not clear whether the samples from the control patients or the patients with the anorectal malformations were derived from exactly the same tissue and region. Some of the samples exhibited degradation, thus may not have been optimal for the analysis. Was SHH picked because it showed the greatest differences compared with the other genes involved in differentiation? It was not clear from the way this article was written exactly how the samples were processed; were they pooled, and how were the chips used? Table 1 in the original article suggests that this may have been the case because only 2 representatives were analyzed for quality assessment. There were apparently 20 samples available from the ARMlo, 20 from the ARMhi-int groups, and 6 controls, so why were only 2 evaluated for quality of DNA from the terminal rectum?

Nevertheless, despite these questions, this is likely an important study. Genetic modifications in DNA sequence or chromosomal aberrations are not easy to fix. With epigenetic modifications, it is possible that environmental factors such as diet may be much more amenable to manipulation, and hence disease prevention is more likely—as long as we understand the mechanism. This study is an interesting early step in understanding epigenetic modification that may lead to anorectal malformations—a step that may eventually indicate a means of preventing them.

J. Neu, MD

FUT 2 polymorphism and outcome in very-low-birth-weight infants
Demmert M, for the German Neonatal Network (Univ at Lübeck, Germany; et al)
Pediatr Res 77:586-590, 2015

Background.—To determine whether the secretor gene fucosyltransferase (FUT)2 polymorphism G428A is predictive for adverse outcomes in a large cohort of very-low-birth weight (VLBW) infants.

Methods.—We prospectively enrolled 2,406 VLBW infants from the population-based multicenter cohort of the German Neonatal network cohort (2009—2011). The secretor genotype (rs601338) was assessed from DNA samples extracted from buccal swabs. Primary study outcomes were clinical sepsis, blood-culture confirmed sepsis, intracerebral hemorrhage (ICH), necrotizing enterocolitis (NEC) or focal intestinal perforation requiring surgery, and death.

Results.—Based on the assumption of a recessive genetic model, AA individuals had a higher incidence of ICH (AA: 19.0% vs. GG/AG: 14.9%, $P = 0.04$) which was not significant in the additive genetic model (multivariable logistic regression analysis; allele carriers: 365 cases, 1,685 controls; OR: 1.2; 95% CI: 0.99—1.4; $P = 0.06$). Other outcomes were not influenced by FUT2 genotype in either genetic model.

Conclusion.—This large-scale multicenter study did not confirm previously reported associations between FUT2 genotype and adverse outcomes in preterm infants.

▶ The fucosyltransferase 2 (FUT2) blood group locus gene is responsible for synthesis of soluble A, B, H, and Lewis B blood group antigens in humans. Approximately 20% of the world's population has a mutation in this gene that results in nonsecretion. As stated in this article, there is a differential response to Norovirus and other infections depending on secretor status. FUT2 genotype was analyzed in a previous study of preterm neonates that evaluated 410 infants.[1] There were more deaths in the nonsecretors than in the heterozygotes or secretor dominant groups. The low-secretor phenotype was also associated with higher necrotizing enterocolitis and Gram negative sepsis even after controlling for multiple clinical factors. Thus, secretor phenotype was considered to be a potentially strong predictive biomarker for these adverse outcomes.

This study, in a considerably larger population that excluded individuals with Asian and African backgrounds, also evaluated various outcomes related to FUT2 secretor status. Of interest, the nonsecretors appeared to have a higher prevalence of preterm labor, but the secretors had a higher prevalence of preeclampsia. In contrast to the study by Morrow et al,[1] there were no differences in sepsis or necrotizing enterocolitis but a higher prevalence of intraventricular hemorrhage in the nonsecretors, which became nonsignificant after adjusting for other well-known risk factors.

It is not clear why there might be discrepancies between these studies, but possible factors may involve the exclusion of Asians and Africans in this study. Another possibility is that buccal swabs were obtained in this study, whereas salivary samples were obtained in the previous study. It will be of interest whether current genome-wide association studies will shed some light on this interesting discrepancy.

J. Neu, MD

Reference

1. Morrow AL, Meinzen-Derr J, Huang P, et al. Fucosyltransferase 2 non-secretor and low secretor status predicts severe outcomes in premature infants. *J Pediatr.* 2011;158:745-751.

Dexamethasone but not the equivalent doses of hydrocortisone induces neurotoxicity in neonatal rat brain
Feng Y, Kumar P, Wang J, et al (Univ of Mississippi Med Ctr, Jackson)
Pediatr Res 77:618-624, 2015

Background.—The use of dexamethasone (Dex) in premature infants to treat or prevent chronic lung disease adversely affects neurodevelopment. Recent clinical studies suggest that hydrocortisone (HC) is a safer alternative to Dex. We compared the effects of Dex and HC on neurotoxicity in newborn rats.

Methods.—Rat pups of a neurodevelopmental stage equivalent to premature human neonates were administered Dex or HC either as a single dose on postnatal day (PD) 6, repeated doses on PD 4 to 6 or tapering doses at PD 3 to 6 by i.p. injection. Brain weight, caspase-3 activity, and apoptotic cells were measured at PD 7; learning capability, memory, and motor function were measured at juvenile age.

Results.—Dex decreased both body and brain weight gain, while HC did not. Tapering and repeated doses of Dex increased caspase-3 activity, cleaved caspase-3 and terminal deoxynucleotidyl transferase dUTP nick end labeling (TUNEL)-positive cells but HC, except at high doses, did not. Dex impaired learning and memory capability at juvenile age, while the rats exposed to HC showed normal cognitive behavior.

Conclusion.—HC is probably safer to use than Dex in the immediate postnatal period in neonatal rats. Cautious extrapolation of these findings to human premature infants is required.

▶ The use of glucocorticoids to prevent or treat bronchopulmonary dysplasia (BPD) in preterm infants has been controversial almost since the therapy began in the 1980s. Dexamethasone, the drug initially chosen, is a powerful, long-acting agent with no mineralocorticoid activity, a feature that seemed attractive. Initial short-term reports were almost uniformly positive, and the therapy became widely adopted. However, as data accumulated regarding its apparent adverse effects on long-term outcomes, the neonatology community retreated, treating far fewer infants. Nonetheless, difficult problems remain: first, many of the most immature infants continue to receive steroid therapy for persistent lung disease, and second, the incidence of BPD has stubbornly persisted or increased, with its own attendant adverse effects on long-term outcomes. Therefore, investigators continue to pursue the elusive goal of using steroid therapy to dampen inflammation without increasing neurodevelopmental risk.

The adverse effects of dexamethasone could be amplified by the large doses previously given to neonates (now generally lower), by its very long half-life compared with native cortisol, or by the imbalance between its glucocorticoid and mineralocorticoid activity. Native cortisol binds primarily to mineralocorticoid receptors in the absence of stress; dexamethasone administration suppresses cortisol production, but does not bind to mineralocorticoid receptors. Feng and colleagues compared the effects of 1 to 4 days of dexamethasone or hydrocortisone treatment at varying doses in a neonatal rat model. They found that dexamethasone, but not the equivalent dose of hydrocortisone, significantly reduced brain and body weight gain and induced apoptosis in neonatal rats. At toxic doses (30 mg/kg/d), hydrocortisone resulted in increased apoptosis versus control, but even at that dose had no other apparent adverse effects. Importantly, these investigators evaluated long-term effects on learning and memory in juvenile rats (postnatal days 25 and 26) and found that dexamethasone impaired learning and memory capability, whereas hydrocortisone did not do so at any dose. Unfortunately, all the dexamethasone regimens which these investigators tested started with a dose of 0.5 mg/kg/d, which is higher than currently prescribed for most infants. However, other investigators have reported similar outcomes (decreased brain and body weights, learning impairment) using a lower starting dose of dexamethasone (0.2 mg/kg/d).[1]

The authors "recommend further animal experiments and also support a large, multicenter, randomized placebo-controlled, prospective trial (RCT) to study the efficacy as well as short and long-term safety of hydrocortisone as a rescue therapy." Happily, 2 such RCTs are underway: one study testing a 10-day hydrocortisone course beginning at 14 to 28 days (NCT01353313), and the other testing a 22-day course starting at 7 to 14 days,[2] both in ventilated infants. Together, these studies should provide a wealth of new information regarding benefits and risks of hydrocortisone therapy for BPD to help guide future therapy.

K. Watterberg

References

1. Ichinohashi Y, Sato Y, Saito A, et al. Dexamethasone administration to the neonatal rat results in neurological dysfunction at the juvenile stage even at low doses. *Early Hum Dev.* 2013;89:283-288.
2. Onland W, Offringa M, Cools F, et al. Systemic hydrocortisone to prevent bronchopulmonary dysplasia in preterm infants (the SToP-BPD study); a multicenter randomized placebo controlled trial. *BMC Pediatr.* 2011;11:102.

4 Labor and Delivery

Endotracheal Suction for Nonvigorous Neonates Born through Meconium Stained Amniotic Fluid: A Randomized Controlled Trial
Chettri S, Adhisivam B, Bhat BV (Jawaharlal Inst of Postgraduate Medical Education and Res (JIPMER), Pondicherry, India)
J Pediatr 166:1208-1213, 2015

Objective.—To assess whether endotracheal suctioning of nonvigorous infants born through meconium stained amniotic fluid (MSAF) reduces the risk and complications of meconium aspiration syndrome (MAS).

Study Design.—Term, nonvigorous babies born through MSAF were randomized to endotracheal suction and no-suction groups (n = 61 in each). Risk of MAS, complications of MAS and endotracheal suction, mortality, duration of neonatal intensive care unit stay, and neurodevelopmental outcome at 9 months were assessed.

Results.—Maternal age, consistency of meconium, mode of delivery, birth weight, sex, and Apgar scores were similar in the groups. In total, 39 (32%) neonates developed MAS and 18 (14.8%) of them died. There were no significant differences in MAS, its severity and complications, mortality, and neurodevelopmental outcome for the 2 groups. One infant had a complication of endotracheal suctioning, which was mild and transient.

Conclusions.—The current practice of routine endotracheal suctioning for nonvigorous neonates born through MSAF should be further evaluated.

Trial Registration.—Clinical Trial Registry of India: CTRI/2013/03/003469.

▶ Even though our focus remains on practicing evidence-based medicine and providing the best possible care for our newborn patients, "standards" that have not been scientifically validated permeate into our daily practice. Intubation of babies born with meconium-stained amniotic fluid (MSAF) represents a prime example. We, who have practiced for some time, have vivid memories of fighting vigorous babies born through MSAF to intubate them. Even as an inexperienced intern, I could never comprehend why a baby who could fight me and a laryngoscope blade would aspirate meconium into the lungs. Over the decades, we had come to believe that meconium can enter the airways and must be cleared to prevent meconium aspiration syndrome (MAS). Attempts were made to suction the mouth and airway at every possible opportunity, starting with the obstetrician at the delivery of the head. Wisewell et al[1] started to dispel some of these age-old myths when their multicenter international collaborative trial concluded that vigorous infants born through MSAF did not need to have their airway suctioned. The Neonatal Resuscitation Program made additional recommendations after Vain et al[2] found in a multicenter randomized study that the oropharynx and nasopharynx suctioning at the perineum did not provide any beneficial protection to the neonate, irrespective of whether it was thick or thin meconium contamination of the amniotic fluid. However, there is still lack of evidence on the current recommendations of tracheal suctioning of nonvigorous neonates. This practice continues to prevail despite studies by Ghindini et al[3] and several other authors indicating that MAS occurs during pregnancy, and the role of obstruction of the airway was largely unsubstantiated.

The practice of continued tracheal suctioning of nonvigorous babies continues to be fiercely debated without the support of well-designed randomized studies. I applaud Chettri and coauthors for their attempt to enhance the evidence base regarding MSAF. Their study found that tracheal suctioning of a nonvigorous infant born through MSAF did not provide any protection against MAS when compared with those who were not suctioned. At the same time, there was no significant difference between the 2 groups with respect to neonatal intensive care unit morbidity and mortality and outcomes at 9 months. The overall incidence of MAS and mortality in both groups is very high, but this study was conducted at a relatively underresourced center and represents what happens in the developing world. In the United States with all the technology including nitric oxide, mechanical ventilation, and extracorporeal membrane oxygenation, if necessary, the mortality from MAS is less than 5%. The mere process of repeated intubations and suctioning is not a benign one and could be fraught with undesirable side effects. We owe it to our patients to examine the risks and benefits of this practice, and this study, I hope, will provide a foundation for future multicenter randomized studies. These studies are needed to guide best practices in the delivery room. I speculate that in the future, this practice of tracheal suctioning in infants born through MSAF will undergo further changes and this study, among others would have led the charge.

M. Bhola, MD

References

1. Wiswell TE, Gannon CM, Jacob J, et al. Delivery room management of the apparently vigorous meconium stained neonate: results of the multicenter, international collaborative trial. *Pediatrics*. 2000;105:1-7.
2. Vain NE, Szyld E, Prudent LM, Wiswell TE, Aguilar AM, Vivas NI. Oropharyngeal and nasopharyngeal suctioning of meconium-stained neonates before delivery of their shoulders: multicenter, randomized controlled trial. *Lancet*. 2004;364:597-602.
3. Ghindini A, Spong CY. Severe meconium aspiration syndrome is not caused by aspiration of meconium. *Am J Obstet Gynecol*. 2001;185:931-938.

Endotracheal Suction for Nonvigorous Neonates Born through Meconium Stained Amniotic Fluid: A Randomized Controlled Trial
Chettri S, Adhisivam B, Bhat BV (Jawaharlal Inst of Postgraduate Med Education and Res (JIPMER), Pondicherry, India)
J Pediatr 166:1208-1213.e1, 2015

Objective.—To assess whether endotracheal suctioning of nonvigorous infants born through meconium stained amniotic fluid (MSAF) reduces the risk and complications of meconium aspiration syndrome (MAS).

Study Design.—Term, nonvigorous babies born through MSAF were randomized to endotracheal suction and no-suction groups (n = 61 in each). Risk of MAS, complications of MAS and endotracheal suction, mortality, duration of neonatal intensive care unit stay, and neurodevelopmental outcome at 9 months were assessed.

Results.—Maternal age, consistency of meconium, mode of delivery, birth weight, sex, and Apgar scores were similar in the groups. In total, 39 (32%) neonates developed MAS and 18 (14.8%) of them died. There were no significant differences in MAS, its severity and complications, mortality, and neurodevelopmental outcome for the 2 groups. One infant had a complication of endotracheal suctioning, which was mild and transient.

Conclusions.—The current practice of routine endotracheal suctioning for nonvigorous neonates born through MSAF should be further evaluated.

Trial Registration.—Clinical Trial Registry of India: CTRI/2013/03/003469.

▶ This small, randomized clinical trial addressed one of the most hotly debated issues in perinatal management: the potential benefits and risks of routine intubation for lower airway suction of infants at risk of meconium aspiration. This study was conducted in the Neonatology Division of Jawaharlal Institute of Postgraduate Medical Education and Research, Pondicherry, India. The authors describe outcomes of 122 term, nonvigorous infants born in the presence of meconium-stained amniotic fluid who were randomized to receiving or withholding endotracheal suctioning. Approximately one-third of the babies develop signs consistent with meconium aspiration syndrome (MAS), and 15% died; 3 deaths followed parental requested redirection of care to comfort measures. No differences in outcomes, including the occurrence or severity of MAS and 9-month neurodevelopmental outcomes, were observed between study groups, except for 1 mild and transient vocal cord injury associated with intubation for meconium suctioning. This is an impressive and difficult study: the first published clinical trial of randomization of intubation and suctioning of nonvigorous infants born through meconium-stained amniotic fluid. Although the trial is of modest size, rates of MAS and mortality are somewhat higher than contemporary rates among infants born in Western countries, and the tool used to assess 9-month neurodevelopmental outcome has not been validated in Western-born populations. All outcomes are impressively equivalent between infants who received or did not receive endotracheal intubation for meconium suctioning. The results are likely to surprise few neonatologists. How many of us can say we have truly spared an infant MAS or death by delivery room intubation? Who among us has not witnessed a complication of intubation to suction meconium-stained fluid? How do we know we are not adding insult to injury by delaying initiation of ventilation to pause to intubate a depressed newborn? Nevertheless, evidence-based approaches require conclusive evidence, not simply anecdote or common sense. Dr Wiswell's important 2000 publication[1] set the stage for abandonment of intubation of vigorous babies for meconium suctioning. Hopefully, Dr Chettri and colleagues' pivotal evidence will set the stage for definitively closing the door on the practice of routine endotracheal intubation of newborn infants at birth for suctioning meconium-stained fluid from the lower airway.

L. J. Van Marter, MD, MPH

Reference

1. Wiswell TE, Gannon CM, Jacob J, et al. Delivery room management of the apparently vigorous meconium-stained neonate: results of the multicenter, international collaborative trial. *Pediatrics.* 2000;105:1-7.

Diagnostic Accuracy of Fetal Heart Rate Monitoring in the Identification of Neonatal Encephalopathy
Graham EM, Adami RR, McKenney SL, et al (Johns Hopkins Univ School of Medicine, Baltimore, MD)
Obstet Gynecol 124:507-513, 2014

Objective.—To estimate the diagnostic accuracy of electronic fetal heart rate abnormalities in the identification of neonates with encephalopathy treated with whole-body hypothermia.

Methods.—Between January 1, 2007, and July 1, 2013, there were 39 neonates born at two hospitals within our system treated with whole-body hypothermia within 6 hours of birth. Neurologically normal control neonates were matched to each case by gestational age and mode of delivery in a two-to-one fashion. The last hour of electronic fetal heart rate monitoring before delivery was evaluated by three obstetricians blinded to outcome.

Results.—The differences in tracing category were not significantly different (neonates in the case group 10.3% I, 76.9% II, 12.8% III; neonates in the control group 9.0% I, 89.7% II, 1.3% III; $P=.18$). Bivariate analysis showed neonates in the case group had significantly increased late decelerations, total deceleration area 30 (debt 30) and 60 minutes (debt 60) before delivery and were more likely to be nonreactive. Multivariable logistic regression showed neonates in the case group had a significant decrease in early decelerations ($P=.03$) and a significant increase in debt 30 (.01) and debt 60 ($P=.005$). The area under the receiver operating characteristic curve, sensitivity, and specificity were 0.72, 23.1%, and 94.9% for early decelerations; 0.66, 33.3%, and 87.2% for debt 30, and 0.68, 35.9%, and 89.7% for debt 60, respectively.

Conclusion.—Abnormalities during the last hour of fetal heart rate monitoring before delivery are poorly predictive of neonatal hypoxic—ischemic encephalopathy qualifying for whole-body hypothermia treatment within 6 hours of birth.
Level of Eviedence.—II.

▶ Over the past decade, we have annually included a comment on electronic fetal heart rate monitoring (EFM) with or without cardiotachography in the YEAR BOOK. Meta-analysis of randomized controlled trials comparing EFM with intermittent auscultation has failed to show that EFM decreases neurologic morbidity or mortality; however, the 12 combined trials have been criticized as containing insufficient subjects to answer that question.[1,2] Chen et al concluded that because of the low prevalence of target conditions (ie, hypoxic—ischemic encephalopathy [HIE]) and mediocre validity (ability to distinguish between those who are diseased and those who are well) that the positive predictive value for infant death and cerebral palsy was near zero percent. However, 89% of the study subjects were monitored, and the mortality was lower in this group.[1] The report from Graham et al does not substantially change the story. Despite the fact that three-quarters of pregnancies in the United States are monitored electronically, its value is extremely limited, mainly because there are nonspecific findings often found in normal pregnancies that obscure the findings in fetuses that are in dire straights. Graham et al began the study as a joint (resident and attending obstetrician) quality improvement project after passing the required course on EFM.[3] The goal was to use this knowledge to identify and quantitate EFM abnormalities in the last hour of labor in encephalopathic neonates who required hypothermia therapy. Thus, picking a clearly defined end point, the standard of care for HIE. If such changes could be identified, perhaps the incidence of HIE could be reduced. Such was not to be the case because the EFM abnormalities that were significantly different when compared with neonates who served as neurologically normal controls were commonly present in normal neonates. This together with the low incidence of HIE limited their ability to identify encephalopathic neonates. EFM is not a precision technology, and it generates many patterns that are not easily fit into defined categories by obstetricians even after specific training. Although Graham et al were unable to measure predictive values in a case—control study, their findings of low sensitivity for any of EFM abnormalities are consistent with the study by Grimes and Peipert,[4] who reported that the positive predictive value of EFM for detecting HIE is near zero. The high frequency of EFM abnormalities in normal neonates, which, coupled with the low prevalence of HIE during the last hour before delivery, does not allow for precision in identifying neonatal encephalopathy qualifying for treatment with hypothermia within 6 hours of birth. So it is back to the drawing board to identify the fetuses likely to become encephalopathic after delivery. In the meantime, the plaintiff's lawyers will rejoice as they present their expert witnesses identifying the precise moment at which the fetus became compromised while pointing to some EFM tracing. Remarkable that in scientific articles, certified maternal fetal specialists cannot tell from an hour of continuous tracing which infants will become encephalopathic, but after the fact, these purported experts can tell to the second when the event happened. That is why there remain so many lawsuits related to injured infants.[5]

A. A. Fanaroff, MBBCh, FRCPE

References

1. Chen HY, Chauhan SP, Ananth CV, Vintzileos AM, Abuhamad AZ. Electronic fetal heart rate monitoring and its relationship to neonatal and infant mortality in the United States. *Am J Obstet Gynecol.* 2011;204:491.e1-491.e10.
2. Alfirevic Z, Devane D, Gyte GM. Continuous cardiotocography (CTG) as a form of electronic fetal monitoring (EFM) for fetal assessment during labour. *Cochrane Database Syst Rev.* 2013;(5):CD006066.
3. Berkowitz RL, D'Alton ME, Goldberg JD, et al. The case for an electronic fetal heart rate monitoring credentialing examination. *Am J Obstet Gynecol.* 2014; 210:204-207.
4. Grimes DA, Peipert JF. Electronic fetal monitoring as a public health screening program: the arithmetic of failure. *Obstet Gynecol.* 2010;116:1397-1400.
5. Klagholz J, Strunk AL. *Overview of the 2012 ACOG Survey on Professional Liability.* Washington, DC: The American Congress of Obstetricians and Gynecologists; 2012, http://www.acog.org/;/media/Departments/Professional%20Liability/2012%20PLSurveyNational.pdf. Accessed May 31, 2015.

Delivery of Breech Presentation at Term Gestation in Canada, 2003–2011
Lyons J, for the Canadian Perinatal Surveillance System (Univ of British Columbia, Vancouver, Canada; Public Health Agency of Canada, Ottawa, Ontario)
Obstet Gynecol 125:1153-1161, 2015

Objective.—To examine neonatal mortality and morbidity rates by mode of delivery among women with breech presentation at term gestation.

Methods.—We carried out a population-based cohort study examining neonatal outcomes among term, nonanomalous singletons in breech presentation among all hospital deliveries in Canada (excluding Quebec) between 2003 and 2011. Mode of delivery was categorized into vaginal delivery, cesarean delivery in labor, and cesarean delivery without labor. Composite neonatal mortality and morbidity (death, assisted ventilation, convulsions, or specific birth injury) was the primary outcome. Logistic regression was used to estimate the independent effects of mode of delivery.

Results.—The study population included 52,671 breech deliveries; vaginal deliveries increased from 2.7% in 2003 to 3.9% in 2011, and cesarean deliveries in labor increased from 8.7% to 9.8%. Composite neonatal mortality and morbidity rates at 37 weeks of gestation or greater after vaginal delivery were significantly higher than those after cesarean without labor (adjusted rate ratio 3.60, 95% confidence interval [CI] 2.50–5.15;

adjusted rate difference 15.8/1,000 deliveries, 95% CI 9.2–25.2). Among women at 40 weeks of gestation or greater, neonatal mortality and morbidity rates after vaginal delivery were significantly higher than those after cesarean delivery without labor (adjusted rate ratio 5.39, 95% CI 2.68–10.8; adjusted rate difference 24.1/1,000 deliveries, 95% CI 9.2–53.8). Neonatal mortality and morbidity rates were also higher after caesarean delivery in labor.

Conclusion.—Among term, nonanomalous singletons in breech presentation at term, composite neonatal mortality and morbidity rates were significantly higher after vaginal delivery and cesarean delivery in labor compared with cesarean delivery without labor.

▶ Who says that you don't have to rediscover the wheel? The Term Breech Trial involving 121 centers from 26 countries unequivocally found that a policy of planned cesarean delivery is superior to that of planned vaginal delivery when the singleton fetus is in the breech position at term. Perinatal death, neonatal death, and serious neonatal morbidity were significantly lower (65%) in the planned cesarean delivery group than in the planned vaginal delivery group. Groups were similar in maternal death and serious maternal morbidity.[1] Statisticians believed that the results were robust, and the number needed to treat to achieve a better outcome was 14 overall, but 7 in countries with low perinatal mortality rate and 39 in countries with a high perinatal mortality rate.

Following the publication of the Term Breech Trial, recommendations for planned cesarean deliveries were promulgated. However, after some European studies that did not find the same differences in outcomes there was a drift to more planned vaginal deliveries. Bear in mind that both planned vaginal deliveries and cesarean deliveries following onset of labor had worse outcomes than a planned cesarean delivery. Furthermore, in 1 of the European studies, mortality was higher but not morbidity and birth trauma.[2]

In an article titled "Once More unto the Breech: Planned Vaginal Delivery Compared with Planned Cesarean Delivery," Joseph et al[3] provided a knowledge-based assessment of the alternatives for a singleton breech at term. They concluded that planned vaginal delivery "continues to be associated with higher rates of adverse perinatal outcomes in these countries. The totality of the evidence therefore unequivocally shows the relatively greater safety of planned cesarean delivery for breech presentation at term gestation."

To reevaluate the situation, Pressey and the Canadian team therefore completed another population-based cohort study with the same outcomes as the original Term Breech Trial. Composite neonatal mortality and morbidity rates were significantly higher after a vaginal delivery and after cesarean delivery in labor compared with cesarean delivery before labor onset. If it were a member of my family at term with the baby in a breech position, the choice would be clear: deliver by cesarean delivery before the onset of labor. I cannot see a rationale for doing otherwise.

A. A. Fanaroff, MBBCh, FRCPE

References

1. Hannah ME, Hannah WJ, Hewson SA, Hodnett ED, Saigal S, Willan AR. Planned caesarean section versus planned vaginal birth for breech presentation at term: a randomized multicentre trial. Term Breech Trial Collaborative Group. *Lancet.* 2000;356:1375-1383.
2. Rietberg CC, Elferink-Stinkens PM, Visser GH. The effect of the Term Breech Trial on medical intervention behaviour and neonatal outcome in The Netherlands: an analysis of 35,453 term breech infants. *BJOG.* 2005;112:205-209.
3. Joseph KS, Pressey T, Lyons J, et al. Once more unto the breech: planned vaginal delivery compared with planned cesarean delivery. *Obstet Gynecol.* 2015;125: 1162-1167.

Delayed cord clamping with and without cord stripping: a prospective randomized trial of preterm neonates
Krueger MS, Eyal FG, Peevy KJ, et al (Univ of South Alabama Children's and Women's Hosp, Mobile)
Am J Obstet Gynecol 212:394.e1-394.e5, 2015

Objective.—Autologous blood transfusion from the placenta to the neonate at birth has been proven beneficial. Transfusion can be accomplished by either delayed cord clamping or cord stripping. Both are equally effective in previous randomized trials. We hypothesized that combining these 2 techniques would further improve outcomes in preterm neonates.

Study Design.—This was a prospective randomized trial for singleton deliveries with estimated gestational ages between 22 and 31 6/7 weeks. The control protocol required a 30-second delayed cord clamping, whereas the test protocol instructed a concurrent cord stripping during the delay. The primary outcome was initial fetal hematocrit. We also examined secondary outcomes of neonatal mortality, length of time on the ventilator, days to discharge, peak bilirubin, number of phototherapy days, and neonatal complication rates.

Results.—Of the 67 patients analyzed, 32 were randomized to the control arm and 35 were randomized to the test arm. The gestational ages and fetal weights were similar between the arms. Mean hematocrit of the control arm was 47.75%, and the mean hematocrit for the test arm was 47.71% ($P=.98$). These results were stratified by gestational age, revealing the infants less than 28 weeks had an average hematocrit of 41.2% in the control arm and 44.7% in the test arm ($P=.12$). In the infants with gestational ages of 28 weeks or longer, the control arm had an average hematocrit of 52.9%, which was higher than the test arm, which averaged 49.5% ($P=.04$). The control arm received an average of 1.53 blood transfusions, whereas the test arm received 0.97 ($P=.33$). The control arm had 3 neonatal deaths, and the test arm had none ($P=.10$). The average number of days until discharge was 71.2 for the control arm and 67.8 for the test arm ($P=.66$). The average number of days on the ventilator was 4.86 for the control arm and 3.06 for the test arm ($P=.34$).

Conclusion.—Adding cord stripping to the delayed cord clamp does not result in an increased hematocrit. Data suggest trends in lower mortality and higher hematocrit in neonates born less than 28 weeks, but these were not statistically significant.

▶ Prior studies with delayed/optimized cord clamping and cord milking/stripping have been analyzed independently and have been shown to be beneficial. The study cited here was designed to see whether the combined method of delayed clamping combined with stripping would further improve outcomes. Such was not to be the case. The evidence on cord milking and delayed clamping continues to be subjected to meta-analyses and Cochrane reviews. The evidence supports both techniques, but there have not been sufficient patients studied to draw firm conclusions on some of the outcomes.

Dang published a meta-analysis that included 6 studies and 292 preterm infants treated with umbilical cord milking (UCM), while 295 received immediate cord clamping (ICC).[1] Compared with ICC, UCM significantly increased initial hemoglobin by 1.84 g/dL and decreased the incidence of transfusion 26%. They concluded that by facilitating the early stabilization of blood pressure, UCM at preterm birth was found to be comparatively safe and associated with lower blood transfusion exposure and lower incidence of intraventricular hemorrhage, necrotizing enterocolitis, and death.

On the other hand, in a meta-analysis designed to evaluate both short- and long-term outcomes, there was a paucity of data on long-term outcomes.[2] The short-term outcomes confirmed the benefits of enhanced placental transfusion strategies on better blood pressure and higher hemoglobin on admission, reduced need for transfusion, and a trend toward reduced intraventricular hemorrhage and episodes of late-onset sepsis. The authors concluded, however, that "paucity of data on neurodevelopmental outcomes and safety concerns tempers enthusiasm for these interventions."[2] Of course, they recommended further randomized controlled trials to fill these gaps in knowledge and address both short- and long-term outcomes.[2] As if on cue, a publication from Sweden appeared at the deadline for the content of the 2015 YEAR BOOK OF NEONATAL PERINATAL MEDICINE. Andersson et al[3] reported on the effect of a randomized controlled trial of a 3-minute delay in cord clamping (CC) on neurodevelopment at 4 years of age. They observed that delayed CC compared with early CC improved scores in the fine-motor and social domains at 4 years of age, especially in boys, indicates that optimizing the time to CC may affect neurodevelopment in a low-risk population of children born in a high-income country.

A. A. Fanaroff, MBBCh, FRCPE

References

1. Dang D, Zhang C, Shi S, Mu X, Lv X, Wu H. Umbilical cord milking reduces need for red cell transfusions and improves neonatal adaptation in preterm infants: meta-analysis. *J Obstet Gynaecol Res.* 2015;41:890-895.

2. Ghavam S, Batra D, Mercer J, et al. Effects of placental transfusion in extremely low birthweight infants: meta-analysis of long- and short-term outcomes. *Transfusion.* 2014;54:1192-1198.
3. Andersson O, Lindquist B, Lindgren M, Stjernqvist K, Domellöf M, Hellström-Westas L. Effect of delayed cord clamping on neurodevelopment at 4 years of age: a randomized clinical trial. *JAMA Pediatr.* 2015 [Epub ahead of print].

Effect of umbilical cord milking on morbidity and survival in extremely low gestational age neonates

Patel S, Clark EAS, Rodriguez CE, et al (Univ of Utah School of Medicine, Salt Lake City; et al)
Am J Obstet Gynecol 211:519.e1-519.e7, 2014

Objective.—Delayed umbilical cord clamping benefits extremely low gestational age neonates (ELGANs) but has not gained wide acceptance. We hypothesized that milking the umbilical cord (MUC) would avoid resuscitation delay but improve hemodynamic stability and reduce rates for composite outcome of severe intraventricular hemorrhage, necrotizing enterocolitis, and/or death before discharge.

Study Design.—We implemented a joint neonatal/maternal-fetal quality improvement process for MUC starting September 2011. The MUC protocol specified that infants who were born at <30 weeks of gestation undergo MUC 3 times over a duration of <30 seconds at delivery. Obstetric and neonatal data were collected until discharge. We compared the MUC group to retrospective ELGAN cohort delivered at our center between January 2010 and August 2011. Analysis was intention-to-treat.

Results.—We identified 318 ELGANs: 158 eligible for MUC and 160 retrospective control neonates. No adverse events were reported with cord milking. There was no difference in neonatal resuscitation, Apgar scores, or admission temperature. Hemodynamic stability was improved in the MUC group with higher mean blood pressures through 24 hours of age, despite less vasopressor use (18% vs 32%; $P < .01$). The initial hematocrit value was higher (50% vs 45%; $P < .01$), and red cell transfusions were fewer (57% vs 79%; $P < .01$) in MUC vs control infants. Presence of the composite outcome was significantly less in MUC vs the historic control infants (22% v 39%; odds ratio, 1.81; 95% confidence interval, 1.06−3.10). There were also reductions in intraventricular hemorrhage, necrotizing enterocolitis, and death before hospital discharge.

Conclusion.—MUC improves early hemodynamic stability and is associated with lower rates of serious morbidity and death among ELGANs (Table 4).

▶ Evidence for benefits of supporting placentofetal transfusion at delivery of preterm infants continues to accrue. Although not a randomized controlled trial, this report describes an experience after implementation of an umbilical cord milking protocol for preterm infants < 30 weeks' gestation (September 2011 through August 2013), compared with historical control infants (January

TABLE 4.—Logistic Regression Model for Composite Outcome of Death, Severe Intraventricular Hemorrhage or Necrotizing Enterocolitis[a]

Variable	Odds ratio	95% CI	P value
Gestation, per week >23	0.70	0.60–0.80	< .001
Clinical chorioamnionitis	2.36	1.32–4.20	.004
Cord milking	0.54	0.31–0.93	.031
Abruption	1.95	1.03–3.69	.041

CI, confidence interval.
[a]Variables also considered but not included in final model: level of resuscitation, dopamine in the first 72 hours of life, preterm rupture of membranes, hematocrit at birth.
Reprinted from Patel S, Clark EAS, Rodriguez CE, et al. Effect of umbilical cord milking on morbidity and survival in extremely low gestational age neonates. Am J Obstet Gynecol. 2014;211:519.e1-519.e7, with permission from Elsevier.

2010 through August 2011). The management strategy for the historical control group is not explicitly described, but the authors note an institutional "reluctance to adopt [delayed cord clamping] ... based on concerns regarding delayed resuscitation," so the comparison apparently is to cord clamping immediately after delivery. After adoption of the cord milking protocol, there were significant reductions in red blood cell transfusions (odds ratio [OR] 0.34, 95% confidence interval [CI] 0.21–0.56, P < .001), use of dopamine in the first hour after birth (OR 0.46, 95% CI 0.27–0.73; P = .004), necrotizing enterocolitis (NEC; OR 5.1, 95% CI 0.28–0.96; P = .045), mortality (OR 0.37, 95% CI 0.17–0.78; P = .011), and in the composite outcome of severe intraventricular hemorrhage, NEC, or death before discharge (OR 0.42, 95% CI 0.26–0.69; P < .001). Regression analysis (Table 4) for the composite outcome to adjust for differences in gestational age, chorioamnionitis, and abruption rates between eras also supported a significant relationship with cord milking (adjusted OR 0.54, 95% CI 0.31–0.93; P = .031). The nonrandomized, sequential assignment of treatments prohibits a strong conclusion that these benefits were caused by the practice change, it seems unlikely that changes of these magnitudes would have resulted simply from secular changes in outcomes over the study period of less than 4 years. It is not clear that these short-term results will translate into improved long-term neurodevelopmental outcomes, whether cord milking will prove superior to simply delaying cord clamping, or how these results might be extrapolated to more mature infants (> 30 weeks' gestation). Those limitations notwithstanding, it is appropriate for the conversation to turn from the matter of whether enhancement of placental transfusion at birth is good for preterm infants to the question of how best to achieve it.

W. E. Benitz, MD

Effect of gravity on volume of placental transfusion: a multicentre, randomised, non-inferiority trial

Vain NE, Satragno DS, Gorenstein AN, et al (Univ of Buenos Aires, Argentina; Foundation for Maternal and Child Health (FUNDASAMIN), Buenos Aires, Argentina; et al)
Lancet 384:235-240, 2014

Background.—Delayed cord clamping allows for the passage of blood from the placenta to the baby and reduces the risk of iron deficiency in infancy. To hold the infant for more than 1 min at the level of the vagina (as is presently recommended), on the assumption that gravity affects the volume of placental transfusion, is cumbersome, might result in low compliance, and interferes with immediate contact of the infant with the mother. We aimed to assess whether gravity affects the volume of placental transfusion

Methods.—We did a multicentre non-inferiority trial at three university-affiliated hospitals in Argentina. We obtained informed consent from healthy mothers with normal term pregnancies admitted early in labour. Vigorous babies born vaginally were randomly assigned in a 1:1 ratio by computer-generated blocks and sequentially numbered sealed opaque envelopes to be held for 2 min before clamping the umbilical cord, at the level of the vagina (introitus group) or on the mother's abdomen or chest (abdomen group). Newborn babies were weighed immediately after birth and after cord clamping. The primary outcome was the difference in weight (as a proxy of placental transfusion volume). The prespecified non-inferiority margin was 18 g (20%). We used t test and χ^2 test for group comparison, and used a multivariable linear regression analysis to control for covariables. This trial is registered with ClinicalTrials.gov, number NCT01497353.

Findings.—Between Aug 1, 2011, and Aug 31, 2012, we allocated 274 newborn babies to the introitus group and 272 to the abdomen group. 77 newborn babies in the introitus group and 78 in the abdomen group were ineligible after randomisation (eg, caesarean section, forceps delivery, short umbilical cord or nuchal cord). Mean weight change was 56 g (SD 47, 95% CI 50–63) for 197 babies in the introitus group compared with 53 g (45, 46–59) for 194 babies in the abdomen group, supporting non-inferiority of the two approaches (difference 3 g, 95% CI −5·8 to 12·8; $p = 0.45$). We did not note any serious adverse events during the study.

Interpretation.—Position of the newborn baby before cord clamping does not seem to affect volume of placental transfusion. Mothers could safely be allowed to hold their baby on their abdomen or chest. This change in practice might increase obstetric compliance with the procedure, enhance maternal-infant bonding, and decrease iron deficiency in infancy.

▶ Recent guidelines from both the American Board of Obstetrics and Gynecology,[1] and the World Health Organization[2] regarding the timing of umbilical cord clamping recommend waiting 1 to 3 minutes before clamping the cord. Evidence supporting this strategy in term infants has accumulated over the past 3 decades, and infants whose umbilical cords are clamped at 1 to 3 minutes have a decreased risk of iron deficiency. Studies of the timing of umbilical cord clamping after preterm delivery have shown that infants whose cords are clamped at 1-3 minutes have less frequent intraventricular hemorrhage and late onset sepsis.

In this study, Nestor Vain and colleagues evaluated the effect of gravity on the volume of placental transfusion to the newborn infant before the umbilical cord is clamped. At delivery, 546 term infants were randomized either to being held at the introitus ($n = 274$) or placed on the mother's chest or abdomen ($n = 272$) for 2 minutes before the umbilical cord was clamped. There was no difference in the mean weight gain between the 197 newborns in the introitus group and 194 newborns in the chest/abdomen group who completed the study: mean weight gain after 2 minutes was 53 grams (SD 47, 95% confidence interval 50—63) and 56 grams (SD 45, confidence interval 46—59), respectively. These results suggest that placing an infant above the introitus does not adversely influence the volume of placental blood that an infant receives before cord clamping and, as such, does not preclude the common practice of placing an infant on a mother's abdomen or chest before clamping the umbilical cord. To date, the practice of waiting several minutes before clamping the umbilical cord has not been widely adopted, despite published guidelines.[3] The data in this study may be useful in encouraging additional practitioners to adopt this practice.

R. Ohls, MD

References

1. Committee on Obstetric Practice, American College of Obstetricians and Gynecologists. Committee opinion no. 543: timing of umbilical cord clamping after birth. *Obstet Gynecol.* 2012;120:1522-1526.
2. World Health Organization. *Guidelines on Basic Newborn Resuscitation, 2012.* Geneva, Switzerland: World Health Organization; 2012.
3. Raju TN. Timing of umbilical cord clamping after birth for optimizing placental transfusion. *Curr Opin Pediatr.* 2013;25:180-187.

Randomized Trial of Occlusive Wrap for Heat Loss Prevention in Preterm Infants

Reilly MC, on behalf of the Vermont Oxford Network Heat Loss Prevention (HeLP) Trial Study Group (Sunnybrook Health Sciences Centre, Toronto, Ontario, Canada)
J Pediatr 166:262-268.e2, 2015

Objective.—To determine whether the application of occlusive wrap applied immediately after birth will reduce mortality in very preterm infants.

Study Design.—This was a prospective randomized controlled trial of infants born 24 0/7 to 27 6/7 weeks' gestation who were assigned randomly to occlusive wrap or no wrap. The primary outcome was all cause mortality at discharge or 6 months' corrected age. Secondary outcomes included temperature, Apgar scores, pH, base deficit, blood pressure and glucose, respiratory distress syndrome, bronchopulmonary dysplasia, seizures, patent ductus arteriosus, necrotizing enterocolitis, gastrointestinal perforation, intraventricular hemorrhage, cystic periventricular leukomalacia, pulmonary hemorrhage, retinopathy of prematurity, sepsis, hearing screen, and pneumothorax.

Results.—Eight hundred one infants were enrolled. There was no difference in baseline population characteristics. There were no significant differences in mortality (OR 1.0, 95% CI 0.7-1.5). Wrap infants had statistically significant greater baseline temperatures (36.3°C wrap vs 35.7°C no wrap, $P < .0001$) and poststabilization temperatures (36.6°C vs 36.2°C, $P < .001$) than nonwrap infants. For the secondary outcomes, there was a significant decrease in pulmonary hemorrhage (OR 0.6, 95% CI 0.3-0.9) in the wrap group and a significant lower mean one minute Apgar score ($P = .007$) in the wrap group. The study was stopped early because continued enrollment would not result in the attainment of a significant difference in the primary outcome.

Conclusion.—Application of occlusive wrap to very preterm infants immediately after birth results in greater mean body temperature but does not reduce mortality (Fig 3).

▶ During the "Golden Hour," the first 60 minutes after the birth of an extremely premature infant, specific attention and a standardized approach to cord management, thermal regulation, respiratory management, and vascular access have positively affected mortality and morbidity. Preventing hypothermia is a major goal so that the babies will be admitted to the neonatal intensive care unit with a temperature above 36°C. Preterm babies are vulnerable to heat loss because they lack insulation (fat), are unable to shiver, and have a relatively large surface area. Furthermore, few centers observe the World Health Organization recommendation to resuscitate these babies in a room heated to 25°C. Many studies, randomized and others, have demonstrated various methods of keeping the infants warm. These include but are not limited to[1-3] plastic wraps, plastic bags (full body and even including the head), radiant warmers, heated humidified gases, heating resuscitation area, skin-to-skin care, and a novel method reported by Horn[4] with active forced-air warming of mothers and newborns immediately after cesarean delivery that reduces the incidence of infant and maternal hypothermia, increases maternal comfort, and reduces maternal shivering.

The study from the Vermont-Oxford Network abstracted here is of considerable interest. The study was discontinued after a 50% enrollment because it was evident that the primary objective could never be accomplished—that is, there was no way that mortality would be reduced 25% in the occlusive wrap group. Whereas the mortality in the lower gestational age group was lower

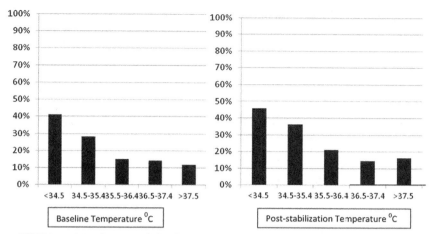

FIGURE 3.—Mortality rates of all infants according to baseline and poststabilization temperature. (Reprinted from Journal Pediatrics Reilly MC, on behalf of the Vermont Oxford Network Heat Loss Prevention (HeLP) Trial Study Group. Randomized trial of occlusive wrap for heat loss prevention in preterm infants. *J Pediatr.* 2015;166:262-268.e2, with permission from Elsevier.)

with the wrap, it was higher, but not statistically significant, in the more mature infants. This may be due in part to the excellent management of the control group at these sophisticated centers. Closer examination of Fig 3 reveals that the infants who did not become hypothermic had higher survival rates. The goal remains to avoid moderate hypothermia, but also hyperthermia. Each center may use its own approach to accomplish this task.

A. A. Fanaroff, MBBCh, FRCPE

References

1. Paris LG, Seitz M, McElroy KG, Regan M. A randomized controlled trial to improve outcomes utilizing various warming techniques during cesarean birth. *J Obstet Gynecol Neonatal Nurs.* 2014;43:719-728.
2. Doglioni N, Cavallin F, Mardegan V, et al. Total body polyethylene wraps for preventing hypothermia in preterm infants: a randomized trial. *J Pediatr.* 2014;16: 261-266.
3. Knobel RB, Wimmer JE, Holbert D. Heat loss prevention for preterm infants in the delivery room. *J Perinatol.* 2005;25:308-312.
4. Horn EP, Bein B, Steinfath M, et al. The incidence and prevention of hypothermia in newborn bonding after cesarean delivery: a randomized controlled trial. *Anesth Analg.* 2014;118:997-1002.

Low Apgar score, neonatal encephalopathy and epidural analgesia during labour: a Swedish registry-based study

Törnell S, Ekéus C, Hultin M, et al (Umeå Univ, Sweden; Karolinska Inst, Stockholm, Sweden; et al)
Acta Anaesthesiol Scand 59:486-495, 2015

Background.—Maternal intrapartum fever (MF) is associated with neonatal sequelae, and women in labour who receive epidural analgesia (EA) are more likely to develop hyperthermia. The aims of this study were to investigate if EA and/or a diagnosis of MF were associated to adverse neonatal outcomes at a population level.

Methods.—Population-based register study with data from the Swedish Birth Register and the Swedish National Patient Register, including all nulliparae ($n = 294{,}329$) with singleton pregnancies who gave birth at term in Sweden 1999−2008. Neonatal outcomes analysed were Apgar score (AS) <7 at 5 min and ICD-10 diagnosis of neonatal encephalopathy (e.g. convulsions or neonatal cerebral ischaemia). Multivariate logistic regression was used to calculate adjusted odds ratios (AOR) with 95% confidence intervals (CI).

Results.—EA was used in 44% of the deliveries. Low AS or encephalopathy was found in 1.26% and 0.39% of the children in the EA group compared with 0.80% and 0.29% in the control group. In multivariate analysis, EA was associated with increased risk with low AS, AOR 1.27 (95% CI 1.16−1.39), but not with diagnosis of encephalopathy, 1.11 (0.96−1.29). A diagnosis of MF was associated with increased risk for both low AS, 2.27 (1.71−3.02), and of neonatal encephalopathy, 1.97 (1.19−3.26).

Conclusion.—Diagnosis of MF was associated with low AS and neonatal encephalopathy, whereas EA was only associated with low AS and not with neonatal encephalopathy. The found associations might be a result of confounding by indication, which is difficult to assess in a registry-based population study.

▶ In this study, investigators attempted to address the effects of maternal fever and the use of epidural anesthesia on Apgar scores and neonatal encephalopathy. Using a retrospective analysis of registry-based data, they found that epidural anesthesia was associated with low Apgar scores but not neonatal encephalopathy, whereas maternal fever was associated with both. The methodology has multiple definitional flaws, as it appears that a 5-minute Apgar score of < 7 was used as a surrogate for "birth depression," rather than using something more objective, such as umbilical cord acid−base balance. Moreover, the *International Classification of Disease (10th Revision)* definition of neonatal encephalopathy (convulsions or cerebral ischemia) is sufficiently vague with respect to timing of injury that I find it difficult to take anything meaningful from this study. Investigations such as this are also subject to significant selection biases, and the most we can conclude is that an interesting hypothesis has been generated to test in a large, prospective clinical observation.

S. M. Donn, MD

Extreme macrosomia – Obstetric outcomes and complications in birthweights >5000 g
Hehir MP, Mchugh AF, Maguire PJ, et al (Natl Maternity Hosp, Dublin, Ireland)
Aust N Z J Obstet Gynaecol 55:42-46, 2015

Objective.—Management of extremely large birthweight infants presents challenges during the period of labour and delivery. We sought to examine outcomes in infants with extreme macrosomia (birthweight >5000 g), at an institution where the management of labour is standardised.

Materials and Methods.—This is a retrospective analysis of prospectively gathered data on all infants with a birthweight >5000 g delivered at a tertiary level institution from 2008 to 2012. Details of labour characteristics and outcomes were examined; these were compared according to parity.

Results.—During the study period, there were 46 128 deliveries at the hospital and 182 infants with a birthweight >5000 g, giving an incidence of 0.4%. The majority of women (133/182) were multiparous. Among nulliparas, 47% (23/49) had a vaginal delivery, while 53% (26/49) had a caesarean delivery. 86% (97/113) of multiparas had a vaginal delivery, and 14% (16/113) had a caesarean delivery. 43% (69/162) required induction of labour. This was more common in nulliparous compared with multiparous women (58% [29/49] vs 30% [40/133], $P = 0.005$, $OR = 3.4$, 95% $CI = 1.7-6.6$). A total of 30% (49/162) of women had their labour accelerated with oxytocin. There were higher rates of oxytocin use in nulliparas than in multiparas (55% [27/49] vs 16.5% [22/133], $P < 0.0001$, $OR = 6.2$, 95% $CI = 3-12.8$). Seventeen of the 120 infants delivered vaginally had a shoulder dystocia (14.2%), with three suffering an Erbs palsy, all of which had resolved before 6 months of age. One baby had a clavicular fracture.

Conclusion.—Extreme macrosomia affects 0.4% of pregnancies in contemporary practice. Multiparas have a low rate of caesarean section. Infants delivered vaginally are at increased risk of shoulder dystocia and associated complications.

▶ Maternal glucose homeostasis is an important determinant of fetal size. Walsh et al[1] have shown that even small variations in fasting glucose concentrations can influence fetal growth and adiposity. The incidence of macrosomia (birth weight > 4.5 kg) was significantly greater for maternal and cord blood glucose levels in the highest quartile compared with the lowest quartile (20.7% vs 11.7%, $P < .05$ in the first trimester, 21.3% vs 7.2%, $P < .05$, at

28 weeks, and 33.3% vs 10%, $P < 0.05$, in cord blood). Hence, the effect endures from the first trimester until delivery.

Demonstrating the medicine is global; investigators from the same center in Ireland published their experience and findings with a cohort of infants with birth weight > 5 kg, in a New Zealand medical journal. It is impressive that 86% of multipara delivered these massive babies vaginally. There is no long-term maternal follow-up, but 2.5% of the mothers experienced sphincteric injury, and significant postpartum hemorrhage occurred in 6% of the deliveries. It is not surprising but highly relevant that 14% of the deliveries were complicated by shoulder dystocia. Fortunately, all 3 infants with brachial plexus injuries recovered fully. This must be taken into consideration when weighing the benefits of vaginal versus operative delivery because there are significant risks of injury to both mother and baby with vaginal delivery of very large babies.

The authors remind us of the multiple risk factors for the development of a macrosomic infant, many of which were present in the above report, including diabetes (5%), post dates beyond 42 weeks' gestation (6%), and high maternal body mass index. Indeed, macrosomia may be constitutional (familial, ethnic, male gender), environmental (maternal diabetes, obesity), or genetic (eg, Beckwith Wiedemann syndrome). Unfortunately, identification by ultrasound is far from precise, and risk modification is extremely limited. Even superb glucose control in an effort to prevent recurrent macrosomia may not be successful.

A. A. Fanaroff, MBBCh, FRCPE

Reference

1. Walsh JM, Mahony R, Byrne J, et al. The association of maternal and fetal glucose homeostasis with fetal adiposity and birthweight. *Eur J Obstet Gynecol Reprod Biol.* 2011;159:338-341.

Between-Hospital Variation in Treatment and Outcomes in Extremely Preterm Infants
Rysavy MA, for the Eunice Kennedy Shriver National Institute of Child Health and Human Development Neonatal Research Network (Univ of Iowa; et al)
N Engl J Med 372:1801-1811, 2015

Background.—Between-hospital variation in outcomes among extremely preterm infants is largely unexplained and may reflect differences in hospital practices regarding the initiation of active lifesaving treatment as compared with comfort care after birth.

Methods.—We studied infants born between April 2006 and March 2011 at 24 hospitals included in the Eunice Kennedy Shriver National Institute of Child Health and Human Development Neonatal Research Network. Data were collected for 4987 infants born before 27 weeks of gestation without congenital anomalies. Active treatment was defined as any potentially lifesaving intervention administered after birth. Survival and neurodevelopmental impairment at 18 to 22 months of corrected age were assessed in 4704 children (94.3%).

Results.—Overall rates of active treatment ranged from 22.1% (interquartile range [IQR], 7.7 to 100) among infants born at 22 weeks of gestation to 99.8% (IQR, 100 to 100) among those born at 26 weeks of gestation. Overall rates of survival and survival without severe impairment ranged from 5.1% (IQR, 0 to 10.6) and 3.4% (IQR, 0 to 6.9), respectively, among children born at 22 weeks of gestation to 81.4% (IQR, 78.2 to 84.0) and 75.6% (IQR, 69.5 to 80.0), respectively, among those born at 26 weeks of gestation. Hospital rates of active treatment accounted for 78% and 75% of the between-hospital variation in survival and survival without severe impairment, respectively, among children born at 22 or 23 weeks of gestation, and accounted for 22% and 16%, respectively, among those born at 24 weeks of gestation, but the rates did not account for any of the variation in outcomes among those born at 25 or 26 weeks of gestation.

Conclusions.—Differences in hospital practices regarding the initiation of active treatment in infants born at 22, 23, or 24 weeks of gestation explain some of the between-hospital variation in survival and survival without impairment among such patients. (Funded by the National Institutes of Health.)

▶ Every major randomized, controlled trial regarding extremely preterm infants has shown marked center-to-center variability in the primary outcome variables and particularly morbidity and mortality. It should come as no surprise that the mortality at the borders of viability should demonstrate marked center variability. For the babies between 22 and 24 weeks of gestation, there is a huge difference in whether active treatment was offered (Fig 1 in the original article). These differences in hospital rates of active treatment among children born at 22, 23, or 24 weeks of gestation explained a large portion of the variation in hospital rates of survival and survival without severe impairment and explained a lesser portion of the variation in hospital rates of survival without moderate or severe impairment. There is a cost to more active treatment, because, in addition to an increased number of survivors, there are more babies with impairment. This has been the pattern over the last 40 years as death is replaced by more intact survivors but also more handicapped babies. In due course the number of intact survivors increases without the burden of an increased number with severe handicap. Reducing intraventricular hemorrhage and sepsis no doubt has played a role (see below).[1] This report is filled with interesting statistics and figures and provides a yardstick for other networks to examine their outcomes.

After the dramatic declines in neonatal mortality among extremely immature infants following the widespread use of antenatal corticosteroics and surfactant therapy, further declines have been slow as evidenced in the National Institute of Child Health and Human Development Neonatal Research Network investigation into the causes and timing in extremely premature infants. They prospectively collected data on 6075 deaths among 22, 248 live births, with gestational ages of 22 0/7 to 28 6/7 weeks, among infants born in study hospitals between 2000 and 2011.[1] Overall, 40.4% of deaths occurred within 12 hours after birth, and 17.3% occurred after 28 days.

There were 275 deaths per 1000 live births from 2000 through 2003 and 285 from 2004 through 2007; the number decreased to 258 in the 2008 to 2011 period ($P=.003$ for the comparison across 3 periods). There were fewer pulmonary-related deaths attributed to the respiratory distress syndrome and bronchopulmonary dysplasia in 2008 to 2011 than in the prior 2 epochs. Similarly, in 2008 to 2011 compared with 2000 to 2003, there were decreases in deaths attributed to immaturity infection or central nervous system injury; however, there were increases in deaths attributed to necrotizing enterocolitis.

In Sweden during 2004 to 2007, the 1-year survival rate of infants born alive at 22 to 26 weeks of gestation was 70% and ranged from 9.8% at 22 weeks to 85% at 26 weeks.[2] This rate followed a more unified approach to babies born at the limits of viability with the presumption that active intervention would decrease mortality and morbidity. Reduced mortality rate was associated with tocolytic treatment, antenatal corticosteroids surfactant treatment within 2 hours after birth, and birth at a level III hospital. Among 1-year survivors, 45% had no major neonatal morbidity. It remains a major challenge to decrease the morbidity and improve the long-term outcome for these infants. As in the study abstracted above, mortality rates in extremely preterm infants varied considerably between Swedish health care regions in the first year after birth, particularly among the most immature infants.[3]

The topic of neonatal death will be discussed in another commentary dealing with the Millennium 2015 goals.

A. A. Fanaroff, MBBCh, FRCPE

References

1. Patel RM, Kandefer S, Walsh MC, et al; Eunice Kennedy Shriver National Institute of Child Health and Human Development Neonatal Research Network. Causes and timing of death in extremely premature infants from 2000 through 2011. *N Engl J Med*. 2015;22:331-340.
2. EXPRESS Group, Fellman V, Hellström-Westas L, Norman M, et al. One-year survival of extremely preterm infants after active perinatal care in Sweden. *JAMA*. 2009;301:2225-2233.
3. Serenius F, Sjörs G, Blennow M, et al; EXPRESS study group. EXPRESS study shows significant regional differences in 1-year outcome of extremely preterm infants in Sweden. *Acta Paediatr*. 2014;103:27-37.

5 Infectious Disease and Immunology

Late-Onset Group B Streptococcal Meningitis Has Cerebrovascular Complications
Tibussek D, Sinclair A, Yau I, et al (Univ of Toronto, Ontario, Canada; et al)
J Pediatr 166:1187-1192.e1, 2015

Objective.—To describe cerebrovascular diseases related to late-onset group B *Streptococcus* (GBS) meningitis.

Study Design.—Retrospective case series. Patients treated for cerebrovascular complication of late-onset GBS meningitis over 5 years were identified through neuroradiology and microbiology databases. Patient charts were reviewed with regard to clinical presentation, laboratory findings, including GBS subtype, treatment, clinical course, and outcome. Cerebral magnetic resonance imaging was reviewed with special emphasis on stroke pattern and cerebrovascular findings.

Results.—Fourteen patients were identified. In 6 out of 9 patients serotype III was causative and positive for surface protein hvgA in 5. Ten had arterial ischemic stroke accompanied by a cerebral sinovenous thrombosis in 2 patients. Evidence of cerebral vasculopathy was found in 4 cases. The stroke pattern was variable with cortical, multifocal ischemia, basal ganglia involvement, or had a clear territorial arterial infarction. Ten patients were treated with anticoagulation. No significant bleeding complications, and no recurrent strokes occurred. Twelve patients had clinical and/or subclinical seizures. Developmental outcome was good in 8 cases. Six patients had moderate to severe developmental delay. Central nervous system complications included subdural empyema, hydrocephalus, epilepsy, microcephaly, and hemiplegia.

Conclusions.—Late-onset GBS meningitis can be complicated by severe cerebrovascular disease, including arterial ischemic stroke and cerebral sinovenous thrombosis. These complications may be underestimated. Were commend a low threshold for cerebral imaging in these cases. Future studies on the exact incidence, the role of GBS subtypes, and on safety and efficiency of preventive anticoagulation therapy are warranted.

▶ In this retrospective case series encompassing infants born during a 5-year period in hospitals in Canada and Germany, the authors describe neurological complications of late-onset group B streptococcal (GBS) meningitis in a subset of patients. Among those with GBS meningitis, 14 patients were identified as having cerebrovascular complications: 10 with arterial ischemic stroke (2 with accompanying sinovenous thrombosis) and 4 with evidence of cerebral vasculopathy. Of this population, 8 had good neurodevelopmental outcome, and 6 experienced moderate-to-severe developmental delay. Other central nervous system complications were noted, including subdural empyema, hydrocephalus, epilepsy, microcephaly, and hemiplegia. In an era in which the occurrence of GBS infection has fallen to low rates due to routine screening and intrapartum prophylaxis, this study serves as a reminder of the potential ravages of GBS infection. Of note, 3 of the 14 patients with cerebrovascular complications had GBS detected only in their cerebrospinal fluid (CSF; 2 by culture, 1 by latex fixation), not in their blood cultures, underscoring prior work indicating that reliance on a positive blood culture as a criterion for evaluating the CSF will lead to missed cases of meningitis. This study serves as a reminder of the importance of evaluating CSF in cases of suspected or known bacteremia and provides a call for neurological and neuroimaging evaluation of infants who experience GBS meningitis.

L. J. Van Marter, MD, MPH

The microbiota regulates neutrophil homeostasis and host resistance to *Escherichia coli* K1 sepsis in neonatal mice

Deshmukh HS, Liu Y, Menkiti OR, et al (Children's Hosp of Philadelphia, PA; et al)
Nat Med 20:524-530, 2014

Acquisition of microbes by the neonate, which begins immediately during birth, is influenced by gestational age and mother's microbiota and modified by exposure to antibiotics. In neonates, prolonged duration of antibiotic therapy is associated with increased risk of sepsis after 4 days of life, known as late-onset sepsis (LOS), a disorder critically controlled by neutrophils, but a role for the microbiota in regulating neutrophil behavior in the neonate has not been described. We exposed pregnant mouse dams to antibiotics in drinking water to limit transfer of maternal microbes to the neonates. Antibiotic exposure of dams decreased the total number of microbes in the intestine, altered the structure of intestinal microbiota and changed the pattern of microbial colonization. These changes were associated with decreased numbers of circulating and bone marrow neutrophils and granulocyte/macrophage restricted progenitor cells in the bone marrow. Antibiotic-exposure of dams attenuated the postnatal granulocytosis by reducing the number of interleukin (IL) 17-producing cells in intestine and consequent production of granulocyte colony stimulating factor (G-CSF). Relative granulocytopenia contributed to increased susceptibility of antibiotic-exposed neonatal mice to *Escherichia coli* K1 and *Klebsiella pneumoniae* sepsis, which could be partially reversed by administration of G-CSF. Restoration of normal microbiota, through TLR4- and MYD88-dependent mechanism, induced accumulation of IL17-producing type 3 innate lymphoid cells (ILC) in the intestine, promoted granulocytosis, and restored the IL17- dependent resistance to sepsis. Specific depletion of ILCs prevented the IL17- and G-CSF-dependent granulocytosis and resistance to sepsis. These data support a role for the intestinal microbiota in regulation of granulocytosis and host resistance to sepsis in the neonates.

▶ Antibiotics are among the most commonly used medications given to pregnant mothers near the time of parturition and in neonates, especially those born preterm. As shown in this study in mice, it is not surprising that this alters the developmental pattern of the intestinal microbiota after birth. Previous epidemiologic studies in human mothers and neonates have suggested that this practice may increase late-onset sepsis and even necrotizing enterocolitis. The mechanism of this effect has been unclear, but this study elegantly shows a relationship between antibiotics and a delayed neutrophil production response. Antibiotic treatment using clinically relevant ampicillin, gentamicin, and vancomycin resulted in increased propensity toward infection with pathogens *Escherichia coli* K1 and *Klebsiella*. The pathways that appear to play a role are toll-like receptor (TLR)-17 induced neutrophil production via granulocyte colony stimulating factor and stimulated by a TLR-4 pathway via MyD88 signaling.

This study is intriguing from the standpoint of its significance in human pregnancy and in neonates. Antibiotics are likely overused in both mothers and neonates, especially preterms neonates. If this practice induces immune hyporesponsiveness in humans as in this study in mice, we have a problem. These antibiotics are clearly harmful, and providing them as we do may not be worth the assumed benefit. Unless we can determine a means to curb antibiotic use, perhaps an approach as the one used in the mice in this study to reverse the delayed granulocyte response by introducing healthy intestinal contents (microbiota) to the antibiotic-treated infants in the form of fecal microbial transplantation analogous to the technique used in older individuals with refractory *Clostridium difficile* infection may be in order. Evidence as provided by this study should increase neonatologists equipoise for a clinical trial.

J. Neu, MD

Effect of Fluconazole Prophylaxis on Candidiasis and Mortality in Premature Infants: A Randomized Clinical Trial

Benjamin DK Jr, for the Fluconazole Prophylaxis Study Team (Duke Clinical Res Inst, Durham, NC; et al)
JAMA 311:1742-1749, 2014

Importance.—Invasive candidiasis in premature infants causes death and neurodevelopmental impairment. Fluconazole prophylaxis reduces candidiasis, but its effect on mortality and the safety of fluconazole are unknown.

Objective.—To evaluate the efficacy and safety of fluconazole in preventing death or invasive candidiasis in extremely low-birth-weight infants.

Design, Setting, and Patients.—This study was a randomized, blinded, placebo-controlled trial of fluconazole in premature infants. Infants weighing less than 750 g at birth (N = 361) from 32 neonatal intensive care units (NICUs) in the United States were randomly assigned to receive either fluconazole or placebo twice weekly for 42 days. Surviving infants were evaluated at 18 to 22 months corrected age for neurodevelopmental outcomes. The study was conducted between November 2008 and February 2013.

Interventions.—Fluconazole (6 mg/kg of body weight) or placebo.

Main Outcomes and Measures.—The primary end point was a composite of death or definite or probable invasive candidiasis prior to study day 49 (1 week after completion of study drug). Secondary and safety outcomes included invasive candidiasis, liver function, bacterial infection, length of stay, intracranial hemorrhage, periventricular leukomalacia, chronic lung disease, patent ductus arteriosus requiring surgery, retinopathy of prematurity requiring surgery, necrotizing enterocolitis, spontaneous intestinal perforation, and neurodevelopmental outcomes—defined as a Bayley-III cognition composite score of less than 70, blindness, deafness, or cerebral palsy at 18 to 22 months corrected age.

Results.—Among infants receiving fluconazole, the composite primary end point of death or invasive candidiasis was 16% (95% CI, 11%-22%) vs 21% in the placebo group (95% CI, 15%-28%; odds ratio, 0.73 [95% CI, 0.43-1.23]; $P = .24$; treatment difference, -5% [95% CI, -13% to 3%]). Invasive candidiasis occurred less frequently in the fluconazole group (3% [95% CI, 1%-6%]) vs the placebo group (9% [95% CI, 5%-14%]; $P = .02$; treatment difference, -6% [95% CI, -11% to -1%]). The cumulative incidences of other secondary outcomes were not statistically different between groups. Neurodevelopmental impairment did not differ between the groups (fluconazole, 31% [95% CI, 21%-41%] vs placebo, 27% [95% CI, 18%-37%]; $P = .60$; treatment difference, 4% [95% CI, -10% to 17%]).

Conclusions and Relevance.—Among infants with a birth weight of less than 750 g, 42 days of fluconazole prophylaxis compared with placebo did not result in a lower incidence of the composite of death or invasive candidiasis. These findings do not support the universal use of prophylactic fluconazole in extremely low-birth-weight infants.

Trial Registration.—clinicaltrials.gov Identifier: NCT00734539.

▶ In a randomized controlled trial conducted between 1998 and 2000, Kaufman et al demonstrated that fluconazole prophylaxis reduced the incidence of invasive fungal infection in babies with birth weights <1000 g from 20% to zero.[1] Reduction in the mortality rate from 20% to 8% was not statistically significant, and rates of the combined outcome of death or invasive fungal infection were not reported. In the intervening years, the incidence of invasive fungal infection in extremely low birth weight (ELBW) infants declined, and some questioned the utility of prophylaxis in the setting of these significantly lower attack rates. This article sets out to address the matter in a well-designed randomized controlled trial, for which the primary endpoint was either death or invasive fungal disease by 49 days of age in infants with birth weights < 750 g. The trial was designed to have adequate power (92%) to detect a reduction in the rate of that primary outcome from 30% to 15%. The primary outcome rate in the placebo arm was only 21% at day 49 and 26% before discharge (vs 16% and 21% in the treatment group), and death contributed equally to outcomes (14% in both groups by day 49 and 18% or 19%, respectively, before discharge). There were statistically significant reductions in the secondary endpoints of rates of invasive disease by day 49 (9% to 3%, $P = .016$) or by discharge (11% to 4%, $P = .015$), however. Infants with candidiasis were more likely to die (pooled odds ratio 4.0, 95% confidence interval 1.6—9.6; $P = .0012$). Although it is correct (as the authors note) that these "findings [absence of effect on the primary outcome] do not support the universal use of prophylactic fluconazole in extremely low-birth-weight infants," those secondary endpoints conversely do not support a complete lack of utility either. The question of whether there is a role for fluconazole prophylaxis in very low birth weight infants therefore remains open. Until better data become available, it may be wise to consider the advice that "In nurseries in which aggressive implementation of infection control policy and judicious antibiotic use still do not reduce risk of invasive candidiasis in ELBW infants to below a few percent, routine fluconazole prophylaxis seems warranted."[2] Whether that approach should be adopted still depends on the magnitude of the problem and the anticipated value of preventing some cases of invasive candidiasis.

W. E. Benitz, MD

References

1. Kaufman D, Boyle R, Hazen KC, Patrie JT, Robinson M, Donowitz LG. Fluconazole prophylaxis against fungal colonization and infection in preterm infants. *N Engl J Med.* 2001;345:1660-1666.
2. Long SS. No long-term adverse effects of fluconazole prophylaxis in ELBW infants. *J Pediatr.* 2011;158:A1.

Blood Transfusion and Breast Milk Transmission of Cytomegalovirus in Very Low-Birth-Weight Infants: A Prospective Cohort Study
Josephson CD, Caliendo AM, Easley KA, et al (Emory Univ, Atlanta, GA; Brown Univ, Providence, RI; et al)
JAMA Pediatr 168:1054-1062, 2014

Importance.—Postnatal cytomegalovirus (CMV) infection can cause serious morbidity and mortality in very low-birth-weight (VLBW) infants. The primary sources of postnatal CMV infection in this population are breast milk and blood transfusion. The current risks attributable to these vectors, as well as the efficacy of approaches to prevent CMV transmission, are poorly characterized.

Objective.—To estimate the risk of postnatal CMV transmission from 2 sources: (1) transfusion of CMV-seronegative and leukoreduced blood and (2) maternal breast milk.

Design, Setting, and Participants.—A prospective, multicenter birth-cohort study was conducted from January 2010 to June 2013 at 3 neonatal intensive care units (2 academically affiliated and 1 private) in Atlanta, Georgia. Cytomegalovirus serologic testing of enrolled mothers was performed to determine their status. Cytomegalovirus nucleic acid testing (NAT) of transfused blood components and breast milk was performed to identify sources of CMV transmission. A total of 539 VLBW infants (birth weight, ≤1500 g) who had not received a blood transfusion were enrolled, with their mothers (n = 462), within 5 days of birth. The infants underwent serum and urine CMV NAT at birth to evaluate congenital infection and surveillance CMV NAT at 5 additional intervals between birth and 90 days, discharge, or death.

Exposures.—Blood transfusion and breast milk feeding.

Main Outcomes and Measures.—Cumulative incidence of postnatal CMV infection, detected by serum or urine NAT.

Results.—The seroprevalence of CMV among the 462 enrolled mothers was 76.2% (n = 352). Among the 539 VLBW infants, the cumulative incidence of postnatal CMV infection at 12 weeks was 6.9%(95% CI, 4.2%-9.2%); 5 of 29 infants (17.2%) with postnatal CMV infection developed symptomatic disease or died. A total of 2061 transfusions were administered among 57.5% (n = 310) of the infants; none of the CMV infections was linked to transfusion, resulting in a CMV infection incidence of 0.0% (95% CI, 0.0%-0.3%) per unit of CMV-seronegative and leukoreduced blood. Twenty-seven of 28 postnatal infections occurred among infants fed CMV-positive breast milk (12-week incidence, 15.3%; 95% CI, 9.3%-20.2%).

Conclusions and Relevance.—Transfusion of CMV-seronegative and leukoreduced blood products effectively prevents transmission of CMV to VLBW infants. Among infants whose care is managed with this transfusion approach, maternal breast milk is the primary source of postnatal CMV infection.

Trial Registration.—clinicaltrials.gov Identifier: NCT00907686.

▶ The use of human milk for preterm neonates in the United States appears to have increased in the past several years, largely due to numerous benefits, including decreases in sepsis and necrotizing enterocolitis, compared with commercial formula use, that have become more evident. However, several concerns regarding human milk use in preterms remain, including the possible transmission of infections, especially cytomegalovirus (CMV). CMV transmission to the preterm infant has the potential to cause serious morbidity. This study evaluates CMV transmission through blood transfusions or breast milk using a prospective multicenter birth cohort design. The authors showed that despite high seroprevalence of 76.2%, the incidence of postnatal CMV infection at 12 weeks was only 6.9%. Of 29 infants with CMV infection, 5 developed symptomatic disease or died. Whether the death could be attributed to CMV was not clear. None of the infections were linked to blood transfusion. The blood used for this study was CMV seronegative and leukoreduced. The majority of infants who developed CMV positivity occurred in infants fed CMV-positive breast milk.

At this juncture, that American Academy of Pediatrics recommendation is that "the value of routinely feeding fresh human milk from CMV seropositive mothers to preterm infants outweighs the risks of clinical disease, especially because no long-term neurodevelopmental abnormalities have been reported."[1] A systematic review of the literature supports low transmission rate and no known evidence of long-term effects; it states that the data "do not support a general approach, either by avoidance or pasteurization of breast milk, in high-risk preterm infants."[2] However, in a more recent study, data from a small number of infants born at 22 to 24 weeks' gestational age suggest that these infants are at high risk of developing a sepsis-like disease and respiratory symptoms.[3] Of the 11 infants who developed this disease in this extremely immature population, 55% failed automated auditory brainstem response testing at discharge. Thus, although we consider the risk to be low and that the usual pasteurization methods should not be used for fresh human milk, additional studies that will lead to complete elimination of this risk are in order.

J. Neu, MD

References

1. Eidelman AI. Breastfeeding and the use of human milk: an analysis of the American Academy of Pediatrics 2012 Breastfeeding Policy Statement. *Breastfeed Med.* 2012;7:323-324.
2. Kurath S, Halwachs-Baumann G, Müller W, Resch B. Transmission of cytomegalovirus via breast milk to the prematurely born infant: a systematic review. *Clin Microbiol Infect.* 2010;16:1172-1178.
3. Mehler K, Oberthuer A, Lang-Roth R, Kribs A. High rate of symptomatic cytomegalovirus infection in extremely low gestational age preterm infants of 22−24 weeks' gestation after transmission via breast milk. *Neonatology.* 2014;105: 27-32.

Blood Transfusion and Breast Milk Transmission of Cytomegalovirus in Very Low-Birth-Weight Infants: A Prospective Cohort Study
Josephson CD, Caliendo AM, Easley KA, et al (Emory Univ, Atlanta, GA; Brown Univ, Providence, RI; et al)
JAMA Pediatr 168:1054-1062, 2014

Importance.—Postnatal cytomegalovirus (CMV) infection can cause serious morbidity and mortality in very low-birth-weight (VLBW) infants. The primary sources of postnatal CMV infection in this population are breast milk and blood transfusion. The current risks attributable to these vectors, as well as the efficacy of approaches to prevent CMV transmission, are poorly characterized.

Objective.—To estimate the risk of postnatal CMV transmission from 2 sources: (1) transfusion of CMV-seronegative and leukoreduced blood and (2) maternal breast milk.

Design, Setting, and Participants.—A prospective, multicenter birth-cohort study was conducted from January 2010 to June 2013 at 3 neonatal intensive care units (2 academically affiliated and 1 private) in Atlanta, Georgia. Cytomegalovirus serologic testing of enrolled mothers was performed to determine their status. Cytomegalovirus nucleic acid testing (NAT) of transfused blood components and breast milk was performed to identify sources of CMV transmission. A total of 539 VLBW infants (birth weight, ≤1500 g) who had not received a blood transfusion were enrolled, with their mothers (n = 462), within 5 days of birth. The infants underwent serum and urine CMV NAT at birth to evaluate congenital infection and surveillance CMV NAT at 5 additional intervals between birth and 90 days, discharge, or death.

Exposures.—Blood transfusion and breast milk feeding.

Main Outcomes and Measures.—Cumulative incidence of postnatal CMV infection, detected by serum or urine NAT.

Results.—The seroprevalence of CMV among the 462 enrolled mothers was 76.2% (n = 352). Among the 539 VLBW infants, the cumulative incidence of postnatal CMV infection at 12 weeks was 6.9% (95% CI, 4.2%-9.2%); 5 of 29 infants (17.2%) with postnatal CMV infection developed symptomatic disease or died. A total of 2061 transfusions were administered among 57.5% (n = 310) of the infants; none of the CMV infections was linked to transfusion, resulting in a CMV infection incidence of 0.0% (95% CI, 0.0%-0.3%) per unit of CMV-seronegative and leukoreduced blood. Twenty-seven of 28 postnatal infections occurred among infants fed CMV-positive breast milk (12-week incidence, 15.3%; 95% CI, 9.3%-20.2%).

Conclusions and Relevance.—Transfusion of CMV-seronegative and leukoreduced blood products effectively prevents transmission of CMV to VLBW infants. Among infants whose care is managed with this transfusion approach, maternal breast milk is the primary source of postnatal CMV infection.

Trial Registration.—clinicaltrials.gov Identifier: NCT00907686.

▶ A number of reports have previously described acquisition of cytomegalovirus (CMV) infection by very low birth weight (VLBW) infants in the first few weeks after birth—in some cases, with devastating consequences. Incomplete data have made it difficult to distinguish among congenital, intrapartum, and postnatal infection, or, in the latter case, infection via transfused blood or from maternal breast milk. This prospective surveillance study, the largest yet reported, provides essential data to elucidate those questions. Only 1 infant had evidence of congenital infection (detection of CMV in blood and urine within 5 days after birth), despite serologic evidence of CMV infection in 76%

of the tested mothers. Exclusive use of leukoreduced blood products from CMV-seronegative donors resulted in elimination of CMV transmission in blood products, despite exposure of VLBW infants to 2061 transfusions from 1038 blood component units. Acquired infection was demonstrated in 28 infants whose initial CMV testing was negative; all of their mothers were CMV seropositive, 27 of these infants had documented exposure to maternal milk that had tested positive by CMV nucleic acid amplification testing before recognition of CMV infection. (The source of infection in the remaining infant was not identified but may have been maternal milk as well; infection was detected at 25 days of age, but milk was tested only during the first week, before CMV shedding would be expected.) The mean time from onset of CMV shedding in milk to recognition of neonatal infection was 36 days (SD ± 22 days). However, transmission of CMV to the infants occurred for only 14% of women whose milk contained CMV. Intrapartum transmission was deemed unlikely because neither cesarean delivery nor prolonged rupture of membranes were significantly associated with transmission of infection. Although still not definitive, these data strongly implicate unpasteurized maternal milk as a source of postnatal CMV infection in VLBW infants. In this series, freezing maternal milk did not appear to be effective because frozen/thawed milk was used exclusively in 78% of infants, and exposure to fresh maternal milk was not associated with an increased risk of CMV infection (18% vs 12% by 12 weeks of age, respectively; $P = .26$). Although the latter lack of statistical significance may reflect the relatively small sample size, it is unlikely that freezing conferred a substantial protective effect. Long-term outcomes, including rates of bronchopulmonary dysplasia, neurosensory, and developmental impairment, were not reported.

The best approach to management of such infants therefore remains far from certain. Pasteurization appears to reduce the risk of CMV transmission but also may inactivate immunoprotective factors and presents substantial logistical challenges. Although early reports suggested efficacy of freezing, this report places that in doubt. National guidelines fro prevention of CMV transmission in breast milk, from North America and Europe, are inconsistent[1] and lack strong evidential foundations. For the moment, the benefits of expressed maternal milk likely outweigh the risks of CMV transmission.

W. E. Benitz, MD

Reference

1. Kurath S, Halwachs-Baumann G, Muller W, Resch B. Transmission of cytomegalovirus via breast milk to the prematurely born infant: a systematic review. *Clin Microbiol Infect.* 2010;16:1172-1178.

Blood Transfusion and Breast Milk Transmission of Cytomegalovirus in Very Low-Birth-Weight Infants: A Prospective Cohort Study

Josephson CD, Caliendo AM, Easley KA, et al (Emory Univ, Atlanta, GA; Brown Univ, Providence, RI; et al)
JAMA Pediatr 168:1054-1062, 2014

Importance.—Postnatal cytomegalovirus (CMV) infection can cause serious morbidity and mortality in very low-birth-weight (VLBW) infants. The primary sources of postnatal CMV infection in this population are breast milk and blood transfusion. The current risks attributable to these vectors, as well as the efficacy of approaches to prevent CMV transmission, are poorly characterized.

Objective.—To estimate the risk of postnatal CMV transmission from 2 sources: (1) transfusion of CMV-seronegative and leukoreduced blood and (2) maternal breast milk.

Design, Setting, and Participants.—A prospective, multicenter birth-cohort study was conducted from January 2010 to June 2013 at 3 neonatal intensive care units (2 academically affiliated and 1 private) in Atlanta, Georgia. Cytomegalovirus serologic testing of enrolled mothers was performed to determine their status. Cytomegalovirus nucleic acid testing (NAT) of transfused blood components and breast milk was performed to identify sources of CMV transmission. A total of 539 VLBW infants (birth weight, ≤1500 g) who had not received a blood transfusion were enrolled, with their mothers (n = 462), within 5 days of birth. The infants underwent serum and urine CMV NAT at birth to evaluate congenital infection and surveillance CMV NAT at 5 additional intervals between birth and 90 days, discharge, or death.

Exposures.—Blood transfusion and breast milk feeding.

Main Outcomes and Measures.—Cumulative incidence of postnatal CMV infection, detected by serum or urine NAT.

Results.—The seroprevalence of CMV among the 462 enrolled mothers was 76.2% (n = 352). Among the 539 VLBW infants, the cumulative incidence of postnatal CMV infection at 12 weeks was 6.9% (95% CI, 4.2%-9.2%); 5 of 29 infants (17.2%) with postnatal CMV infection developed symptomatic disease or died. A total of 2061 transfusions were administered among 57.5% (n = 310) of the infants; none of the CMV infections was linked to transfusion, resulting in a CMV infection incidence of 0.0% (95% CI, 0.0%-0.3%) per unit of CMV-seronegative and leukoreduced blood. Twenty-seven of 28 postnatal infections occurred among infants fed CMV-positive breast milk (12-week incidence, 15.3%; 95% CI, 9.3%-20.2%).

Conclusions and Relevance.—Transfusion of CMV-seronegative and leukoreduced blood products effectively prevents transmission of CMV to VLBW infants. Among infants whose care is managed with this transfusion approach, maternal breast milk is the primary source of postnatal CMV infection.

Trial Registration.—clinicaltrials.gov Identifier: NCT00907686.

▶ It is rather sobering, but not surprising, to take home the messages from this prospective study on the transmission of cytomegalovirus (CMV) infection from blood transfusions and human milk. The data on blood transfusions are very encouraging. No cases were acquired from transfusions. All transfused red blood cell and apheresis platelet units were CMV seronegative, leukoreduced before storage, and irradiated (some before and some after storage); residual leukocyte quantitation and CMV nucleic acid testing were performed on samples. It would appear as if this should become the standard of care for blood and platelet transfusions in neonates. On the other hand, CMV was acquired from human milk. This can cause serious long-term consequences affecting hearing, cognitive, and other neurodevelopmental disabilities.[1]

CMV is the most frequently contracted virus in preterm infants. Postnatal infection is mostly asymptomatic but is sometimes associated with severe disease. Turner et al[2] reported that whereas congenital CMV infection was associated with significant hearing loss and neurodevelopmental problems, acquired CMV infection did not have long-term sequelae, but they studied a very small cohort.

To diagnose an infection, urine or saliva samples can be tested for CMV DNA by real-time polymerase chain reaction. Gunkel et al determined that urine is superior to saliva when screening for postnatal CMV infections in preterm infants.[3]

Some neonatal centers freeze maternal milk (MM) to prevent CMV transmission; however, this practice is controversial. Omarsdottir et al[4] found that routine freezing did not affect the rate of CMV transmission from mother's milk. Because the benefits of human milk far outweigh the risks, it is necessary to find a technique of treating the milk that will get rid of CMV but still preserve the many beneficial features of human milk.

A. A. Fanaroff, MBBCh, FRCPE

References

1. Brecht KF, Goelz R, Bevot A, et al. Postnatal human cytomegalovirus infection in preterm infants has long-term neuropsychological sequelae. *J Pediatr.* 2015;166: 834-839.e1.
2. Turner KM, Lee HC, Boppana SB, Carlo WA, Randolph DA. Incidence and impact of CMV infection in very low birth weight infants. *Pediatrics.* 2014;133: e609-e615.
3. Gunkel J, Wolfs TF, Nijman J, et al. Urine is superior to saliva when screening for postnatal CMV infections in preterm infants. *J Clin Virol.* 2014;61:61-64.
4. Omarsdottir S, Casper C, Navér L, et al. Cytomegalovirus infection and neonatal outcome in extremely preterm infants after freezing of maternal milk. *Pediatr Infect Dis J.* 2015;34:482-489.

Oropharyngeal Colostrum Administration in Extremely Premature Infants: An RCT

Lee J, Kim H-S, Jung YH, et al (Seoul Natl Univ College of Medicine, Korea; et al)
Pediatrics 135:e357-e366, 2015

Objective.—To determine the immunologic effects of oropharyngeal colostrum administration in abstract extremely premature infants.

Methods.—We conducted a double-blind, randomized, placebo-controlled trial involving 48 preterm infants born before 28 weeks' gestation. Subjects received 0.2 mL of their mother's colostrum or sterile water via oropharyngeal route every 3 hours for 3 days beginning at 48 to 96 hours of life. To measure concentrations of secretory immunoglobulin A, lactoferrin, and several immune substances, urine and saliva were obtained during the first 24 hours of life and at 8 and 15 days. Clinical data during hospitalization were collected.

Results.—Urinary levels of secretory immunoglobulin A at 1 week (71.4 vs 26.5 ng/g creatinine, $P=.04$) and 2 weeks (233.8 vs 48.3 µg/g creatinine, $P=.006$), and lactoferrin at 1 week (3.5 vs 0.9 µg/g creatinine, $P=.01$) were significantly higher in colostrum group. Urine interleukin-1β level was significantly lower in colostrum group at 2 weeks (55.3 vs 91.8 µg/g creatinine, $P=.01$). Salivary transforming growth factor-β1 (39.2 vs 69.7 µg/mL, $P=.03$) and interleukin-8 (1.2 vs 4.9 ng/mL, $P=.04$) were significantly lower at 2 weeks in colostrum group. A significant reduction in the incidence of clinical sepsis was noted in colostrum group (50% vs 92%, $P=.003$).

Conclusions.—This study suggests that oropharyngeal administration of colostrum may decrease clinical sepsis, inhibit secretion of pro-inflammatory cytokines, and increase levels of circulating immune-protective factors in extremely premature infants. Larger studies to confirm these findings are warranted.

▶ The old wives' tale was that all babies regurgitated human milk, including through their nose, so that the upper respiratory tract would be lined and protected by secretory immunoglobulin A and other factors from the milk. Indeed, cytokines applied to the oropharynx may stimulate the lymphoid tissue enhancing the immune system. Colostrum is rich in cytokines and other immune agents that provide bacteriostatic bactericidal, antiviral, antiinflammatory, and immunomodulatory protection against infection. Rodriguez postulated that own mother's colostrum (OMC) may be especially protective for the extremely low birth weight (ELBW) infant in the first days of life. Because enteral feeding may be impossible in the first days of life, they postulated that the oropharyngeal route would be an alternative method of providing OMC.[1] This was put to the test in a pilot study of 5 patients. They concluded that "Oropharyngeal administration of own mother's colostrum is easy, inexpensive, and well-tolerated by even the smallest and sickest ELBW infants. Future research should continue to examine the optimal procedure for measuring the direct immune effects of this therapy, as well as the clinical outcomes such as infections, particularly ventilator-associated pneumonia."[2] Seigel et al[3] from Duke University completed a retrospective cohort study that confirmed the safety and suggested nutritional benefits as well.

The study from Korea is more comprehensive, prospective, and randomized. The findings with regard to immunoglobulin A, lactoferrin, and the inflammatory cytokines are impressive. However, it is disappointing to note a 92% clinical sepsis rate in the controls and 50% in the colostrum-treated group because there were only 48 babies in the study. Whereas I unequivocally accept the evidence on the pro- and antiinflammatory cytokines and the numbers reveal a reduction in clinical sepsis, I am concerned by the high rates in both groups and would probe into this in more depth. Nonetheless, the procedure is harmless, the quantities minute, the potential benefits immense, and it is easy enough to place a small amount of colostrum in the cheeks of preterm infants, even if they are on the ventilator. It is a process worth exploring further.

A. A. Fanaroff, MBBCh, FRCPE

References

1. Rodriguez NA, Meier PP, Groer MW, Zeller JM. Oropharyngeal administration of colostrum to extremely low birth weight infants: theoretical perspectives. *J Perinatol.* 2009;29:1-7.
2. Rodriguez NA, Meier PP, Groer MW, Zeller JM, Engstrom JL, Fogg L. A pilot study to determine the safety and feasibility of oropharyngeal administration of own mother's colostrum to extremely low-birth-weight infants. *Adv Neonatal Care.* 2010;10:206-212.
3. Seigel JK, Smith PB, Ashley PL, et al. Early administration of oropharyngeal colostrum to extremely low birth weight infants. *Breastfeed Med.* 2013;8: 491-495.

Oropharyngeal Colostrum Administration in Extremely Premature Infants: An RCT

Lee J, Kim H-S, Jung YH, et al (Seoul Natl Univ College of Medicine, Korea; et al)

Pediatrics 135:e357-e366, 2015

Objective.—To determine the immunologic effects of oropharyngeal colostrum administration in abstract extremely premature infants.

Methods.—We conducted a double-blind, randomized, placebo-controlled trial involving 48 preterm infants born before 28 weeks' gestation. Subjects received 0.2 mL of their mother's colostrum or sterile water via oropharyngeal route every 3 hours for 3 days beginning at 48 to 96 hours of life. To measure concentrations of secretory immunoglobulin A, lactoferrin, and several immune substances, urine and saliva were obtained during the first 24 hours of life and at 8 and 15 days. Clinical data during hospitalization were collected.

Results.—Urinary levels of secretory immunoglobulin A at 1 week (71.4 vs 26.5 ng/g creatinine, $P=.04$) and 2 weeks (233.8 vs 48.3 ng/g creatinine, $P=.006$), and lactoferrin at 1 week (3.5 vs 0.9 μg/g creatinine, $P=.01$) were significantly higher in colostrum group. Urine interleukin-1β level was significantly lower in colostrum group at 2 weeks (55.3 vs 91.8 μg/g creatinine, $P=.01$). Salivary transforming growth factor-β1 (39.2 vs 69.7 μg/mL, $P=.03$) and interleukin-8 (1.2 vs 4.9 ng/mL, $P=.04$) were significantly lower at 2 weeks in colostrum group. A significant reduction in the incidence of clinical sepsis was noted in colostrum group (50% vs 92%, $P=.003$).

Conclusions.—This study suggests that oropharyngeal administration of colostrum may decrease clinical sepsis, inhibit secretion of pro-inflammatory cytokines, and increase levels of circulating immune-protective factors in extremely premature infants. Larger studies to confirm these findings are warranted.

▶ Although oropharyngeal administration of colostrum is already being used in several neonatal centers, validation of its use in a controlled study has been needed. This is one of the first randomized trials to determine the effects of oropharyngeal administration of colostrum in very preterm infants (≤28 weeks' gestational age). The authors used a design similar to a pilot study previously used by another group.[1] In the current study, administration of 0.2 mL colostrum every 3 hours for 3 days starting at 48 to 72 hours after birth resulted in several alterations in potentially protective immune markers (immunoglobulin (Ig)A and lactoferrin) in urine along with a decrease in interleukin (IL)-1β at 2 weeks. There was also a decrease in salivary tumor growth factor-β1 and IL-8 in the saliva at 2 weeks. Those infants who received colostrum also had a decrease in clinical sepsis (nonculture proven). No differences in necrotizing enterocolitis or other morbidities were found between the 2 groups.

Overall, this study was well designed and provides encouraging data on safety and possible efficacy of providing oropharyngeal colostrum to this population of infants. Although the groups were randomized, the control group had a higher baseline incidence of histologic chorioamnionitis. Whether this could have affected some of the outcomes remains a question.

The mechanism of colostrum-mediated changes in the concentrations of several of these agents (eg, IgA and IL-1 β) in the urine 1 week after the last administration of the colostrum is of interest because this is no longer likely to be a direct effect of higher levels of these agents being administered to the patient during the time of measurement but rather from early colostrum stimulation of a continuing mechanism of production of these agents. Whether the increased levels of these agents in saliva and urine are due to direct stimulation of buccal mechanisms compared with intestinal mechanisms remains unclear. It is likely that some of the colostrum would have gotten into the intestinal tract.

Although additional studies are needed to better understand the mechanisms as well as to further validate this technique, it appears to be safe, and there are few if any contraindications to its use.

J. Neu, MD

Reference

1. Rodriguez NA, Meier PP, Groer MW, Zeller JM, Engstrom JL, Fogg L. A pilot study to determine the safety and feasibility of oropharyngeal administration of own mother's colostrum to extremely low-birth-weight infants. *Adv Neonatal Care*. 2010;10:206-212.

Effect of emollient therapy on clinical outcomes in preterm neonates in Pakistan: a randomised controlled trial

Salam RA, Darmstadt GL, Bhutta ZA (The Aga Khan Univ, Karachi, Sindh, Pakistan; Bill & Melinda Gates Foundation, Seattle, WA; et al)
Arch Dis Child Fetal Neonatal Ed 100:F210-F215, 2015

Importance.—Newborn oil massage, a traditional community practice, could potentially benefit thermoregulation and skin barrier function, and prevent serious infections, morbidity and mortality in high-risk preterm infants, but has only been evaluated in limited studies in low income settings.

Objectives.—To assess the efficacy of topical coconut oil applications among a cohort of hospital-born preterm infants.

Design.—A prospective, individually randomised controlled clinical trial.

Setting.—Nursery and neonatal intensive care unit at Aga Khan University Hospital, Pakistan.

Participants.—Of 270 eligible neonates, a consecutive cohort of 258 hospital-born preterm infants (gestational age ≤ 26 weeks and ≤ 37 weeks).

Intervention.—Twice daily topical application of coconut oil by nurses from birth until discharge and continued thereafter by mothers at home until completion of the 28th day of life.

Primary Outcome Measures.—Incidence of hospital acquired bloodstream infections.

Secondary Outcome Measures.—Weight gain, skin condition and neonatal mortality.

Results.—23% of the enrolled neonates developed clinically suspected sepsis while 14% developed blood culture proven infection. The unadjusted hazard for developing hospital-acquired infection in the control group was 4.7 (95% CI 1.8 to 12.4) compared with the intervention group. After adjusting for gestational age, birth weight, duration of intubation and duration of hospitalisation for possible confounding, the hazard for hospital-acquired infection in the control group was 6.0 (95% CI 2.3 to 16) compared with the intervention group. The rate of hospital-acquired infections in the control and intervention groups was 219.1 and 39.5 per 1000 patient-days, respectively. Mean weight gain was 11.3 g/day higher (95% CI 8.1 to 14.6, $p < 0.0001$) and average skin condition was significantly better in the intervention group when compared with controls. There was no significant impact on duration of hospitalisation or neonatal mortality. No adverse effects such as local irritation or local infection were observed among newborns receiving coconut oil applications.

Conclusions.—Topical emollient therapy was effective in maintaining skin integrity and reducing the risk of bloodstream infection in preterm infants in a tertiary hospital setting in Pakistan. The effectiveness of this approach in primary care settings needs to be further explored.

Trial Registration Number.—NCT01396642.

▶ Maintaining integrity of the skin is a priority to prevent sepsis. When examining the literature, it is abundantly clear that there are large regional differences and that although emollients did not prevent infection in the United States,[1] they were lifesaving in the developing world.[2] Salam[2] reviewed 7 studies and an unpublished report on emollient use in the developing world and concluded that topical emollient therapy significantly reduced neonatal mortality by 27% and hospital acquired infection by 50%. An added benefit was better weight gain without affecting length or head circumference. Darmstadt explored the relationship between skin integrity and infection and noted that the rate of deterioration of the skin condition was lower with emollients and emollients only reduced the incidence of infection when there were no signs of skin deterioration.[3] They recommended use of emollients immediately after birth to preserve skin integrity and reduce the risk of infection.

Ponnusamy et al[4] wrote, "There are no convincing roles for routine application of emollient creams on the skin, topical antiseptics on the umbilical stump, or maternal vaginal washes with chlorhexidine for the prevention of neonatal infection." They added the inevitable plea for large multicenter trials to address these issues. Their wish is partially granted by this publication from Salam et al abstracted here. They confirm the benefits of an emollient—in this case, coconut oil—on a population of preterm infants in Pakistan. Improved skin integrity and reduced number of infections are statistically significant in the treated versus the control group. Nonetheless, they plea for more studies. It is time that these studies are sufficiently powered to answer the question once and for all time. Just wishful thinking.

A. A. Fanaroff, MBBCh, FRCPE

References

1. Edwards WH, Conner JM, Soll RF; Vermont Oxford Network Neonatal Skin Care Study Group. The effect of prophylactic ointment therapy on nosocomial sepsis rates and skin integrity in infants with birth weights of 501 to 1000 g. *Pediatrics.* 2004;113:1195-1203.
2. Salam RA, Das JK, Darmstadt GL, Bhutta ZA. Emollient therapy for preterm newborn infants—evidence from the developing world. *BMC Public Health.* 2013;13: S31.
3. Darmstadt GL, Ahmed S, Ahmed AS, Saha SK. Mechanism for prevention of infection in preterm neonates by topical emollients: a randomized, controlled clinical trial. *Pediatr Infect Dis J.* 2014;33:1124-1127.
4. Ponnusamy V, Venkatesh V, Clarke P. Skin antisepsis in the neonate: what should we use? *Curr Opin Infect Dis.* 2014;27:244-250.

Presepsin for the Detection of Late-Onset Sepsis in Preterm Newborns
Poggi C, Bianconi T, Gozzini E, et al (Careggi Univ Hosp of Florence, Italy)
Pediatrics 135:68-75, 2015

Background.—Late-onset sepsis (LOS) is among the leading causes of morbidity and mortality in preterm newborns, and currently available diagnostic tools are inadequate. The objective of this study was to evaluate the accuracy of presepsin (P-SEP) as novel biomarker of bacterial infection for the diagnosis of LOS in preterm newborns.

Methods.—We prospectively studied newborns ≤32 weeks' gestational age with LOS ($n=19$) and noninfected controls ($n=21$) at 4 to 60 days' postnatal age. At enrollment, and 1, 3, and 5 days later, we ascertained the C-reactive protein, procalcitonin, and P-SEP in the LOS group, whereas P-SEP alone was ascertained in the control group.

Results.—P-SEP at enrollment was higher in the LOS than the control group (median 1295 vs 562 ng/L, $P=.00001$) and remained higher throughout the study period. In the LOS group, P-SEP had a borderline reduction at day 1 versus values at enrollment (median 1011 vs 1295 ng/L, $P=.05$), whereas C-reactive protein and procalcitonin at day 1 did not differ from baseline values. The receiver operating characteristic curve of P-SEP at enrollment shows an area under the curve of 0.972. The best calculated cutoff value was 885 ng/L, with 94% sensitivity and 100% specificity. Negative likelihood ratio was 0.05, and positive likelihood ratio was infinity.

Conclusions.—We demonstrated for the first time in a cohort of preterm newborns that P-SEP is an accurate biomarker for the diagnosis of possible LOS and may also provide useful information for monitoring the response to therapeutic interventions.

▶ Diagnostic tests for neonatal sepsis have utility for 2 distinct purposes. The first relies on development of negative predictive value over time to enable discontinuation of antibiotic therapy with confidence that the baby does not have serious bacterial infection. Several diagnostic parameters, including blood cultures, blood cell counts, C-reactive protein [CRP], and absence or resolution of physical findings suggestive of sepsis, currently are used in that way. Tools for the second objective—reliable identification of at-risk or symptomatic infants who are not infected—have been more elusive. (Tests that identify infants who appear to be well but are nonetheless infected would be of less value because the low risk of sepsis in such babies likely makes their positive predictive value quite low, as well.) For such a test to be useful, it must meet a few critical criteria. There should be a short interval from onset of infection to development of an abnormal result, so the measured analyte cannot be something that requires de novo synthesis after the infection develops (eg, C-reactive protein, calcitonin, cytokines). It should be highly sensitive, consistently demonstrating abnormal results in all infected babies (unlike white blood cell counts and CRP at the onset of illness). It should be specific for infection, distinguishing infected babies from sick ones (not simply sick from well), and it should not be confounded by artifactual effects of immune cell activation (such as increased CD11b expression on granulocytes activated by exposure to plastic at room temperature). Finally, a blood test should require a minimal volume of blood, and the analytic turnaround time must be short enough to inform decisions about treatment without imposing inordinate delays.

Presepsin, or soluble CD14 subtype (sCD14-ST), is emerging as an attractive candidate for use in this second category. As a specific cell-surface receptor for complexes of bacterial lipopolysaccharide (LPS) and LPS binding protein (LBP), CD14 is an early component of the TLR4-mediated innate immune response to bacterial products. The CD14-LPS-LBP complex is shed from monocytes, macrophages, and neutrophils as soluble CD14 (sCD14), from which presepsin is derived as a cleavage product. Because it is derived from a constitutively expressed substrate, no new protein synthesis is required in its production, resulting in a short response time between onset of infection and elevation of plasma levels. Studies in adults and preliminary evaluations in neonates suggest that elevated levels are highly sensitive and specific for sepsis, even when the control group consists of subjects with systemic inflammatory response syndrome. The measurement can be performed at the point of care on as little as 50 µL of blood, producing diagnostic results in 15 minutes.

This small but provocative study compares presepsin levels in 19 infants with late-onset sepsis (15 with positive cultures) to those in 21 similar controls. All subjects were preterm (≤32 weeks' gestation) without major malformations or hydrops. The extremely high sensitivity, specificity, and area under the receiving operator characteristic curve for presepsin levels at the time of the initial sepsis evaluation, as noted in the abstract, are similar to preliminary results reported from Egypt [1] and Poland.[2] Reproduction in larger cohorts, more data for infants with suspected early-onset sepsis, and confirmation of the ability to distinguish infants with bacterial sepsis from those with SIRS are still needed. Nonetheless, this methodology promises to become an important component of the neonatologist's diagnostic toolkit in the near future.

W. E. Benitz, MD

References

1. AbdElaziz H. Diagnosis of neonatal sepsis using different sepsis markers. *J Mol Biomark Diagn.* 2013;4:134.
2. Kwiatkowska-Gruca M, Behrendt J, Sonsala A, Wiśniewska-Ulfik D, Mazur B, Godula-Stuglik U. Presepsin (soluble CD14-ST) as a biomarker for sepsis in neonates. *Pediatria Polska.* 2013;88:392-397.

Timely empiric antimicrobials are associated with faster microbiologic clearance in preterm neonates with late-onset bloodstream infections
Natarajan G, Monday L, Scheer T, et al (Wayne State Univ, Detroit, MI; Hutzel Women's Hosp, Detroit, MI)
Acta Paediatr 103:e418-e423, 2014

Aim.—The impact of timely empiric antimicrobial therapy on neonates is unclear. Our aim was to examine rates of effective timely empiric antimicrobial therapy on preterm neonates, together with the associated outcomes.

Methods.—We performed a single-centre retrospective study of preterm infants (<32 weeks of gestational age) with a late-onset (>72 h of age) bloodstream infection (BSI). Empiric antimicrobial administration took place before the results of blood culture were available and its timing was determined by the electronic medical records.

Results.—Our cohort (n = 105) was predominantly female (59%) and black (83%) with a mean (SD) gestational age of 27.4 (2.3) weeks and birthweight of 948 (335) g. Effective empiric antimicrobials were initiated in 114 (69%) of 165 BSI episodes, and a third of the BSIs without empiric antimicrobials were found to be fungal. Both antimicrobial timing ($r = 0.27$, $p = 0.002$) and fungal organism ($r = 0.35$, $p = 0.0001$) showed significant correlations and were independently associated with time to clearance. Neither variable was associated with survival or length of stay.

Conclusion.—Two-thirds of preterm infants with late-onset BSIs received effective empiric antimicrobials. Timely empiric antimicrobials were associated with shorter time to microbiologic clearance. These data suggest the need for standardised guidelines and quality improvement initiatives.

▶ Belief in the necessity for prompt administration of antimicrobial therapy to infants with suspected sepsis is deeply ingrained in the culture of neonatal medicine, but there is little empiric evidence to allow assessment of impacts of longer intervals between onset of illness and administration of effective treatment. Because it cannot be ethically addressed in the context of controlled trials, the best estimates of this relationship must be derived from retrospective analyses such as those presented in this report. Interpretation of such data is quite challenging, however, because timing of treatment may be confounded by differences in severity of illness and causative organisms between treatment groups. In this report, for example, infants for whom treatment was deferred until after culture results were available were much more likely to have been infected with coagulase-negative *Staphylococci* (CONs; including *Staphylccoccus epidermidis*) or yeast, suggesting that the typically incolent course of these infections did not motivate early treatment. The predominance of those less virulent organisms in the deferred treatment group may account for the observation that delayed treatment was not associated with a higher mortality rate or longer hospital stay. Similarly, the longer interval between the first positive culture and clearance of the bacteremia/fungemia (89 ± 59 vs

55 ± 40 hours) may be attributable to delay in initiation of effective treatment alone, without a contribution from a longer interval between treatment and response. At least for CONS and yeast, therefore, it is not clear that delayed treatment results in worse outcomes. Because the numbers of other Gram-positive cocci (*Enterococcus*, *Staphylococcus aureus*, *Streptococcus*) and Gram-negative bacilli (organisms not further described) were small and few cases were associated with delayed or ineffective treatment, the expectation of uncompromised outcomes must not be generalized to infants infected with those organisms, however.

Delays in administration of effective antimicrobial therapy may be placed into 3 categories: 1) decisions not to order treatment, 2) selection of ineffective treatment, and 3) delays between orders for and delivery of effective treatments. In this report, no treatment was ordered within 24 hours after obtaining blood cultures in 43 of the 165 infected infants (26%). Among the 25 infants with fungal infection, 17 (68%) did not receive immediate treatment, prompting the authors to advocate consideration of empiric antifungal therapy. That measure is only necessary in settings in which yeast infection is relatively common and will only be effective if coupled with a low threshold for initiation of empiric treatment. Selection of an ineffective antibiotic regimen was relatively uncommon (8 infants, or 5% of the cases), and was associated with empiric use of ampicillin rather than vancomycin in the 5 cases of Gram-positive sepsis; antibiotic susceptibilities in the 3 cases of Gram-negative sepsis (*Serratia*, *Acinetobacter*, *Enterobacter*) were not further specified. Perhaps the most worrisome finding in this report is that the mean time from physician order to antimicrobial administration was nearly 2 hours, with only 25% of infants receiving treatment within 1 hour and 66% within 2 hours after entry of orders for treatment. While we await development of rapid, specific diagnostic tests for late-onset neonatal sepsis, there is a substantial opportunity for process improvement to optimize intervention on behalf of these at-risk babies.

W. E. Benitz, MD

The Role of Coagulase-Negative Staphylococci in Early Onset Sepsis in a Large European Cohort of Very Low Birth Weight Infants

Mularoni A, Madrid M, Azpeitia A, et al (Istituto Giannina Gaslini, Genova, Italy; Hospital de Cruces, Barakaldo-Bilbao, Spain)
Pediatr Infect Dis J 33:e121-e125, 2014

Background.—Early Onset Sepsis (EOS) is associated with increased major morbidity and mortality rates among very low birth weight (VLBW) infants. The epidemiology is changing in response to evolving medical practice. The objective of the study was to evaluate EOS epidemiology, risk factors, mortality and major morbidity rates among VLBW infants within a European cohort.

Methods.—Data from VLBW infants born from 2006 through 2009 was collected by neonatal units participating in the EuroNeoNet initiative. Univariate and multivariate analyses were performed to assess the independent association of EOS with VLBW infant's perinatal characteristics, morbidity and mortality rates.

Results.—The cohort included 14,719 infants, 391 developed EOS (2.7%). The most common pathogen responsible for EOS was Gram-positive bacteria (53.9%). Coagulase-negative staphylccocci (CoNS) were isolated in 22.5% of episodes. Antenatal steroids exposure, single gestation, very low gestational age and birth weight, low 5 minute Apgar score and delivery room resuscitation were independently associated with EOS. EOS was also associated with a longer hospital stay, increased risk of mortality [adjusted odd ratio (aOR): 2.4; 95% Confidence Interval (CI): 1.9—3.1], respiratory distress syndrome (OR: 1.4; 95% CI: 1.1—1.9), severe intraventricular haemorrhage (aOR: 2.1; 95% CI: 1.6—2.8) and severe retinopathy of prematurity (aOR: 5; 95% CI: 1.9—13.3). Morbidity and mortality rates of infants with EOS caused by CoNS were similar to those of infants with EOS caused by other pathogens.

Conclusions.—VLBW infants with EOS are at an increased risk of mortality and major morbidities. CoNS was a significant cause of sepsis, infants with CoNS were at a similarly high risk of complication of prematurity and mortality as those with EOS caused by other organisms.

▶ For many years, it has been the convention to consicer isolation of coagulase-negative *Staphylococci* (CONS) in blood cultures from newborn infants <72 hours of age to represent contamination of the specimen by commensal skin organisms. Nearly 20 years ago, Stoll and Fanaroff, using data from the Eunice Kennedy Shriver National Institute of Child Health and Human Development Neonatal Research Network, suggested that a substantial proportion of such early-onset sepsis episodes in very low birth weight (VLBW) infants might actually reflect genuine sepsis caused by CONS.[1] More recently, national laboratory surveillance data from England and Wales for 2006 to 2008 indicated that CONS was the isolate in 21.5% of cases of sepsis in infants <48 hours of age,[2] second in frequency only to group B streptococcus. (No breakdown by gestational age or birth weight was provided.) In that series, 80% of the CONS isolates tested were sensitive to the combination of penicillin and gentamicin. Although most such isolates would be covered by standard empirical treatment, those authors questioned the adequacy of current strategies. The high rates of antimicrobial resistance characteristic of CONS in most other reports suggest that this skepticism is well justified.

This report is one of a growing collection of population-based case series that should prompt further consideration of that concern. These authors report data from a large European cohort of VLBW infants in which 22.5% of the cases of early-onset sepsis in 2006 to 2009 were attributed to CONS. In a multivariate analysis, they found no differences in rates of several important morbidities between infants with sepsis caused by CONS and those infected by other organisms. One interpretation might be that CONS is as much a pathogen as those more traditionally accepted pathogens. Another possibility is that effective treatment reduced the adverse effects associated with pathogenic infections to a level indistinguishable from background rates, which are not altered by CONS bacteremia or by incidental isolation of contaminating commensals. This will be a difficult dilemma to resolve, at least until reliable biomarkers of sepsis are defined. In the meantime, some circumspection should be applied before dismissal of CONS isolation from blood cultures as a contaminant just because the source is an infant < 72 hours of age, especially those who are VLBW.

W. E. Benitz, MD

References

1. Stoll BJ, Fanaroff A. Early-onset coagulase-negative staphylococcal sepsis in preterm neonate. National Institute of Child Health and Human Development (NICHD) Neonatal Research Network. *Lancet.* 1995;345:1236-1237.
2. Muller-Pebody B, Johnson AP, Heath PT, Gilbert RE, Henderson KL, Sharland M. Empirical treatment of neonatal sepsis: are the current guidelines adequate? *Arch Dis Child Fetal Neonatal Ed.* 2011;96:F4-F8.

Incidence, Etiology, and Outcome of Bacterial Meningitis in Infants Aged <90 Days in the United Kingdom and Republic of Ireland: Prospective, Enhanced, National Population-Based Surveillance
Okike IO, for the neoMen Study Group (Univ of London, UK)
Clin Infect Dis 59:e150-e157, 2014

Background.—Bacterial meningitis remains a major cause of morbidity and mortality in young infants. Understanding the epidemiology and burden of disease is important.

Methods.—Prospective, enhanced, national population-based active surveillance was undertaken to determine the incidence, etiology, and outcome of bacterial meningitis in infants aged <90 days in the United Kingdom and Ireland.

Results.—During July 2010–July 2011, 364 cases were identified (annual incidence, 0.38/1000 live births; 95% confidence interval [CI], .35–.42). In England and Wales, the incidence of confirmed neonatal bacterial meningitis was 0.21 (n = 167; 95% CI, .18–.25). A total of 302 bacteria were isolated in 298 (82%) of the cases. The pathogens responsible varied by route of admission, gestation at birth, and age at infection. Group B *Streptococcus* (GBS) (150/302 [50%]; incidence, 0.16/1000 live births; 95% CI, .13–.18) and *Escherichia coli* (41/302 [14%]; incidence, 0.04/1000; 95% CI, .03–.06) were responsible for approximately two-thirds of identified bacteria. Pneumococcal (28/302 [9%]) and meningococcal (23/302 [8%]) meningitis were rare in the first month, whereas *Listeria* meningitis was seen only in the first month of life (11/302 [4%]). In hospitalized preterm infants, the etiology of both early- and late-onset meningitis was more varied. Overall case fatality was 8% (25/

329) and was higher for pneumococcal meningitis (5/26 [19%]) than GBS meningitis (7/135 [5%]; $P =.04$) and for preterm (15/90 [17%]) compared with term (10/235 [4%]; $P =.0002$) infants.

Conclusions.—The incidence of bacterial meningitis in young infants remains unchanged since the 1980s and is associated with significant case fatality. Prevention strategies and guidelines to improve the early management of cases should be prioritized.

▶ Changes in obstetrical practices over the past 2 decades have produced a sustained reduction in the rate of early-onset neonatal sepsis in the United States. Along with recent observations that infection rates are low in late-preterm and term infant who appear to be well, a more restrained approach to treatment of asymptomatic babies ascertained on the basis of exposure to putative risk factors is now evolving. This culture shift may be overgeneralized to assumption that neonatal meningitis is no longer a matter of concern. This population-based report stands as a warning against that error. The data presented require careful parsing because some results are reported for the United Kingdom and Republic of Ireland, some for England and Wales, and some for England alone, but the effort to get beyond the summary data presented in the abstract is well rewarded. In the full survey of 954 189 live births over a 13-month period early in this decade, there were 282 cases (0.23 cases per 1000 live births) of culture-proven meningitis (bacteria isolated from cerebrospinal fluid); an additional 65 infants had cerebrospinal fluid pleocytosis and a positive blood culture (0.07 cases per 1000 births), for a total rate of "confirmed" meningitis (by those criteria) of 0.30 cases per 1000 live births in infants < 90 days of age. Meningitis has clearly not gone away. Cases of culture-proven, probable, and possible meningitis were almost equally divided among the age strata of 0 to 6, 7 to 28, and 29 to 89 days, corresponding to daily incidence rates of 0.017, 0.006, and 0.002 cases per day per 1000 live births in those age intervals; the rate of neonatal meningitis (age ≤28 days) was 0.25 per 1000. There was a steep gradient of risk of "confirmed" meningitis with decreasing birth weight and gestational age (incidence rate ratios of 3.1 and 16.3 for infants 1500 to 2499 g and <1500 g, respectively, versus those ≥2500 g, and 3.4 and 7.1 for infants 32 to 36 and <32 weeks' gestation versus those ≥37 weeks; $P < .0001$ for all comparisons), but more than 70% of the cases occurred in term infants and in those ≥2500 g. Only 56% of the infants with a positive CSF culture had a positive blood culture, affirming previous observations that blood culture alone is not sufficient for diagnosis of neonatal meningitis. Clinical vigilance and specific investigation remain essential for timely detection and appropriate management of this disease.

Comparing these results with their previous report, the authors also note that "the GBS [Group B *Streptococcus*] meningitis incidence is unchanged from UK rates from a decade ago, suggesting little impact of the national GBS prevention policy introduced in 2003." UK recommendations for GBS prevention do not include antepartum screening for maternal GBS colonization, which have been in place in the US since 2002. Absence of this benefit in the UK therefore should not undermine confidence in the substantial reduction in rates of early-onset GBS sepsis (and presumably meningitis, although empirical data are difficult to find) in the United States since 1995.

W. E. Benitz, MD

Clinical and laboratory characteristics of central nervous system herpes simplex virus infection in neonates and young infants

Kotzbauer D, Andresen D, Doelling N, et al (Children's Healthcare of Atlanta, GA)
Pediatr Infect Dis J 33:1187-1189, 2014

We reviewed the characteristics of infants <3 months of age with central nervous system herpes simplex virus infection at our institution. Twenty-six cases were identified. The age range was 4–73 days. Most infants presented with fever, seizure activity and skin lesions. The blood herpes simplex virus polymerase chain reaction was positive in 91% of patients tested. Suppressive oral acyclovir therapy was likely helpful in preventing disease recurrence.

▶ This article reviews clinical and laboratory findings of herpes simplex meningitis/encephalitis in newborns and young infants over a 9-year period in Atlanta. Although the information presented is not really novel, it does serve as a useful reminder of the presentation and epidemiological manifestations of this devastating disease. The authors used a positive polymerase chain reaction of the cerebrospinal fluid (CSF) as the gold standard of diagnosis. They found 26 cases in babies ranging from 4 to 73 days of age, although 80% occurred between the ages of 10 and 28 days at diagnosis. Only 4 cases were associated with a positive maternal history. Fever, seizures, and skin lesions were the most common presenting features. Liver enzymes were normal in all patients in whom it was tested. MRI findings and CSF pleocytosis were variable, although the majority (20 of 24) displayed abnormal diffusion and/or signal enhancement. All but 1 patient survived.

Herpes simplex virus has, like syphilis, been called "the great imitator" because of the many ways in which it may present. This study, which focused solely on central nervous system involvement, suggests that this form of the disease does have a fairly consistent presentation, although a negative maternal history is commonly encountered. Like many relatively rare neonatal conditions, the key to early diagnosis is to consider it in the differential diagnosis, and to this effect, this short article is worthwhile.

S. M. Donn, MD

Valganciclovir for Symptomatic Congenital Cytomegalovirus Disease
Kimberlin DW, for the National Institute of Allergy and Infectious Diseases Collaborative Antiviral Study Group (Univ of Alabama at Birmingham; et al)
N Engl J Med 372:933-943, 2015

Background.—The treatment of symptomatic congenital cytomegalovirus (CMV) disease with intravenous ganciclovir for 6 weeks has been shown to improve audiologic outcomes at 6 months, but the benefits wane over time.

Methods.—We conducted a randomized, placebo-controlled trial of valganciclovir therapy in neonates with symptomatic congenital CMV disease, comparing 6 months of therapy with 6 weeks of therapy. The primary end point was the change in hearing in the better ear ("best-ear" hearing) from baseline to 6 months. Secondary end points included the change in hearing from baseline to follow-up at 12 and 24 months and neurodevelopmental outcomes, with each end point adjusted for central nervous system involvement at baseline.

Results.—A total of 96 neonates underwent randomization, of whom 86 had follow-up data at 6 months that could be evaluated. Best-ear hearing at 6 months was similar in the 6-month group and the 6-week group (2 and 3 participants, respectively, had improvement; 36 and 37 had no change; and 5 and 3 had worsening; $P = 0.41$). Total-ear hearing (hearing in one or both ears that could be evaluated) was more likely to be improved or to remain normal at 12 months in the 6-month group than in the 6-week group (73% vs. 57%, $P = 0.01$). The benefit in total-ear hearing was maintained at 24 months (77% vs. 64%, $P = 0.04$). At 24 months, the 6-month group, as compared with the 6-week group, had better neurodevelopmental scores on the Bayley Scales of Infant and Toddler Development, third edition, on the language-composite component ($P = 0.004$) and on the receptive-communication scale ($P = 0.003$). Grade 3 or 4 neutropenia occurred in 19% of the participants during the first 6 weeks. During the next 4.5 months of the study, grade 3 or 4 neutropenia occurred in 21% of the participants in the 6-month group and in 27% of those in the 6-week group ($P = 0.64$).

Conclusions.—Treating symptomatic congenital CMV disease with valganciclovir for 6 months, as compared with 6 weeks, did not improve hearing in the short term but appeared to improve hearing and developmental outcomes modestly in the longer term. (Funded by the National Institute of Allergy and Infectious Diseases; ClinicalTrials.gov number, NCT00466817.)

▶ In 2003, the National Institute of Allergy and Infectious Diseases Collaborative Antiviral Study Group reported results of a randomized controlled trial of ganciclovir treatment of congenital cytomegalovirus (CMV) disease.[1] That trial enrolled newborn infants (<1 month of age) from whom CMV had been isolated from the urine and who had evidence of central nervous system (CNS) involvement (microcephaly, intracranial calcifications, abnormal cerebrospinal fluid [CSF], chorioretinitis, or hearing deficit). Infants who were < 32 weeks' gestation or weighed < 1500 g at birth, and those with impending death, prior treatment (antiviral agents or immune globulin), renal impairment (creatinine > 1.5 mg/dL), human immunodeficiency virus infection, or hydranencephaly were excluded. Infants were randomized to receive intravenous ganciclovir for 6 weeks or to receive no treatment. That trial demonstrated significant treatment benefits. In particular, treatment increased the proportion of infants whose hearing in the best ear improved between baseline and age ≥1 year from 0% to 17% (number needed to treat [NNT] = 6) and reduced the proportion in whom hearing deteriorated from 68% to 21% (NNT = 2). However, the requirement for twice-daily intravenous dosing has been a significant barrier to adoption of this treatment, and the observation that improvements in hearing observed at 6 months were often not sustained beyond 1 year has led to doubts about the utility of this treatment.

In this follow-up trial, the same consortium evaluated effects of valganciclovir in a different population of neonates with congenital CMV. This study enrolled infants ≤30 days of age with CMV infection demonstrated by culture or polymerase chain reaction of urine, throat swab, or CSF, as well as clinical signs of infection (petechiae, thrombocytopenia, hepatomegaly, splenomegaly, intrauterine growth retardation, hepatitis, or CNS involvement as above). All subjects were ≥32 weeks' gestation and weighed at least 1800 g at enrollment. Because of the previously demonstrated benefit of ganciclovir, infants were randomly assigned to treatment for either 6 weeks or 6 months, with no nontreatment arm. (This trial design does not permit calculation of NNT vs nontreatment.) There were no differences between groups in unadjusted analyses of hearing outcomes at 6, 12, or 24 months, but outcomes in both groups were much better than in the nontreatment arm of the earlier trial. Adjustment for CNS involvement revealed better hearing outcomes and improved Bayley-III scores at 12 and 24 months of age with the longer treatment. This may reflect a greater relative benefit in subjects with CNS involvement, for whom the likelihood of improvement from baseline to 12 and 24 months increased by 65% and 46%, respectively, compared with 22% and 19% in those without CNS disease. The longer treatment arm was made feasible by oral administration of the drug, which obviates the need to maintain prolonged intravenous access. These results support treatment of symptomatic infants with congenital CMV, particularly if there is CNS involvement. It is therefore incumbent on neonatologists to recognize and confirm the diagnosis in these infants so that this treatment can be initiated.

W. E. Benitz, MD

Reference

1. Kimberlin DW, Lin CY, Sanchez PJ, et al. Effect of ganciclovir therapy on hearing in symptomatic congenital cytomegalovirus disease involving the central nervous system: a randomized, controlled trial. *J Pediatr.* 2003;143:16-25.

Valganciclovir for Symptomatic Congenital Cytomegalovirus Disease
Kimberlin DW, for the National Institute of Allergy and Infectious Diseases Collaborative Antiviral Study Group (Univ of Alabama at Birmingham, TX; et al)
N Engl J Med 372:933-943, 2015

Background.—The treatment of symptomatic congenital cytomegalovirus (CMV) disease with intravenous ganciclovir for 6 weeks has been shown to improve audiologic outcomes at 6 months, but the benefits wane over time.

Methods.—We conducted a randomized, placebo-controlled trial of valganciclovir therapy in neonates with symptomatic congenital CMV disease, comparing 6 months of therapy with 6 weeks of therapy. The primary end point was the change in hearing in the better ear ("best-ear" hearing) from baseline to 6 months. Secondary end points included the change in hearing from baseline to follow-up at 12 and 24 months and neurodevelopmental outcomes, with each end point adjusted for central nervous system involvement at baseline.

Results.—A total of 96 neonates underwent randomization, of whom 86 had follow-up data at 6 months that could be evaluated. Best-ear hearing at 6 months was similar in the 6-month group and the 6-week group (2 and 3 participants, respectively, had improvement; 36 and 37 had no change; and 5 and 3 had worsening; $P = 0.41$). Total-ear hearing (hearing in one or both ears that could be evaluated) was more likely to be improved or to remain normal at 12 months in the 6-month group than in the 6-week group (73% vs. 57%, $P = 0.01$). The benefit in total-ear hearing was maintained at 24 months (77% vs. 64%, $P = 0.04$). At 24 months, the 6-month group, as compared with the 6-week group, had better neurodevelopmental scores on the Bayley Scales of Infant and Toddler Development, third edition, on the language-composite component ($P = 0.004$) and on the receptive-communication scale ($P = 0.003$). Grade 3 or 4 neutropenia occurred in 19% of the participants during the first 6 weeks. During the next 4.5 months of the study, grade 3 or 4 neutropenia occurred in 21% of the participants in the 6-month group and in 27% of those in the 6-week group ($P = 0.64$).

Conclusions.—Treating symptomatic congenital CMV disease with valganciclovir for 6 months, as compared with 6 weeks, did not improve hearing in the short term but appeared to improve hearing and developmental outcomes modestly in the longer term. (Funded by the National Institute of Allergy and Infectious Diseases; ClinicalTrials.gov number, NCT00466817.)

▶ Cytomegalovirus (CMV) infection is relatively common throughout the world. Congenital CMV represents the top nongenetic cause of sensorineural hearing loss and the most common viral cause of mental retardation. In neonates with symptomatic congenital CMV disease, intravenous ganciclovir for 6 weeks improves audiologic outcomes at 6 months of life. However, the benefit at 2 years of life may be negligible. To explore the potential benefits of extended therapy, Kimberlin and colleagues randomized 96 neonates with symptomatic congenital CMV disease to 6 months of oral valganciclovir therapy or placebo after 6 weeks of standard therapy. Although outcomes were similar between groups at 6 months of age, infants treated for 6 months were more likely to have improved hearing or maintained normal hearing at 12 months of age (73% vs 57%, $P=.01$) and 24 months of age (77% vs 64%, $P=.04$). Additionally, infants treated for 6 months had superior Bayley III scores in language ($P=.004$) and receptive-communication ($P=.003$) at 24 months of age. All other outcomes assessed by the Bayley III trended toward superiority for infants treated for 6 months. The incidence of neutropenia during prolonged therapy was not different between groups. This trial represents a major forward step in the treatment of neonates with symptomatic congenital CMV disease. The treatment of neonates with asymptomatic disease remains controversial and represents an ongoing research need.

C. McPherson

Anaerobic Antimicrobial Therapy After Necrotizing Enterocolitis in VLBW Infants

Autmizguine J, Best Pharmaceuticals for Children Act—Pediatric Trials Network Administrative Core Committee (Duke Univ Med Ctr, Durham, NC; et al)
Pediatrics 135:e117-e125, 2015

Objective.—To evaluate the effect of anaerobic antimicrobial therapy for necrotizing enterocolitis (NEC) on clinical outcomes in very low birth weight ($\leq$1500 g) infants.

Methods.—We identified very low birth weight infants with NEC from 348 US NICUs from 1997 to 2012. Anaerobic antimicrobial therapy was defined by antibiotic exposure on the first day of NEC. We matched (1:1) infants exposed to anaerobic antimicrobial therapy with infants who were not exposed by using a propensity score stratified by NEC severity (medical and surgical). The primary composite outcome was in-hospital death or intestinal stricture. We assessed the relationship between anaerobic antimicrobial therapy and outcome by using a conditional logistic regression on the matched cohort.

Results.—A total of 1390 infants exposed to anaerobic antimicrobial therapy were matched with 1390 infants not exposed. Mean gestational age and birth weight were 27 weeks and 946 g, respectively, and were similar in both groups. We found no significant difference in the combined outcome of death or strictures, but strictures as a single outcome were more common in the anaerobic antimicrobial therapy group (odds ratio 1.73; 95% confidence interval, 1.11–2.72). Among infants with surgical NEC, mortality was less common with anaerobic antimicrobial therapy (odds ratio 0.71; 95% confidence interval, 0.52–0.95).

Conclusions.—Anaerobic antimicrobial therapy was not associated with the composite outcome of death or strictures but was associated with an increase in intestinal strictures. This higher incidence of intestinal strictures may be explained by the fact that death is a competing outcome for intestinal strictures, and mortality was slightly lower in the anaerobic cohort. Infants with surgical NEC who received anaerobic antimicrobial therapy had lower mortality.

▶ The potential role of anaerobic bacteria in neonatal infections has been a source of puzzlement for decades. Although babies typically become colonized with anaerobic flora by the second week after birth, some early data suggested that infections are rare. As a result, neonatologists have often chosen not to use antimicrobial drugs effective against anaerobes, but pediatric surgeons have been more likely to advocate their use, particularly for suspected intra-abdominal infections. This landmark article now provides empirical evidence to inform this discussion. Using the multicenter database accumulated by Pediatrix Medical Group from 348 nurseries over a 15-year interval, these authors identified 6737 infants ≤1500 g with necrotizing enterocolitis, about half of whom had treatment that included anaerobic antibiotic therapy. From that population, pairs of cases, in which one subject did and the other did not receive anaerobic treatment, were selected using propensity score matching. This analytical strategy uses a multivariable logistic regression model to match subjects based on predicted risk of the outcome of interest; in this instance, the model included postnatal age, mechanical ventilation, fraction of inspired oxygen, use of inotropes in the first day after diagnosis, gestational age, small for gestational age, sex, race, 5-minute Apgar score, discharge year, and site. The propensity-matched analysis revealed no differences between groups in the primary outcome of death or stricture. Strictures were more common among survivors after anaerobic therapy. Stratification into medical and surgical necrotizing enterocolitis (NEC) cases demonstrated a lower mortality rate in infants who received anaerobic antimicrobials (see abstract). There was no benefit from anaerobic therapy in medical cases (odds ratio [OR] for death 0.99, 95% confidence interval [CI] 0.78-1.26; OR for death or stricture 1.09, 95% CI 0.87-1.37). Multivariate logistic regression modeling based on the entire cohort found no difference in the rate of death or stricture as a combined outcome (OR 0.90, 95% CI 0.76-1.07), a decrease in mortality rate (OR 0.80, 95% CI 0.67-0.97), and an increase in strictures (OR 1.67, 95% CI 1.16-2.39). Collectively, these results suggest that infants with surgical NEC, but not those with medical disease, may benefit from additional anaerobic antimicrobial coverage. With respect to treatment of the patients they are primarily responsible for, it therefore appears that neonatologists and pediatric surgeons have both been right about their antibiotic preferences.

W. E. Benitz, MD

Mortality Due to Bloodstream Infections and Necrotizing Enterocolitis in Very Low Birth Weight Infants

Schwab F, Zibell R, Piening B, et al (Charité Univ Medicine Berlin, Germany; et al)
Pediatr Infect Dis J 34:235-240, 2015

Background.—We evaluated the mortality due to nosocomial bloodstream infection (BSI) and necrotizing enterocolitis (NEC) in very low birth weight (VLBW) infants in 229 neonatal departments participating in the German national neonatal infection surveillance system between 2000 and 2011.

Methods.—For each infection type, we conducted a retrospective cohort study and a case—control study. In the cohort studies, the mortality risk due to BSI and/or NEC was estimated by calculating adjusted hazard ratios (AHRs) with 95% confidence intervals (CIs) using Cox proportional hazard regression with time the dependent variable infection. In the matched case—control studies, the attributable mortality was calculated.

Results.—A total of 43,116 VLBW infants, of which 6911 patients had at least 1 BSI and 1271 patients had at least 1 NEC, were analyzed. Overall mortality was 6.6%. Patients with at least 1 BSI had a mortality of 5.6%, and patients with at least 1 NEC had a mortality of 19.2%. The cohort studies revealed that BSI (AHR = 1.83; 95% CI: 1.61—2.08) and NEC (AHR = 6.35; 95% CI: 5.47—7.37) are independently associated with increased mortality. In the case—control study for BSI, 5187 (75.1%) patients with BSI were matched. Attributable mortality was 1.4% (95% CI: 0.7—2.2). In the case—control study for NEC, 1092 (85.9%) patients with NEC were matched. Attributable mortality was 14.7% (95% CI: 12.2—17.1).

Conclusions.—Nosocomial BSI and NEC increased mortality in VLBW infants. BSI, however, was associated with a relatively small attributable mortality of 1.4%, whereas NEC had a high attributable mortality of 14.7%.

▶ This extensive review of nosocomial infections and necrotizing enterocolitis (NEC) from 229 units in Germany over an 11-year period serves as the background for a smorgasbord of articles relating to neonatal sepsis. The good news overall is that the rates of infection and mortality are declining. The bad news is that there are still too many cases and very virulent bacteria, fungi, and viruses that need to be dealt with. Furthermore, it is revealing to witness the effect of the UK National Institute for Health Care Excellence (NICE) guideline on the evaluation of early-onset sepsis.

The review by Schwab et al is an impressive compilation of in excess of 40 000 patients from 229 neonatal units, which no doubt represents this as probably the largest study to date investigating increased mortality risk and attributable mortality due to primary bloodstream infections (BSI) and NEC in very low birth weight (VLBW) infants. The mortality rate is lower than reports from Vermont Oxford,[1] between 14.3% and 12.4%, in the period from 2000 to 2009. The Swiss Neonatal Network described a stable mortality of 13% in the VLBW infants group in the time period from 1996 to 2008.[2] Over the past decade with closer attention to the placement and management of central line catheters, there have been dramatic declines in the incidence of nosocomial sepsis attributable to these lines. Whereas sepsis was considered inevitable in VLBW infants, this concept is no longer applicable, and zero line infections are the attainable target. Limitations of the study are outlined by the authors and include the fact that early-onset sepsis was not taken into consideration; follow-up was restricted to a weight of 1800 g; and matching was not possible for all patients, and unmatched patients had a higher mortality. The mortality from NEC remains higher than from BSI so that the focus should shift to prevention of NEC as well as BSI.

There was an interesting and evidently first time report from Tsai et al,[3] who investigated the incidence, risk factors, and outcomes of breakthrough bacteremia in the neonatal intensive care unit (NICU). An episode of breakthrough bacteremia was defined as positive blood cultures despite appropriate antibiotic therapy. These authors documented that breakthrough bacteremia was not a rare event in the NICU, was more often caused by Gram-negative pathogens or fungi, and was more likely to occur in infants previously treated with broad-spectrum antibiotics within 1 month. In this study, 7.6% (72 of 942) of neonatal bacteremia, and 43 (59.7%) occurred as recurrent episodes. Gram-negative organisms (41.7%) and fungi (15.3%) accounted for more than half of all microorganisms in breakthrough bacteremia. Compared with non-breakthrough bacteremia, breakthrough bacteremia was significantly associated with more severe disease, was more likely to require aggressive therapies, and had a higher rate of infectious complications. Some particular pathogens, including *Pseudomonas aeruginosa* and fungi, were independent risk factors for developing breakthrough bacteremia. Breakthrough bacteremia is associated with more severe disease and a higher rate of sepsis-attributable mortality.

Regarding early onset sepsis there is an illuminating report from the United Kingdom.[4] In August 2012, a new national guidance from NICE for management of early-onset sepsis (EOS) was introduced in the United Kingdom. The guidance outlined a consistent approach for septic screens in newborn infants based on risk factors, and suggested biochemical and clinical parameters to guide management. In particular, it advised a second C-reactive protein level (CRP) 18 to 24 hours into treatment to help determine length of antibiotic course, need for lumbar puncture (LP), and suggested review of blood culture at 36 hours. In contrast to what had been anticipated—namely that is the new guideline would shorten hospital stay as a result of the call for a second CRP—the opposite was observed. Before NICE guidance, 38.1% of screened babies stayed < 72 hours. This reduced to 18.4% following guidance. However, before guidance, 20.9% babies stayed > 5 days, which increased to 27.7% by applying NICE recommendations. Repeat CRP measurements, which greatly influenced management and length of stay, increased from 45% to 97% and resulted in an increase in LPs performed from 14% to 23%. There were no positive blood cultures or LP results. More babies had longer courses of antibiotics and longer stays. The net effect was that the new guidelines not only affected workload and cost, without identifying more cases of EOS, but also changed the parental experience in the first days of life.

A. A. Fanaroff, MBBCh, FRCPE

References

1. Horbar JD, Carpenter JH, Badger GJ, et al. Mortality and neonatal morbidity among infants 501 to 1500 grams from 2000 to 2009. *Pediatrics.* 2012;129: 1019-1026.
2. Rüegger C, Hegglin M, Adams M, Bucher HU, Swiss Neonatal Network. Population based trends in mortality, morbidity and treatment for very preterm- and very low birth weight infants over 12 years. *BMC Pediatr.* 2012;12:17.
3. Tsai MH, Chu SM, Hsu JF, et al. Breakthrough bacteremia in the neonatal intensive care unit; incidence, risk factors and attributable mortality. *Am J Infect Control.* 2015;43:20-25.
4. Mukherjee A, Davidson L, Anguvaa L, Duffy DA, Kennea N. NICE neonatal early onset sepsis guidance: greater consistency, but more investigations, and greater length of stay. *Arch Dis Child Fetal Neonatal Ed.* 2015;100:F248-F249.

Role of Guidelines on Length of Therapy in Chorioamnionitis and Neonatal Sepsis

Kiser C, Nawab U, McKenna K, et al (Thomas Jefferson Univ/Nemours, Philadelphia, PA)

Pediatrics 133:992-998, 2014

Background and Objective.—Chorioamnionitis (CAM) is a major risk factor for neonatal sepsis. At our institution, neonates exposed to CAM and intrapartum antibiotics are treated with prolonged antimicrobial therapy if laboratory values are abnormal despite a sterile blood culture. Recently, the Committee on the Fetus and Newborn (COFN) recommended a similar strategy for treating neonates exposed to CAM. Our objective was to determine the frequency of abnormal laboratory parameters in term and late-preterm neonates exposed to CAM and evaluate the implication of recent COFN guidelines.

Methods.—This retrospective data analysis included late-preterm and term neonates exposed to CAM. Laboratory parameters, clinical symptoms and the number of infants treated with prolonged antibiotics were determined.

Results.—A total of 554 infants met the inclusion criteria. Eighty-three infants (14.9%) had an abnormal immature to total neutrophil ratio (>0.2) and 121 infants (22%) had an abnormal C-reactive protein level (>1 mg/dL) at 12 hours of age. A total of 153 infants (27.6%) had an abnormal immature to total neutrophil ratio and/or abnormal C-reactive protein level at 12 hours of age. Only 4 (0.7%) of 554 infants had a positive blood culture result. A total of 134 (24.2%) infants were treated with prolonged antibiotics (112 [20.2%] were treated solely based on abnormal laboratory data). Lumbar puncture was performed in 120 (21.6%) infants.

Conclusions.—When managed by using a strategy similar to recent COFN guidelines, a large number of term and late-preterm infants exposed to CAM who had sterile blood culture findings were treated with prolonged antibiotic therapy due to abnormal laboratory findings. They were also subjected to additional invasive procedures and had a longer duration of hospitalization.

▶ For at least 15 years, chorioamnionitis has been identified as a major predictor of risk for early-onset neonatal sepsis. To at least some extent, the impetus for evaluation and empiric treatment of babies born to women with chorioamnionitis was the observation that nearly 90% of the reported instances of early-onset sepsis following intrapartum antibiotic prophylaxis occurred in infants exposed to chorioamnionitis, as I summarized in a review of risk factors for sepsis in 1999. From a frequentist perspective, that association was not likely to have been simply coincidental. This important paper provides compelling evidence that chorioamnionitis is not a reliable predictor of risk in late-preterm and term infants; however, only 4 of the 554 chorioamnionitis-exposed babies (0.7%) in this series had culture-proven early-onset sepsis. Similarly, low rates of early-onset sepsis in late-preterm and term infants have been reported by others, so this result is not anomalous. How can these observations be reconciled? The key lies in stratification by gestational age, which was not available in the older reports. In contrast to late-preterm and term infants, those who are more immature (< 33 weeks' gestation) or very low birth weight (< 1500 g) are much more likely to develop early-onset sepsis in association with chorioamnionitis, with reported attack rates ranging from 5% to 17%. Because chorioamnionitis is a frequent cause of prematurity, those babies are overrepresented in cohorts of infants exposed to that risk factor, driving the strong association in the population at large. That relationship does not apply among more mature newborns, however. Furthermore, these authors report that abnormal neutrophil ratios (immature:total) or C-reactive protein levels are quite common in these infants, indicating that those laboratory tests also have a poor positive predictive value in this setting, but abnormal results often led to prolonged courses (≥7 days) of antibiotic treatment. These authors correctly question the value of treatment of large numbers of babies based on a history of chorioamnionitis and abnormal laboratory results and suggest revision of the Committee on Fetus and Newborn recommendation of prolongation of treatment of neonates with negative blood cultures and abnormal hematological or C-reactive protein results. Recognition of the low risk of early-onset sepsis in asymptomatic late-preterm and term newborns, even in association with chorioamnionitis, might allow omission of unnecessary diagnostic and therapeutic interventions for those infants. That would go much further to obviate the "health care costs and risks associated with an extended course of antibiotics, prolonged hospitalization, lumbar puncture, intravenous access, and separation of infant from mother" than simply shortening the course of an unnecessary treatment.

W. E. Benitz, MD

Newborn Screening for Severe Combined Immunodeficiency in 11 Screening Programs in the United States

Kwan A, Abraham RS, Currier R, et al (Univ of California, San Francisco; Mayo Clinic, Rochester, MN; California Dept of Public Health, Richmond; et al)
JAMA 312:729-738, 2014

Importance.—Newborn screening for severe combined immunodeficiency (SCID) using assays to detect T-cell receptor excision circles (TRECs) began in Wisconsin in 2008, and SCID was added to the national recommended uniform panel for newborn screened disorders in 2010. Currently 23 states, the District of Columbia, and the Navajo Nation conduct population-wide newborn screening for SCID. The incidence of SCID is estimated at 1 in 100 000 births.

Objectives.—To present data from a spectrum of SCID newborn screening programs, establish population-based incidence for SCID and other conditions with T-cell lymphopenia and document early institution of effective treatments.

Design.—Epidemiological and retrospective observational study.

Setting.—Representatives in states conducting SCID newborn screening were invited to submit their SCID screening algorithms, test performance data and deidentified clinical and laboratory information regarding infants screened and cases with nonnormal results. Infants born from the start of each participating program from January 2008 through the most recent evaluable date prior to July 2013 were included. Representatives from 10 states plus the Navajo Area Indian Health Service contributed data from 3 030 083 newborns screened with a TREC test.

Main Outcomes and Measures.—Infants with SCID and other diagnoses of T-cell lymphopenia were classified. Incidence and, where possible, etiologies were determined. Interventions and survival were tracked.

Results.—Screening detected 52 cases of typical SCID, leaky SCID, and Omenn syndrome, affecting 1 in 58 000 infants (95% CI, 1/46 000-1/80 000). Survival of SCID-affected infants through their diagnosis and immune reconstitution was 87% (45/52), 92% (45/49) for infants who received transplantation, enzyme replacement, and/or gene therapy. Additional interventions for SCID and non-SCID T-cell lymphopenia included immunoglobulin infusions, preventive antibiotics, and avoidance of live vaccines. Variations in definitions and follow-up practices influenced the rates of detection of non-SCID T-cell lymphopenia.

Conclusions and Relevance.—Newborn screening in 11 programs in the United States identified SCID in 1 in 58 000 infants, with high survival. The usefulness of detection of non-SCID T-cell lymphopenias by the same screening remains to be determined (Table 5).

▶ Just as postmarketing surveillance is essential to establish the safety of new drugs, postimplementation surveillance is a critical step in evaluating efficacy of new strategies for disease screening. This report provides the first description of results of newborn screening for severe combined immune deficiencies (SCID)

TABLE 5.—Diagnoses of 411 Infants With Non-SCID T-Cell Lymphopenia Identified by Newborn Screening

Condition	No. of Infants
Syndromes with T-cell impairment[a]	136
DiGeorge	78[b]
Trisomy 21	21
Ataxia telangiectasia	4
Trisomy 18	4
CHARGE	3
Jacobsen	2
CLOVES	1
ECC	1
Fryns	1
Nijmegen breakage	1
Noonan	1
Rac2 defect	1[c]
Renpenning	1
TAR	1
Not specified	10
Cytogenetic abnormalities[d]	6
Secondary T-cell impairment	117
Cardiac anomalies	30
Multiple congenital anomalies	23
Loss into third space	15
Gastrointestinal anomalies	15
Neonatal leukemia	4
Not specified	30
Preterm birth alone	29
Variant SCID	12[e]
Unspecified T-cell lymphopenia[f]	117

Abbreviations: CHARGE, coloboma, heart defect, atresia choanae, retarded growth and development, genital and ear abnormality; CLOVES, congenital lipomatous overgrowth, vascular malformations, epidermal nevi, and spinal/skeletal anomalies; ECC, ectodermal dysplasia, ectrodactyly, and clefting; SCID, severe combined immunodeficiency; TAR, thrombocytopenia and absent radius.

Editor's Note: Please refer to original journal article for full references.

[a]Eponymous syndromes: DiGeorge, cardiac defects, hypocalcemia, thymus dysplasia, and other anomalies, most often with chromosome 22q11.2 interstitial deletion; Jacobsen, growth and psychomotor retardation and congenital anomalies with chromosome 11qter deletion; Fryns, diaphragmatic hernia and other congenital anomalies; Noonan, multiple congenital anomalies; Renpenning, X chromosome—linked mental retardation with distinctive facies.
[b]Included 3 infants with complete DiGeorge syndrome and absent T cells, 2 of whom received a thymus transplant.
[c]Eventual hematopoietic cell transplant performed.[17]
[d]Included chromosome 6p deletion, ring chromosome 14, ring chromosome 17, chromosome 17q duplication, and 2 siblings with unspecified chromosome abnormalities.
[e]Eventual hematopoietic cell transplant performed for 1 case.
[f]Includes infants from Michigan (46), New York (30), Massachusetts (25), Wisconsin (13), Connecticut (2), and Delaware (1); further information was not available for these infants, although those from New York were reported to require ongoing monitoring or treatment for a deficiency of T cells.[30]

Reprinted from Kwan A, Abraham RS, Currier R, et al. Newborn Screening for Severe Combined Immunodeficiency in 11 Screening Programs in the United States. JAMA. 2014;312:729-738. Copyright 2014, American Medical Association. All rights reserved.

using T-cell receptor excision circle (TREC) counts in a large population of more than 3 million infants.

Screening strategies can fail because of either excessive false-negative or false-positive results. In this population, SCID was detected in 52 infants (1 in 58 000 screened infants). No missed cases were recognized. Although it is difficult to estimate precisely, these results suggest a very low false-negative rate. Conversely, identification of more cases than expected based on the priori prevalence estimate of 1 in 100 000 live births suggests that reliance on clinical presentation may have resulted in underdiagnosis of SCID, possibly because some affected infants died of overwhelming infection without recognition of their underlying disease. These results were achieved with remarkably few false-positive results given that only 1265 infants were referred for confirmatory flow cytometry (42 per 100 000 screened infants). Only 1 in 42 infants with a positive screening result was subsequently found to have SCID, reflecting the low positive predictive value of TREC counts for SCID (2.4%).

Exclusion of SCID in infants with positive screening tests did not imply absence of any disease, however. Subgroup analysis demonstrated a positive predictive value of 36% for prediction of lymphopenia (<1500/µL) by a low TREC count. Among 411 infants with low TREC counts, results of evaluation for underlying diagnoses were reported for 296 infants (Table 5). Because most babies with these conditions will have been admitted to a neonatal intensive care unit (NICU), this listing provides a useful differential diagnosis for evaluation of NICU patients with positive TREC screening results. Among the third who have confirmed lymphopenia, roughly 20% will have lymphopenia due to prematurity (10%), hydrops (5%; listed as "loss into third space"), or gastrointestinal anomalies including gastroschisis (5%); their lymphopenia can be expected to resolve with maturation or management of the associated condition. About 13% of cases did not have a specified diagnosis, but the remainder had conditions for which attention to an associated immune deficiency may contribute substantially to accurate diagnosis or overall management. Accordingly, a low TREC count should not be dismissed once SCID is excluded.

Most important, 45 of the 52 infants with SCID identified by screening have survived with specific treatment. Two of the 7 infants who died did so because of associated major congenital anomalies, so 90% of the affected infants may have accrued substantial benefit from the screening program. These initial results are a substantial achievement resulting from application of recent advances in molecular immunology and stem cell biology.

W. E. Benitz, MD

First Pertussis Vaccine Dose and Prevention of Infant Mortality
Tiwari TSP, Baughman AL, Clark TA (Ctrs for Disease Control and Prevention, Atlanta, GA)
Pediatrics 135:990-999, 2015

Background.—American infants are at highest risk of severe pertussis and death. We investigated the role of ≥1 pertussis vaccinations in preventing pertussis-related deaths and risk markers for death among infants aged <42 days.

Methods.—We analyzed characteristics of fatal and nonfatal infant pertussis cases reported nationally during 1991−2008. Infants were categorized into 2 age groups on the basis of eligibility to receive a first pertussis vaccine dose at age 6 weeks; dose 1 was considered valid if given ≥14 days before illness onset. Multivariable logistic regression was used to estimate the effect of ≥1 pertussis vaccine doses on outcome and risk markers.

Results.—Pertussis-related deaths occurred among 258 of 45 404 cases. Fatal and nonfatal cases were confirmed by culture (54% vs 49%) and polymerase chain reaction (31% vs 27%). All deaths occurred before age 34 weeks at illness onset; 64% occurred before age 6 weeks. Among infants aged ≥42 days, receiving ≥1 doses of vaccine protected against death (adjusted odds ratio [aOR]: 0.28; 95% confidence interval [CI]: 0.11–0.74), hospitalization (aOR: 0.69; 95% CI: 0.63–0.77), and pneumonia (aOR: 0.80; 95% CI: 0.68–0.95). Risk was elevated for Hispanic ethnicity (aOR: 2.28; 95% CI: 1.36–3.83) and American Indian/Alaska Native race (aOR: 5.15; 95% CI: 2.37–11.2) and lower for recommended antibiotic treatment (aOR: 0.28; 95% CI: 0.16–0.47). Among infants aged <42 days, risk was elevated for Hispanic ethnicity and lower with recommended antibiotic use.

Conclusions.—The first pertussis vaccine dose and antibiotic treatment protect against death, hospitalization, and pneumonia.

▶ Indelibly etched in my memory is one of the first sick patients whom I cared for in internship: a tiny baby who had acquired pertussis in the first weeks of life. I'll never forget the anxiety in the eyes of this little baby as she struggled, deeply cyanotic, through every wheezy, airway-obstructing cough. Mercifully, she survived, and the experience reinforced my advocacy for immunization against pertussis and other potentially lethal childhood diseases. In this study, Tiwari and colleagues analyzed data reported to the National Notifiable Diseases Surveillance System between 1991 and 2008, finding that pertussis-related deaths occurred among 258 of 45 404 cases, all among infants who were younger than 8.5 months of age. Among infants at 42 days or more, ≥1 dose of pertussis vaccine protected against death. Tiwari and colleagues' data provide justification, in the absence of contraindications, for moving forward with Pertussis immunization according to schedule, even for babies who remain hospitalized in the NICU.

L. J. Van Marter, MD, MPH

6 Cardiovascular System

Natural evolution of patent ductus arteriosus in the extremely preterm infant
Rolland A, Shankar-Aguilera S, Diomandé D, et al (CHI Poissy Saint-Germain-en-Laye, France; Hôpital Antoine-Béclère, Clamart, France; et al)
Arch Dis Child Fetal Neonatal Ed 100:F55-F58, 2014

Objective.—The persistence of the patent ductus arteriosus (PDA) is frequently encountered in very preterm infants. Neither preventive nor curative treatments of PDA have been shown to improve the outcome of these infants. Since no consensus on optimal treatment of PDA is established, we evaluated the rate of spontaneous PDA closure in infants born before 28 weeks of gestation.

Patients and Methods.—We studied a retrospective cohort of 103 infants (gestational age 24–27 weeks) admitted to our neonatal intensive care unit from 1 June 2008 to 31 July 2010. Maternal and neonatal characteristics were collected. The PDA was defined by the persistence of ductal patency after 72 h and was followed up by regular echocardiography.

Results.—Twelve infants died within the first 72 h and were excluded from the analysis. Among 91 infants analysed, 8 (9%) closed their ductus arteriosus before 72 h and the ductus could not be determined patent in 13. Of the 70 infants with a PDA still persistent, one underwent surgical ligation and echocardiography showed spontaneous closure in 51 (73%) of them. In the remaining 18 infants, the date of PDA closure could not be determined either because of their death (n = 11) or due to discharge (n = 7). Overall, a spontaneous closure of the ductus arteriosus was observed in 59 of the 91 infants.

Conclusions.—We have to question whether exposure to the risks of therapeutic interventions targeted for ductal closure is warranted since a PDA closes spontaneously in at least 73% of infants born before 28 weeks (Fig 1).

▶ Increasing recognition that early, routine treatment to close the persistently patent ductus arteriosus (PDA) in preterm infants does not produce improved long-term outcomes has resulted in a substantial shift in strategies for management of that condition over the past 5 years or so. Evidence from many randomized controlled trials makes it clear that early treatment has no advantages, but

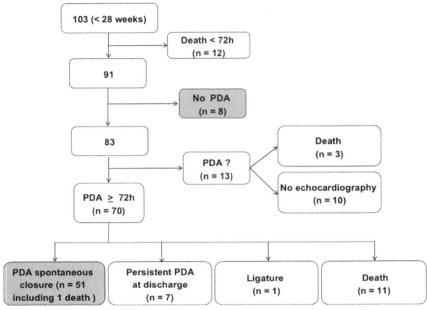

FIGURE 1.—Natural evolution of patent ductus arteriosus in a population of infants born before 28 weeks of gestation. (Reprinted from Rolland A, Shankar-Aguilera S, Diomandé D, et al. Natural evolution of patent ductus arteriosus in the extremely preterm infant. *Arch Dis Child Fetal Neonatal Ed.* 2014;100:F55-F58, with permission from the BMJ Publishing Group Ltd.)

high rates of crossover to "rescue" treatment in the "control" arms of those trials leave room for doubt about the utility (or lack of same) of later treatment. Similarly, frequent use of cyclooxygenase (COX) inhibitors or surgical ligation has, in most instances, compromised data on rates and timing of spontaneous ductal closure because neither the probability of later closure nor potential adverse consequences of continued patency can be assessed after treatment. This small series from France begins to address that uncertainty. In a cohort of 103 consecutively admitted infants less than 28 weeks gestational age (24-0/7 to 27-6/7 weeks), in whom COX inhibitors were not used for prophylaxis or treatment of PDA, ductal patency was assessed by echocardiography by the fourth day after birth. In infants with PDA at ≥72 hours of age, echocardiography was repeated once or twice weekly until ductal closure was demonstrated. The progression of those findings is shown in Fig 1. These data can also be expressed as a mortality rate of 26% (27 of 103), confirmed spontaneous PDA closure in 56% (58 of 103), likely but unconfirmed PDA closure in 10% (10 of 103), persistent PDA at discharge in 7% (7 of 103), and ligation in 1% (1 of 103). Among surviving infants, ductal closure was confirmed or probable in 89% (68 of 76). Of the 7 infants discharged with persistent PDA, 3 had no heart murmur at follow-up, and 4 were lost to follow-up. Among the 51 infants whose PDA closed after 72 hours of age, the mean age at documentation of closure was 61 ± 37 days (range 4–165 days). (These data are therefore not inconsistent with the other reports of high rates of ductal patency at 30 days of age.[1]) Spontaneous closure rates were not significantly different between infants born at 24 to 25 weeks' or at 26 to 27 weeks' gestation (60% and 80%, respectively), nor among the groups with significant, insignificant, or indeterminate hemodynamic effects of PDA (78, 73, and 65%, respectively). These data from a high-risk population provide considerable reassurance that omission of (as opposed to only deferral of) treatment of PDA in small preterm infants is not greatly harmful. The authors note that these data cannot exclude the possibility that some deaths might have been prevented by PDA treatment. Although that question can only be answered by future randomized controlled trials, it is evident that such cases must be relatively unusual, and they currently are not prospectively identifiable.

W. E. Benitz, MD

Reference

1. Smith A, Maguire M, Livingstone V, Dempsey EM. Peak systolic to end diastolic flow velocity ratio is associated with ductal patency in infants below 32 weeks of gestation. *Arch Dis Child Fetal Neonatal Ed.* 2015;100:F132-F136.

Use of ultrasound in the haemodynamic assessment of the sick neonate
Kluckow M (Univ of Sydney, St Leonards, Australia)
Arch Dis Child Fetal Neonatal Ed 99:F332-F337, 2014

Clinician performed ultrasound (CPU) by the clinician caring for a sick patient is increasingly used in critical care specialties. The real-time haemodynamic information obtained helps the clinician to understand underlying physiology, target treatment and refine clinical decision-making. Neonatologists are increasingly using ultrasound to assess sick neonates with a range of clinical presentations and demand for training and accreditation programmes is increasing. This review discusses the current expanded uses for CPU in the haemodynamic assessment of the sick neonate.

▶ Various terminologies are in use by neonatologists for bedside hemodynamic assessment. This includes targeted neonatal echocardiography, neonatologist performed cardiac ultrasound, and point of care echocardiography.[1] Although its usefulness is increasingly recognized, its widespread utilization is still limited by lack of standardized training and accreditation of neonatologists and the reluctance of pediatric cardiologists to transfer this skill to neonatologists.[2] As a result, neonatologists are trying to find nomenclature for bedside functional echocardiography that separates it from assessing structural heart defects. Additionally, in the absence of a standardized assessment tool and variation in skills and practices, there is an inherent risk of overdiagnosing normal transitional changes or false reassurance of normality when there is hemodynamic instability.

Key opinion leaders in the field have suggested what to assess during transition to diagnose deviation from the norm, but further evidence is required to prove the benefits of routine bedside functional echocardiography for intensive care and management of the sick newborn infants compared to routine clinical care. In the review by Kluckow, various indications for functional echocardiography and the table of uses of clinician performed ultrasound (CPU) in several neonatal clinical dilemmas are summarized. There is, however, continued lack of standardization of techniques suggested for assessment. For example, different groups have proposed various assessment tools for diagnosing patent ductus arteriosus, myocardial function, and pulmonary hypertension. This has a potential to lead to a greater degree of intraobserver and interobserver variability and thus undermine the usefulness of investigation. There is an urgent need to standardize the techniques and use a basic set of assessments for various disease states. Newer techniques and tools can then be assessed for their potential to improve diagnosis and guide treatment.

One such example is superior vena cava flow, widely studied in the 1990s and reported to be a standard to assess systemic venous return. Although this group reported its usefulness in decision making and prognosticating outcomes, there was a large variation when other investigators tried to use it. Further data from magnetic resonance imaging highlighted the limitations of assessments given that superior vena cava is elliptical rather than circular, and the point of measurement can multiply errors while calculating cross-sectional area and thus over- or underestimate the flow.[3] The assessment of preload has also remained subjective, and crude assessments such as "eyeballing" end-diastolic volume have been suggested and continue to have poor repeatability between observers.

CPU has improved the understanding of transition and the recognition of a potentially significant patent ductus arteriosus (PDA) before it is symptomatic, but it may lead to overdiagnosis of a hemodynamically significant PDA by the injudicious use of bedside echocardiography. This has created uncertainty among clinicians in managing PDA and a shift to nonintervention rather than an evidence-based approach for management.[4]

Understanding of transition and assessment of cardiac function in preterm infants can potentially select and titrate inotropes rather than using vasopressors injudiciously. Understanding transitional changes using bedside functional echocardiography has highlighted the limitations of targeting therapy based solely on blood pressure measurements.[5] This is a significant change in approach that has helped to reduce short-term morbidity, but further studies are now required to study long-term outcomes.

In the present review, a discussion of limitations of assessments and pitfalls of functional echocardiography with examples of misadventures in novice hands could have helped the reader in understanding that functional echocardiography is a tool that should not be used without appropriate training and supervision. The authors highlighted the uses of such hemodynamic assessments but did not provide a balanced argument of current limitations. In expert hands, information from bedside CPU seems to be of benefit to sick and premature infants.

S. Gupta, DM, MRCP, MD, FRCPCH, FRCPI

References

1. Evans N, Gournay V, Cabanas F, et al. Point-of-care ultrasound in the neonatal intensive care unit: international perspectives. *Semin Fetal Neonatal Med.* 2011; 16:61-68.
2. Roehr CC, te Pas AB, Dold SK, et al. Investigating the European perspective of neonatal point-of-care echocardiography in the neonatal intensive care unit—a pilot study. *Eur J Pediatr.* 2013;172:907-911.
3. Ficial B, Finnemore AE, Cox DJ, et al. Validation study of the accuracy of echocardiographic measurements of systemic blood flow volume in newborn infants. *J Am Soc Echocardiogr.* 2013;26:1365-1371.
4. Benitz WE. Patent ductus arteriosus: to treat or not to treat? *Arch Dis Child Fetal Neonatal Ed.* 2012;97:F80-F82.
5. Gupta S, Donn SM. Neonatal hypotension: dopamine or dobutamine? *Semin Fetal Neonatal Med.* 2014;19:54-59.

Vasopressin versus Dopamine for Treatment of Hypotension in Extremely Low Birth Weight Infants: A Randomized, Blinded Pilot Study
Rios DR, Kaiser JR (Baylor College of Medicine and Texas Children's Hosp, Houston)
J Pediatr 166:850-855, 2015

Objective.—To evaluate vasopressin vs dopamine as initial therapy in extremely low birth weight (ELBW) infants with hypotension during the first 24 hours of life.

Study Design.—ELBW infants with hypertension ≤30 weeks' gestation and ≤24 hours old randomly received treatment with vasopressin or dopamine in a blinded fashion. Normotensive infants not receiving vasopressor support served as a comparison group.

Results.—Twenty ELBW infants with hypertension received vasopressin (n = 10) or dopamine (n = 10), and 50 were enrolled for comparison. Mean gestational age was 25.6 ± 1.4 weeks and birth weight 705 ± 154 g. Response to vasopressin paralleled that of dopamine in time to adequate mean blood pressure (Kaplan-Meier curve, $P = .986$); 90% of infants in each treatment group responded with adequate blood pressure. The vasopressin group received fewer doses of surfactant ($P < .05$), had lower $PaCO_2$ values ($P < .05$), and were not tachycardic ($P < .001$) during vasopressin administration, compared with the dopamine group.

Conclusions.—Vasopressin in ELBW infants as the initial agent for early hypotension appeared safe. This pilot study supports a larger randomized controlled trial of vasopressin vs dopamine therapy in ELBW infants with hypotension.

▶ Although the definition of hypotension in preterm infants is controversial, treatment with vasopressors remains common. Standard therapies to treat hypotension fail to reduce the incidence of short-term morbidities and fail to improve long-term neurodevelopmental outcomes. Clinicians traditionally use dopamine as first-line therapy for hypotension because of its inotropic and vasoconstrictive actions (including pulmonary vasoconstriction). Vasopressin has emerged as an alternative to dopamine with potent systemic vasoconstrictive effects in the setting of hypoxia and acidosis, minimal inotropic effects, and vasodilatory effects on the pulmonary vasculature. Vasopressin has previously been described in extremely low birth weight infants in case reports and series; Rios and colleagues performed the first randomized, blinded trial of vasopressin compared to dopamine in this population. The authors randomized 20 extremely low birth weight infants with hypotension in the first 24 hours of life. Of importance, the authors demonstrated the feasibility of this trial design including willingness of clinicians and parents to consent and ability to randomize to blinded vasopressor in a timely fashion. The response to therapy was similar between groups (time to goal mean arterial pressure and percent responders). Compared with dopamine, vasopressin-treated patients had lower $PaCO_2$ values ($P < .05$) and had less tachycardia ($P < .001$). Although limited by a small sample size, the results of this trial highlight potential undesirable pulmonary effects of dopamine. This pilot trial demonstrates the importance of continued investigation of alternative strategies for addressing hypotension in extremely low birth weight infants. Larger trials focusing on long-term outcomes, in addition to short-term effects, continue to be a top priority in neonatal research.

C. McPherson

Do small doses of atropine (<0.1 mg) cause bradycardia in young children?
Eisa L, Passi Y, Lerman J, et al (Women and Children's Hosp of Buffalo, NY)
Arch Dis Child 100:684-688, 2015

Objective.—To determine the heart rate response to atropine (<0.1 mg) in anaesthetised young infants.
Design.—Prospective, observational and controlled.
Setting.—Elective surgery.
Patients.—Sixty unpremedicated healthy infants less than 15 kg were enrolled. Standard monitoring was applied. Anaesthesia was induced by mask with nitrous oxide (66%) and oxygen (33%) followed by sevoflurane (8%).
Interventions.—Intravenous (IV) atropine (5 µg/kg) was flushed into a fast flowing IV. The ECG was recorded continuously from 30 s before the atropine until 5 min afterwards.
Main Outcome Measures.—The incidence of bradycardia and arrhythmias was determined from the ECGs by a blinded observer.
Results.—The median (IQR) age was 6.5 (4—12) months and the mean (95% CI) weight was 8.6 (8.1 to 9.1) kg. The mean (95% CI) dose of atropine was 40.9 (37.3 to 44) µg. Bradycardia did not occur. Two infants developed premature atrial contractions and one developed a premature ventricular contraction. When compared with baseline values, heart rate increased by 7% 30 s after atropine, 14% 1 min after atropine and 25% 5 min after atropine. Twenty-nine infants (48%) experienced tachycardia

(>20% above baseline rate) after atropine lasting 222.7 s (range 27.9—286). The change in heart rate 5 min after atropine was inversely related to the baseline heart rate.

Conclusions.—The upper 95% CI for the occurrence of bradycardia in the entire population of infants based on a zero incidence in this study is 5%. These results rebut the notion that atropine <0.1 mg IV causes bradycardia in young infants.

Trial Registration Number.—ClinicalTrials.gov #NCT01819064.

▶ Atropine is frequently used in neonates to prevent bradycardia and decrease bronchial and salivary secretions during intubation. Many references (including the Pediatric Advanced Life Support course) caution against dose of atropine <0.1 mg due to a risk of paradoxical bradycardia. This minimum dose is based on 1 human study in which infants and children receiving small doses of atropine experience neither bradycardia nor sequelae of arrhythmia. No premature infants were included in this study. Eisa et al performed a prospective, observational study in 60 healthy infants <15 kg given intravenous atropine 0.005 mg/kg. The mean dose of atropine was 0.041 mg. No infants experienced bradycardia. Two infants developed premature atrial contractions, and 1 developed a premature ventricular contraction. These minor arrhythmias did not compromise cardiovascular indices. These findings support prospective studies demonstrating prevention of laryngoscopy-induced bradycardia with no paradoxical bradycardia using 0.01 to 0.02 mg/kg even in small, preterm infants.[1] A 0.1-mg minimum dose of intravenous atropine poses a significant risk to infants less than 5 kg, with progressive increase in risk for smaller infants. Several reports have described cholinergic syndrome and death after atropine overdose. Given the documented risks of overdose and the growing body of evidence refuting the historic minimum dose, this minimum should be removed from guidelines and dosing references.

C. McPherson

Reference

1. Barrington KJ. The myth of a minimum dose for atropine. *Pediatrics.* 2011;127: 783-784.

Antidepressant Use Late in Pregnancy and Risk of Persistent Pulmonary Hypertension of the Newborn

Huybrechts KF, Bateman BT, Palmsten K, et al (Brigham and Women's Hosp, Boston, MA; Massachusetts General Hosp, Boston; et al)
JAMA 313:2142-2151, 2015

Importance.—The association between selective serotonin reuptake inhibitor (SSRI) antidepressant use during pregnancy and risk of persistent pulmonary hypertension of the newborn (PPHN) has been controversial since the US Food and Drug Administration issued a public health advisory in 2006.

Objective.—To examine the risk of PPHN associated with exposure to different antidepressant medication classes late in pregnancy.

Design and Setting.—Cohort study nested in the 2000-2010 Medicaid Analytic eXtract for 46 US states and Washington, DC. Last follow-up date was December 31, 2010.

Participants.—A total of 3 789 330 pregnant women enrolled in Medicaid from 2 months or fewer after the date of last menstrual period through at least 1 month after delivery. The source cohort was restricted to women with a depression diagnosis and logistic regression analysis with propensity score adjustment applied to control for potential confounders.

Exposures for Observational Studies.—SSRI and non-SSRI monotherapy use during the 90 days before delivery vs no use.

Main Outcomes and Measures.—Recorded diagnosis of PPHN during the first 30 days after delivery.

Results.—A total of 128 950 women (3.4%) filled at least 1 prescription for antidepressants late in pregnancy: 102 179 (2.7%) used an SSRI and 26 771 (0.7%) a non-SSRI. Overall, 7630 infants not exposed to antidepressants were diagnosed with PPHN (20.8; 95% CI, 20.4-21.3 per 10 000 births) compared with 322 infants exposed to SSRIs (31.5; 95% CI, 28.3-35.2 per 10 000 births), and 78 infants exposed to non-SSRIs (29.1; 95% CI, 23.3-36.4 per 10 000 births). Associations between antidepressant use and PPHN were attenuated with increasing levels of confounding adjustment. For SSRIs, odds ratios were 1.51 (95% CI, 1.35-1.69) unadjusted and 1.10 (95% CI, 0.94-1.29) after restricting to women with depression and adjusting for the high-dimensional propensity score. For non-SSRIs, the odds ratios were 1.40 (95% CI, 1.12-1.75) and 1.02 (95% CI, 0.77-1.35), respectively. Upon restriction of the outcome to primary PPHN, the adjusted odds ratio for SSRIs was 1.28 (95% CI, 1.01-1.64) and for non-SSRIs 1.14 (95% CI, 0.74-1.74).

Conclusions and Relevance.—Evidence from this large study of publicly insured pregnant women may be consistent with a potential increased risk of PPHN associated with maternal use of SSRIs in late pregnancy. However, the absolute risk was small, and the risk increase appears more modest than suggested in previous studies.

▶ To examine the association of antidepressant use and persistent pulmonary hypertension of the newborn (PPHN), Huybrechts et al analyzed more than 3.7 million mother-infant pairs from a Medicaid dataset (Medicate Analytic eXtract) from 2000 to 2010. The exposures were either selective serotonin reuptake inhibitor (SSRI) or other non-SSRI antidepressant use during the 90 days before delivery. The prevalence of antidepressant use late in pregnancy was 3.4% (2.7% for SSRI and 0.7% for non-SSRI). The incidence of PPHN was 20.8 per 10 000 among infants not exposed to antidepressants compared to 31.5 per 10 000 among infants exposed to SSRIs and 29.1 per 10 000 for non-SSRI antidepressants. The odds ratio of PPHN among SSRI users versus nonusers was 1.51 (95% confidence interval [CI] 1.35-1.69). When the investigators restricted to women with depression, the OR was attenuated to 1.36 (95% CI 1.18-1.57) or as low as 1.10 (95% CI 0.94-1.29) when high-dimensional propensity score stratification was used. This attenuation suggests that depressed women have a baseline increased risk of offspring PPHN. The authors conclude that the absolute risk of PPHN remains small with SSRI use. However, these data support a small, but potentially important, effect of SSRIs on PPHN risk. Thoughtful continuation and selective discontinuation of SSRIs in pregnancy should be a priority for perinatal providers. In other words, it seems to be time to consider efforts to create antidepressant stewardship programs as a part of prenatal care.

H. H. Burris, MD, MPH

Fetal Thrombotic Vasculopathy and Perinatal Thrombosis: Should all Placentas be Examined?
Magnetti F, Bagna R, Botta G, et al (Università degli Studi di Torino, Italy; Città della Scienza e della Salute, Torino, Italy)
Am J Perinatol 31:695-700, 2014

Objective.—Numerous fetal placenta vascular lesions seem to be a predisposing condition for some types of perinatal disease. Placental disease and newborn thromboses might be both manifestations of the same underlying disorder. Objective of this study is to describe pathological lesions of the placenta in newborns with perinatal thrombosis.

Study Design.—We present retrospective data review and analysis regarding neonates admitted at our neonatal intensive care unit and diagnosed with an episode of thromboembolic events (TE) in the period from 2009 to 2013; among them we report three cases of perinatal thrombosis in newborns whose placentas demonstrated fetal thrombotic vasculopathy (FTV).

Results.—In all the three cases a prothrombotic maternal condition was found, and in one patient a maternal infection with chorioamnionitis; the histological examination of placenta, required soon after birth for maternal pathological conditions, was important in confirming and explaining the clinical diagnosis of neonatal thrombosis and for the management of future pregnancies.

Conclusion.—It is proposed that placenta of newborns with TE in first days of life should always be examined, for its association with FTV and thus the storage of placentas for a week after birth should be routinely implemented.

▶ Multiple environmental and genetic factors play a role in the pathogenesis of neonatal thrombosis. These factors differ depending on the vascular beds involved, the gestational age of the newborn, and several factors affecting the pregnancy. Known environmental factors for neonatal thrombosis include gestational age, presence of indwelling vascular catheters, and infection. The role of genetic factors in neonatal thrombosis is poorly understood and often extrapolated from underpowered studies or from adult studies of venous thromboembolism.[1] Furthermore, the role of placental pathology in the pathogenesis of neonatal thrombosis is unclear.

Although the systematic review of placental pathology detailed in the article allowed the authors to make connections between abnormal placental pathology and clinical thrombosis, there were several weaknesses that limited the strength of the conclusions. The primary weaknesses of the article are low numbers and missing data. If the focus was to provide a justification for placental pathologic examinations, a critical piece of data is missing: the incidence of fetal thrombotic vasculopathy in all placentas examined, not just those with thromboembolic events. The authors found 13 neonates with thrombosis. Nine of these had placentas available for examination, and 6 were abnormal. Three of the 9 placental exams documented fetal thrombotic vasculopathy. How many placentas had fetal thrombotic vasculopathy without neonatal thrombosis? Even without these data, more infants with thrombosis had placentas without fetal vasculopathy than those that had fetal vasculopathy.

Clinical details of the mothers and infants in this study should be considered noted with caution. Large genome-wide association studies of thrombosis have demonstrated that many previously published single-gene association studies claiming to connect common polymorphisms with thrombosis suffered from statistical errors.[3] In particular, genetic associations with a common polymorphism in methylenetetrahydrofolate reductase (MTHFR) (C677T), allele frequency of 31% in Europeans, have been shown to have no valid associations with thrombosis. Although the large genetic study did not include pregnant women, readers should not connect the presence MTHFR polymorphisms in mothers to neonatal thrombosis. Furthermore, the coagulation system develops throughout gestation and the levels of procoagulant, anticoagulant, and fibrinolytic proteins often do not reach adult levels until the first year after birth.[2] Additionally, during a thrombotic process or severe illness, the levels of these proteins change in the acute phase response or due to consumption in a thrombosis. Therefore, the interpretation of the levels of components of the procoagulant and anticoagulant system are extremely difficult and may have no relationship with thrombophilia, neonatal thrombosis, or fetal thrombotic vasculopathy.

K. Desch, MD

References

1. Nowak-Gottl U, Kurnik K, Manner D, Kenet G. Thrombophilia testing in neonates and infants with thrombosis. *Semin Fetal Neonatal Med.* 2011;16:345-348.
2. Cantor AB. *Developmental Hemostasis: Relevence to Hematology of Infancy and Childhood.* 7th ed. Philadelphia, PA: Saunders; 2009.
3. Germain M, Chasman DI, de Haan H, et al. Meta-analysis of 65,734 individuals identifies TSPAN15 and SLC44A2 as two susceptibility loci for venous thromboembolism. *Am J Hum Genet.* 2015;96:532-542.

Transplantation-Free Survival and Interventions at 3 Years in the Single Ventricle Reconstruction Trial

Newburger JW, for the Pediatric Heart Network Investigators (Boston Children's Hosp and Harvard Med School, MA; et al)
Circulation 129:2013-2020, 2014

Background.—In the Single Ventricle Reconstruction (SVR) trial, 1-year transplantation-free survival was better for the Norwood procedure with right ventricle—to—pulmonary artery shunt (RVPAS) compared with a modified Blalock-Taussig shunt (MBTS). At 3 years, we compared transplantation-free survival, echocardiographic right ventricular ejection fraction, and unplanned interventions in the treatment groups.

Methods and Results.—Vital status and medical history were ascertained from annual medical records, death indexes, and phone interviews. The cohort included 549 patients randomized and treated in the SVR trial. Transplantation-free survival for the RVPAS versus MBTS groups did not differ at 3 years (67% versus 61%; $P = 0.15$) or with all available follow-up of 4.8 ± 1.1 years (log-rank $P = 0.14$). Pre-Fontan right ventricular ejection fraction was lower in the RVPAS group than in the MBTS group ($41.7 \pm 5.1\%$ versus $44.7 \pm 6.0\%$; $P = 0.007$), and right ventricular ejection fraction deteriorated in RVPAS ($P = 0.004$) but not MBTS ($P = 0.40$) subjects (pre-Fontan minus 14-month mean, $-3.25 \pm 8.24\%$ versus $0.99 \pm 8.80\%$; $P = 0.009$). The RVPAS versus MBTS treatment effect had nonproportional hazards ($P = 0.004$); the hazard ratio favored the RVPAS before 5 months (hazard ratio $= 0.63$; 95% confidence interval, $0.45-0.88$) but the MBTS beyond 1 year (hazard ratio $= 2.22$; 95% confidence interval, $1.07-4.62$). By 3 years, RVPAS subjects had a higher incidence of catheter interventions ($P < 0.001$) with an increasing HR over time ($P = 0.005$): <5 months, 1.14 (95% confidence interval, $0.81-1.60$); from 5 months to 1 year, 1.94 (95% confidence interval, $1.02-3.69$); and >1 year, 2.48 (95% confidence interval, $1.28-4.80$).

Conclusions.—By 3 years, the Norwood procedure with RVPAS compared with MBTS was no longer associated with superior transplantation-free survival. Moreover, RVPAS subjects had slightly worse right ventricular ejection fraction and underwent more catheter interventions with increasing hazard ratio over time.

Clinical Trial Registration.—URL: http://www.clinicaltrials.gov. Unique identifier: NCT00115934 (Fig 1).

▶ Hypoplastic left heart syndrome is among the most common severe congenital heart malformations, affecting approximately 1 in 5000 liveborn infants. Until development of the 3-stage palliative surgery by Norwood in 1981, this condition was uniformly and rapidly lethal. With growing experience with that procedure, survival rates have improved substantially. This report describes a multicenter randomized controlled trial comparing 2 surgical techniques for the first stage in that surgical sequence. The 12-month survival advantage for infants managed with a right ventricle to pulmonary artery

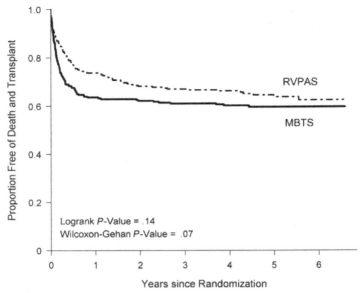

FIGURE 1.—Comparison of the shunt types by intention-to-treat analysis in their freedom from the composite end point of death or cardiac transplantation (ie, transplantation-free survival). MBTS indicates modified Blalock-Taussig shunt; and RVPAS, right ventricle–to–pulmonary artery shunt. (Reprinted from Newburger JW, for the Pediatric Heart Network Investigators. Transplantation-free survival and interventions at 3 years in the single ventricle reconstruction trial. *Circulation*. 2014;129:2013-2020, with permission from American Heart Association, Inc.)

shunt, compared with the traditional modified Blalock-Taussig shunt, found in the initial analysis from this trial, is lost over the next 24 months, so that no significant differences in outcomes were sustained. This observation has implications regarding selection of surgical technique by cardiac surgeons and also illuminates the pathophysiological evolution of cardiac performance after Norwood surgeries. The message for neonatologists, however, is simpler but equally important: no matter which shunt method is used, rates of survival without transplantation are only 61% to 67% at 3 years (Fig 1) and 60% to 64% at 5 years. Death and heart transplantation are not equivalent outcomes, with very different implications for the patient, but a detailed breakdown of those events is not provided. By the age of 3 years, however, 36% of all infants in the trial had died. Thus, the long-term survival rate for patients with hypoplastic left heart syndrome falls far short of ideal. Unless outcomes at a particular center are known to deviate substantially from these results, parents of babies with this condition deserve to know that one-third (or more) of the infants who embark on this pathway do not survive to the age of 3 years.

W. E. Benitz, MD

7 Respiratory Disorders

Spontaneously Breathing Preterm Infants Change in Tidal Volume to Improve Lung Aeration Immediately after Birth

Mian Q, Cheung P-Y, O'Reilly M, et al (Royal Alexandra Hosp, Edmonton, Canada; et al)

J Pediatr, 2015 [Epub ahead of print]

Objective.—To examine the temporal course of lung aeration at birth in preterm infants <33 weeks gestation.

Study Design.—The research team attended deliveries of preterm infants <33 weeks gestation at the Royal Alexandra Hospital. Infants who received only continuous positive airway pressure were eligible for inclusion. A combined carbon dioxide (CO_2) and flow-sensor was placed between the mask and the ventilation device. To analyze lung aeration patterns during spontaneous breathing, tidal volume (V_T), and exhaled CO_2 (ECO_2) were recorded for the first 100 breaths.

Results.—Thirty preterm infants were included with a total of 1512 breaths with mask leak <30%. Mean (SD) gestational age and birth weight was 30 (1) weeks and 1478 (430) g. Initial V_T and ECO_2 for the first 30 breaths was 5-6 mL/kg and 15-22 mm Hg, respectively. V_T and ECO_2 increased over the next 20 breaths to 7-8 mL/kg and 25-32 mm Hg, respectively. For the remaining observation period V_T decreased to 4-6 mL/kg and ECO_2 continued to increase to 35-37 mm Hg.

Conclusions.—Preterm infants begin taking deeper breaths approximately 30 breaths after initiating spontaneous breathing to inflate their lungs. Concurrent CO_2 removal rises as alveoli are recruited. Lung aeration occurs in 2 phases: initially, large volume breaths with poor alveolar aeration followed by smaller breaths with elimination of CO_2 as a consequence of adequate aeration.

▶ Drs Mian and Schmölzer in Edmonton, Canada; Davis of Melbourne, Australia; Pichler of Graz, Austria; and their colleagues have collaborated on 2 recently published interesting physiological studies of pulmonary adaptation at birth. This study evaluated a subset of 30 spontaneously breathing infants born before 33 weeks of gestation at the Royal Alexandria Hospital, Edmonton, describing changes in tidal volume and exhaled carbon dioxide (CO_2) over the first 100 breaths. Tidal volumes began at 5 to 6 mL/kg, increased over 20 breaths or so to 7 to 8 mL/kg, then settled out at 4 to 6 mL/kg. Interestingly, despite relatively large initial tidal volumes, end-tidal CO_2 initially was low (15 to 22) and later increased as ventilation became more effective. The latter finding mirrors a finding of Schmölzer's earlier study[1] of more mature infants: the first breaths of healthy spontaneously breathing term infants did not contain detectable CO_2. This work is fascinating, and these and related findings might well be useful in designing optimally effective and protective strategies for perinatal lung recruitment and respiratory support.

L. J. Van Marter, MD, MPH

Reference

1. Schmölzer GM, Hooper SB, Wong C, Kamlin CO, Davis PG. Exhaled carbon dioxide in healthy term infants immediately after birth. *J Pediatr.* 2015;166: 844-849.

Sustained Lung Inflation at Birth for Preterm Infants: A Randomized Clinical Trial
Lista G, for the SLI Trial Investigators ("V. Buzzi" Children's Hosp, ICP, Milan, Italy; et al)
Pediatrics 135:e457-e464, 2015

Background.—Studies suggest that giving newly born preterm infants sustained lung inflation abstract (SLI) may decrease their need for mechanical ventilation (MV) and improve their respiratory outcomes.

Methods.—We randomly assigned infants born at 25 weeks 0 days to 28 weeks 6 days of gestation to receive SLI (25 cm H_2O for 15 seconds) followed by nasal continuous positive airway pressure (nCPAP) or nCPAP alone in the delivery room. SLI and nCPAP were delivered by using a neonatal mask and a T-piece ventilator. The primary end point was the need for MV in the first 72 hours of life. The secondary end points included the need for respiratory supports and survival without bronchopulmonary dysplasia (BPD).

Results.—A total of 148 infants were enrolled in the SLI group and 143 in the control group. Significantly fewer infants were ventilated in the first 72 hours of life in the SLI group (79 of 148 [53%]) than in the control group (93 of 143 [65%]); unadjusted odds ratio: 0.62 (95% confidence interval: 0.38−0.99; $P=.04$). The need for respiratory support and survival without BPD did not differ between the groups. Pneumothorax occurred in 1% ($n=2$) of infants in the control group compared with 6% ($n=9$) in the SLI group, with an unadjusted odds ratio of 4.57 (95% confidence interval: 0.97−21.50; $P=.06$).

Conclusions.—SLI followed by nCPAP in the delivery room decreased the need for MV in the first 72 hours of life in preterm infants at high risk of respiratory distress syndrome compared with nCPAP alone but did not decrease the need for respiratory support and the occurrence of BPD.

▶ Strategies to decrease the incidence of bronchopulmonary dysplasia (BPD) in preterm infants remain a continuing challenge for neonatologists. Evidence over the years has established that BPD has a multipronged etiology. Barotrauma/ventilator-induced lung injury is one of the key factors in the pathogenesis of BPD. Efforts to minimize this injury have shifted from the Neonatal Intensive Care Unit toward different strategies used during resuscitation soon after delivery. It is imperative that all measures to minimize lung injury, including oxygen and respiratory support, be precisely controlled from the moment of birth. Optimizing the functional residual capacity (FRC) of the lung and use of sustained lung inflation by noninvasive methods are key maneuvers. This fact was first pointed out by Tony Milner's group in term infants 34 years ago.[1] The concept was "reinvented and reexamined" decades later in a preterm rabbit model and preterm infants by several investigators led by te Pas et al[2,3] and Linder et al.[4] In a study in infants younger than 29 weeks, a sustained inflation at birth was not effective unless infants breathed. Although large mask leak accounted for one-third of the failures as functional residual capacity gain was only associated with breathing, the authors speculated that active glottis adduction may have been responsible for most failures.[5]

In the Italian randomized trial cited above, the authors, headed by Lista, mimicked the basic model from the previous studies but enrolled smaller preterm infants. They randomly selected almost 300 neonates, and as had been seen in the previous studies, they elegantly showed the importance of establishing FRC and optimal lung expansion on decreasing the need for mechanical ventilation in the first 72 hours. Unfortunately, this did not translate into reduction of BPD, and there was also a slight increase in the incidence of pneumothorax in this group. The "magic bullet" for reducing the incidence of BPD remains elusive, but this body of work definitely emphasizes the role of establishing FRC in the delivery room. We no doubt need further studies to establish the optimal level of lung inflation in the delivery room, which is not only safe but also has a sustained effect and translates into reduction of the incidence of BPD. Don't hold your breath on this one yet.

M. Bhola, MD

References

1. Vyas H, Milner AD, Hopkin IE, Boon AW. Physiologic responses to prolonged and slow-rise inflation in the resuscitation of the asphyxiated newborn infant. *J Pediatr.* 1981;99:635-639.
2. te Pas AB, Walther FJ. A randomized, controlled trial of delivery-room respiratory management in very preterm infants. *Pediatrics.* 2007;120:322-329.
3. te Pas AB, Siew M, Wallace MJ, et al. Establishing functional residual capacity at birth: the effect of sustained inflation and positive end-expiratory pressure in a preterm rabbit model. *Pediatr Res.* 2009;65:537-541.
4. Lindner W, Högel J, Pohlandt F. Sustained pressure-controlled inflation or intermittent mandatory ventilation in preterm infants in the delivery room? A randomized, controlled trial on initial respiratory support via nasopharyngeal tube. *Acta Paediatr.* 2005;94:303-309.
5. van Vonderen JJ, Hooper SB, Hummler HD, Lopriore E, te Pas AB. Effects of sustained inflation in preterm infants at birth. *J Pediatr.* 2014;165:903-908.

Safe oxygen saturation targeting and monitoring in preterm infants: can we avoid hypoxia and hyperoxia?
Sola A, Golombek SG, Montes Bueno MT, et al (Ibero American Society of Neonatology (SIBEN), Dana Point, CA; Hosp La Paz, Madrid, Spain; et al)
Acta Paediatr 103:1009-1018, 2014

Oxygen is a neonatal health hazard that should be avoided in clinical practice. In this review, an international team of neonatologists and nurses assessed oxygen saturation (SpO_2) targeting in preterm infants and evaluated the potential weaknesses of randomised clinical trials.

Conclusion.—SpO_2 of 85–89% can increase mortality and 91–95% can cause hyperoxia and ill effects. Neither of these ranges can be recommended, and wider intermediate targets, such as 87–94% or 88–94%, may be safer.

▶ This article is a thoughtful consensus piece on pulse oximetry monitoring. It was written by experienced clinicians, many of whom have participated in various clinical trials. The article was obviously written in light of recent investigations (SUPPORT, COT, BOOST II, etc) and reached an opinion that is best described as regression to the mean. Eliminate the upper tail to reduce retinopathy of prematurity and eliminate the lower tail to reduce death. But is it that simple? Can we make sense of the disparate results? In my mind, there is a question of biological plausibility. Do we have enough information and data to believe (1) that there is enough separation of high and low target groups (confounded by the algorithm problem discovered in the midst of the trials); (2) that despite the relatively large sample sizes, we have adequately controlled for other variables, including hemoglobin concentration, mix (Hb F/Hb A), transfusions, average pH, cardiac function, and average carbon dioxide tension; and (3) that other clinical confounders have been accounted for. It is difficult to imagine that a 1% to 2% difference in SpO_2 can result in clinically different outcomes given the adaptive abilities of even the most preterm baby to respond to brief periods of desaturation or "hypersaturation." Something else has to explain this. Until we have that information, as the authors of this review have concluded, it is probably wise to take a middle-of-the-road approach.

S. M. Donn, MD

Oxygen Saturation Target Range for Extremely Preterm Infants: A Systemic Review and Meta-analysis
Manja V, Lakshminrusimha S, Cook DJ (Veterans Affairs Med Ctr, Buffalo, NY; State Univ of New York, Buffalo; McMaster Univ, Hamilton, Ontario, Canada; et al)
JAMA Pediatr 169:332-340, 2015

Importance.—The optimal oxygen saturation (SpO_2) target for extremely preterm infants is unknown.

Objective.—To systematically review evidence evaluating the effect of restricted vs liberal oxygen exposure on morbidity and mortality in extremely preterm infants.
Data Sources.—MEDLINE, PubMed, CENTRAL, and CINAHL databases from their inception to March 31, 2014, and abstracts submitted to Pediatric Academic Societies from 2000 to 2014.
Study Selection.—All published randomized trials evaluating the effect of restricted (SpO_2, 85%-89%) vs liberal (SpO_2, 91%-95%) oxygen exposure in preterm infants (<28 weeks' gestation at birth).
Data Extraction and Synthesis.—All meta-analyses were performed using Review Manager 5.2. The Cochrane risk-of-bias tool was used to assess study quality. The summary of the findings and the level of confidence in the estimate of effect were assessed using GRADEpro. Treatment effect was analyzed using a random-effects model.
Main Outcomes and Measures.—Death before hospital discharge, death or severe disability before 24 months, death before 24 months, neurodevelopmental outcomes, hearing loss, bronchopulmonary dysplasia, necrotizing enterocolitis, and severe retinopathy of prematurity.
Results.—Five trials were included in the final synthesis. These studies had a similar design with a prespecified composite outcome of death/disability at 18 to 24 months corrected for prematurity; however, this outcome has not been reported for 2 of the 5 trials. There was no difference in the outcome of death/disability before 24 months (risk ratio [RR], 1.02 [95% CI, 0.92-1.14]). Mortality before 24 months was not different (RR, 1.13 [95% CI, 0.97-1.33]); however, a significant increase in mortality before hospital discharge was found in the restricted oxygen group (RR, 1.18 [95% CI, 1.03-1.36]). The rates of bronchopulmonary dysplasia, neurodevelopmental outcomes, hearing loss, and retinopathy of prematurity were similar between the 2 groups. Necrotizing enterocolitis occurred more frequently in infants on restricted oxygen (RR, 1.24 [95% CI, 1.05-1.47]). Using the Grades of Recommendation, Assessment, Development, and Evaluation (GRADE) criteria, we found that the quality of evidence for these outcomes was moderate to low.
Conclusions and Relevance.—Although infants cared for with a liberal oxygen target had significantly lower mortality before hospital discharge than infants cared for with a restricted oxygen target, the quality of evidence for this estimate of effect is low. Necrotizing enterocolitis occurred less frequently in the liberal oxygen group. We found no significant differences in death or disability at 24 months, bronchopulmonary dysplasia, retinopathy of prematurity, neurodevelopmental outcomes, or hearing loss at 24 months.

▶ Between 2005 and 2007, 5 randomized trials were initiated to identify an optimal oxygen saturation target range in extremely preterm infants (85%-89% vs 91%-95%). In the last year, there have been 2 meta-analyses of the trials, including the one above. The authors of the earlier meta-analysis recommended oxygen saturation ranges of 90% to 95% for preterm infants born at less than 28 weeks' gestation until 36 weeks' postmenstrual age.[1] However, the authors of the above meta-analysis concluded that the level of confidence for many of the estimates was low and that there is still significant uncertainty about the optimal target range for blood oxygen saturation in extremely preterm babies. A novel aspect of the above meta-analysis is the incorporation of the Grades of Recommendation, Assessment, Development, and Evaluation (GRADE) criteria to evaluate the quality of the evidence. With the use of the GRADE criteria, the confidence in the data was downgraded. Outcomes graded as moderate or low (eg retinopathy of prematurity and death before hospital discharge in the oxygen therapy trials) are interpreted as indicating that research may or will likely change the estimate.

Thus, it seems that the definitive answer to the optimal oxygen saturation level for preterm infants remains elusive. During the planning phase of the trials, the different study teams agreed to perform an individual patient data meta-analysis after completion and publication of all 5 trials. Hopefully, information from the analysis will be useful and can help inform clinical decision making regarding the optimal oxygen therapy for an individual infant.

L. A. Papile, MD

Reference

1. Saugstad OD, Aune D. Optimal oxygenation of extremely low birthweight infants: a meta-analysis and systemic review of the oxygen saturation target studies. *Neonatology.* 2014;105:55-63.

PaCO$_2$ in Surfactant, Positive Pressure, and Oxygenation Randomised Trial (SUPPORT)
Ambalavanan N, For the SUPPORT Study Group of the NICHD Neonatal Research Network (Univ of Alabama at Birmingham, et al)
Arch Dis Child Fetal Neonatal Ed 100:F145-F149, 2015

Objective.—To determine the association of arterial partial pressure of carbon dioxide PaCO$_2$ with severe intraventricular haemorrhage (sIVH), bronchopulmonary dysplasia (BPD), and neurodevelopmental impairment (NDI) at 18—22 months in premature infants.

Design.—Secondary exploratory data analysis of Surfactant, Positive Pressure, and Oxygenation Randomised Trial (SUPPORT).

Setting.—Multiple referral neonatal intensive care units.

Patients.—1316 infants 24 0/7 to 27 6/7 weeks gestation randomised to different oxygenation (SpO$_2$ target 85—89% vs 91—95%) and ventilation strategies.

Main Outcome Measures.—Blood gases from postnatal day 0 to day 14 were analysed. Five PaCO$_2$ variables were defined: minimum (Min), maximum (Max), SD, average (time-weighted), and a four level categorical variable (hypercapnic (highest quartile of Max PaCO$_2$), hypocapnic (lowest quartile of Min PaCO$_2$), fluctuators (hypercapnia and hypocapnia), and normocapnic (middle two quartiles of Max and Min $PaCO_2$)). $PaCO_2$ variables were compared for infants with and without sIVH, BPD and NDI (±death). Multivariable logistic regression models were developed for adjusted results.

Results.—sIVH, BPD and NDI (±death) were associated with hypercapnic infants and fluctuators. Association of Max $PaCO_2$ and outcomes persisted after adjustment (per 10 mm Hg increase: sIVH/death: OR 1.27 (1.13 to 1.41); BPD/death: OR 1.27 (1.12 to 1.44); NDI/death: OR 1.23 (1.10 to 1.38), death: OR 1.27 (1.12 to 1.44), all $p < 0.001$). No interaction was found between $PaCO_2$ category and SpO_2 treatment group for sIVH/death, NDI/death or death. Max $PaCO_2$ was positively correlated with maximum FiO_2 ($r_s 0.55$, $p < 0.0001$) and ventilator days ($r_s 0.61$, $p < 0.0001$).

Conclusions.—Higher $PaCO_2$ was an independent predictor of sIVH/death, BPD/death and NDI/death. Further trials are needed to evaluate optimal $PaCO_2$ targets for high-risk infants.

▶ In 1999, Mariani et al[1] reported that "a ventilatory strategy of permissive hypercapnia in preterm infants who receive assisted ventilation is feasible, seems safe, and may reduce the duration of assisted ventilation." As recently as 2012, Ryu et al,[2] after a literature review, concluded: "Experimental and clinical data indicate that ventilator strategies with permissive hypercapnia may reduce lung injury by a variety of mechanisms. Seven randomized controlled trials in preterm neonates suggest that permissive hypercapnia started early, before the initiation of mechanical ventilation (in conjunction with continuous positive airway pressure), followed by prolonged permissive hypercapnia if mechanical ventilation is needed as an alternative to early ventilation and surfactant. Permissive hypercapnia may improve pulmonary outcomes and survival." It is thus somewhat sobering to read this secondary exploratory analysis from the SUPPORT trial, authored by Ambalavanan and colleagues. They noted that severe intraventricular hemorrhage, bronchopulmonary dysplasia, death, and impaired neurodevelopment occurred statistically more frequently in infants classified as hypercapnic during the first 2 weeks of life or those with increased carbon dioxide fluctuations. Lacking some of the ventilator parameters cause and effect could not be established, but the extent of the morbidity and mortality are beyond questioning.

Van Kaam et al[3] used the Neovent study group to determine the incidence of hypocapnia and hypercapnia in a cross-sectional cohort of ventilated newborns, using 173 neonatal intensive care units. Among 508 patients, including more than 1500 blood gas measurements, P_{CO_2} was significantly higher in preterm infants; hypocapnia (P_{CO_2} < 30 mm Hg or 4 kPa) was documented in 4% (69), usually in the first 3 days of life; and hypercapnia (P_{CO_2} > 52 mm Hg or 7 kPa) was present in 492 (31%) of the blood gases. They concluded that permissive hypercapnia "has found its way into clinical practice." In light of the findings reported by Ambalavanan, this practice needs to be seriously reconsidered.

A. A. Fanaroff, MBBCh, FRCPE

References

1. Mariani G, Cifuentes J, Carlo WA. Randomized trial of permissive hypercapnia in preterm infants. *Pediatrics*. 1999;104:1082-1088.
2. Ryu J, Haddad G, Carlo WA. Clinical effectiveness and safety of permissive hypercapnia. *Clin Perinatol*. 2012;39:603-612.
3. van Kaam AH, De Jaegere AP, Rimensberger PC, Neovent Study Group. Incidence of hypo- and hyper-capnia in a cross-sectional European cohort of ventilated newborn infants. *Arch Dis Child Fetal Neonatal Ed*. 2013;98:F323-F326.

A randomised controlled trial of an automated oxygen delivery algorithm for preterm neonates receiving supplemental oxygen without mechanical ventilation

Zapata J, Gómez JJ, Araque Campo R, et al (Centro Medico Imbanaco, Cali, Colombia; et al)
Acta Paediatr 103:928-933, 2014

Aim.—Providing consistent levels of oxygen saturation (SpO_2) for infants in neonatal intensive care units is not easy. This study explored how effectively the Auto-Mixer® algorithm automatically adjusted fraction of inspired oxygen (FiO_2) levels to maintain SpO_2 within an intended range in extremely low birth weight infants receiving supplemental oxygen without mechanical ventilation.

Methods.—Twenty extremely low birth weight infants were randomly assigned to the Auto- Mixer® group or the manual intervention group and studied for 12 h. The SpO_2 target was 85–93%, and the outcomes were the percentage of time SpO_2 was within target, SpO_2 variability, SpO_2 >95%, oxygen received and manual interventions.

Results.—The percentage of time within intended SpO_2 was 58 ± 4% in the Auto-Mixer® group and 33.7 ± 4.7% in the manual group, SpO_2 >95% was 26.5% vs 54.8%, average SpO_2 and FiO_2 were 89.8% vs 92.2% and 37% vs 44.1%, and manual interventions were 0 vs 80 ($p < 0.05$). Brief periods of SpO_2 <85% occurred more frequently in the Auto- Mixer® group.

Conclusion.—The Auto-Mixer® effectively increased the percentage of time that SpO_2 was within the intended target range and decreased the time with high SpO_2 in spontaneously breathing extremely low birth weight infants receiving supplemental oxygen (Fig 2).

▶ The optimal target range for adjustments of oxygen supplementation remains elusive. Recent trials targeting higher or lower pulse oximetry values (SUPPORT, BOOST II, and COT) have indicated that lower pulse oximetry target ranges are associated with less retinopathy of prematurity but increased mortality, but these trials have significant limitations in application to practice. All trials incorporated algorithms for display of offset values for SpO_2, allowing blinding of care providers to the true oxygen saturations. This strategy may have minimized the impact of human factors that might affect oxygen adjustments, but devices with these "jiggered" displays are not available, so the better strategy (whichever that may be) cannot actually be replicated in routine practice. In addition, the range of achieved oxygen saturations in both target groups was quite broad, with extensive overlap between groups, in all 3 trials. Recent observations have suggested that attempts to achieve tighter control (ie, less variability) of saturation levels may actually make the situation worse because adjustments in response to brief desaturations may be followed by long periods with saturations above the upper limit of the target range.

This article adds to a growing set of small, randomized trials that provide hope for a better option. Like a similar trial in babies on mechanical ventilation,[1] these authors found that automated adjustment of the inspired oxygen concentration increased the proportion of time with SpO_2 readings within the target range, reduced the time with readings above the target range, and increased the time with readings below the target range compared with infants managed using manual adjustments (Fig 2), but in this trial, the infants were receiving oxygen by nasal cannula without positive pressure support. During the study period, infants in the automated adjustment group had lower mean SpO_2 readings and oxygen concentrations in blended cannula gas (the effective inspired oxygen concentration was not directly measured, and flow rates were not specified or standardized), as noted in the abstract, as well as less variability in SpO_2 readings. The article does not describe how the latter was calculated, however, and the magnitude of the difference appears to be small. That is disappointing because reduction in the variance of SpO_2 levels would seem to be a primary objective of automated control. Those limitations notwithstanding, these pilot observations suggest that automated control of oxygen delivery may reduce periods of excessive oxygen exposure. The cost of formally studying the

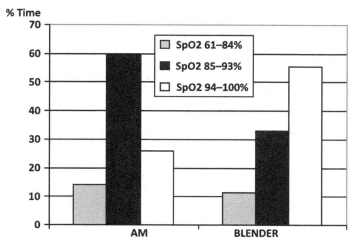

FIGURE 2.—Percentage of time spent below, within and above the intended oxygen saturation (SpO_2) range with the Auto-Mixer (AM) and manual routine care (blender). (Reprinted from Zapata J, Gómez JJ, Araque Campo R, et al. A randomised controlled trial of an automated oxygen delivery algorithm for preterm neonates receiving supplemental oxygen without mechanical ventilation. *Acta Paediatr.* 2014;103:928-933, with permission from Acta Paediatrica and John Wiley and sons, www.interscience.wiley.com.)

impact of this technology in adequately powered randomized trials is likely to be prohibitive, so careful postmarketing surveillance will be essential to determine optimal goals for oxygen therapy as these devices come to market.

W. E. Benitz, MD

Reference

1. Claure N, Bancalari E, D'Ugard C, et al. Multicenter crossover study of automated control of inspired oxygen in ventilated preterm infants. *Pediatrics*. 2011;127: e76-e83.

Unbound Unconjugated Hyperbilirubinemia Is Associated with Central Apnea in Premature Infants

Amin SB, Wang H (Univ of Rochester School of Medicine and Dentistry, NY)
J Pediatr 166:571-575, 2015

Objective.—To evaluate whether jaundice, indexed by unbound bilirubin (UB), is associated with central apnea in premature infants.

Study Design.—A prospective observational study was performed with 27-33 weeks' gestational age infants who were not requiring either mechanical ventilation or noninvasive ventilation with continuous positive airway pressure beyond 24 hours after birth. Infants with congenital infections, chromosomal disorders, craniofacial anomalies, and/or family history of hearing loss were excluded. Total serum bilirubin and UB were measured twice daily during the first postnatal week and then when clinically indicated. Central apnea was evaluated by visual inspection of continuous, electronic cardiorespiratory recordings until 2 weeks of age.

Results.—One hundred infants were subdivided into 2 groups via median peak UB level: the high UB group (greater than median) and low UB group (less than median). The high UB group had an increased frequency of apnea events during the first 2 weeks compared with infants in the low UB group. After we controlled for confounders, the high UB group had more events of apnea during the first 2 postnatal weeks compared with the low UB group (incidence rate ratio: 1.9, 95% CI 1.2-3.2).

Conclusions.—Our findings suggest that jaundice, as indexed by UB, is associated with central apnea in premature infants.

▶ Unconjugated unbound bilirubin is a known toxin that can cause brainstem injury and dysfunction, and Sanjiv Amin has provided extensive documentation of this important relationship in premature infants.[1-4] In this latest study, Amin and Wang provide prospective documentation of the relationship between unbound bilirubin (UB) and central apnea in preterm infants. Although this relationship has been observed in retrospective studies, this is the first prospective confirmation of this important association. Although there was a strong relationship between UB and central apnea, there was no association between total serum bilirubin and apnea. These investigators also found that these infants required prolonged respiratory support and methylxanthine therapy. These observations confirm both the pivotal role of UB in bilirubin toxicity and an important association between unconjugated hyperbilirubinemia and a prolonged adverse effect on brainstem-mediated respiratory control.

M. J. Maisels, MB, BCh, DSc

References

1. Amin SB, Bhutani VK, Watchko JF. Apnea in acute bilirubin encephalopathy. *Semin Perinatol.* 2014;38:407-411.
2. Amin SB, Ahlfors CE, Orlando MS, Dalzell LE, Merle KS, Guillet R. Bilirubin and serial auditory brainstem responses in premature infants. *Pediatrics.* 2001;107: 664-670.
3. Amin SB, Charafeddine L, Guillet R. Transient bilirubin encephalopathy and apnea of prematurity in 28 to 32 weeks gestational age infants. *J Perinatol.* 2005;25:386-390.
4. Amin SB. Clinical assessment of bilirubin-induced neurotoxicity in premature infants. *Semin Perinatol.* 2004;28:340-347.

Very long apnea events in preterm infants
Mohr MA, Vergales BD, Lee H, et al (College of William and Mary, Williamsburg, VA; Univ of Virginia, Charlottesville; et al)
J Appl Physiol 118:558-568, 2015

Apnea is nearly universal among very low birth weight (VLBW) infants, and the associated bradycardia and desaturation may have detrimental consequences. We describe here very long (>60 s) central apnea events (VLAs) with bradycardia and desaturation, discovered using a computerized detection system applied to our database of over 100 infant years of electronic signals. Eighty-six VLAs occurred in 29 out of 335 VLBW infants. Eighteen of the 29 infants had a clinical event or condition possibly related to the VLA. Most VLAs occurred while infants were on nasal continuous positive airway pressure, supplemental oxygen, and caffeine. Apnea alarms on the bedside monitor activated in 66% of events, on average 28 s after cessation of breathing. Bradycardia alarms activated late, on average 64 s after cessation of breathing. Before VLAs oxygen saturation was unusually high, and during VLAs oxygen saturation and heart rate fell unusually slowly. We give measures of the relative severity of VLAs and theoretical calculations that describe the rate of decrease of oxygen saturation. A clinical conclusion is that very long apnea (VLA) events with bradycardia and desaturation are not rare. Apnea alarms failed to activate for about one-third of VLAs. It appears that neonatal intensive care unit (NICU) personnel respond quickly to bradycardia alarms but not consistently to apnea alarms. We speculate that more reliable apnea detection systems would improve patient safety in the NICU. A physiological conclusion is that the slow decrease of oxygen saturation is consistent with a physiological model based on assumed high values of initial oxygen saturation.

▶ Our technical ability to quantify apnea episodes in neonates is limited by dependence on impedance monitoring, which assesses chest wall and abdominal motion rather than airflow. As a result, we rely on heart rate and oxygen saturation monitors to detect cardiorespiratory events and trigger alarms. Preterm infants have low lung volumes and limited oxygen stores and, as a result, short respiratory pauses (even periodic breathing) may cause oxygen desaturation below 80% and trigger frequent resultant reflex bradycardia below 80 beats per minute. It is these events (rather than apnea > 20 seconds) that typically trigger monitor alarms and delay hospital discharge.

In the accompanying article, Mohr and colleagues alert us to an infrequent, but new, problem: very long central apneic events that may go undetected, especially if they do not trigger bradycardia or desaturation monitors. These episodes are often preceded by a rise in oxygen saturation, which may provide a buffer against early desaturation and bradycardia. An alternate possibility is that a rise in oxygen saturation inhibits peripheral chemosensitivity and prolongs the episode by delaying onset of breathing. I hope the authors are incorrect in their speculation that members of the nursing staff are more likely to ignore apnea compared with bradycardia or desaturation alarms. Meanwhile, several investigators continue to explore the feasibility of directly or indirectly documenting airflow as an alternative to impedance for monitoring breathing.

R. J. Martin, MD

Less invasive surfactant administration is associated with improved pulmonary outcomes in spontaneously breathing preterm infants
Göpel W, for the German Neonatal Network (GNN) (Univ of Lübeck, Germany; et al)
Acta Paediatr 104:241-246, 2015

Aim.—Providing less invasive surfactant administration (LISA) to spontaneously breathing preterm infants has been reported to reduce mechanical ventilation and bronchopulmonary dysplasia (BPD) in randomised controlled trials. This large cohort study compared these outcome measures between LISA-treated infants and controls.

Methods.—Infants receiving LISA, who were born before 32 gestational weeks and enrolled in the German Neonatal Network, were matched to control infants by gestational age, umbilical cord pH, Apgar-score at 5 min, small for gestational age status, antenatal treatment with steroids, gender and highest supplemental oxygen during the first 12 h of life. Outcome data were compared with chi-square and Mann–Whitney U-tests and adjusted for multiple comparisons.

Results.—Between 2009 and 2012, 1103 infants were treated with LISA at 37 centres. LISA infants had lower rates of mechanical ventilation (41% versus 62%, $p < 0.001$), postnatal dexamethasone treatment (2.5% versus

7%, $p < 0.001$), BPD (12% versus 18%, $p = 0.001$) and BPD or death (14% versus 21%, $p < 0.001$) than the controls.

Conclusion.—Surfactant treatment of spontaneously breathing infants was associated with lower rates of mechanical ventilation and BPD. Additional large-scale randomised controlled trials are needed to assess the possible long-term benefits of LISA.

▶ This large German network cohort study compared the use of less invasive surfactant administration (LISA) to spontaneously breathing preterm infants. Compared with a matched control group, the rates of mechanical ventilation, postnatal steroid use, bronchopulmonary dysplasia (BPD), and death or BPD were lower.

The authors of this article are indeed correct in calling for a large multicenter, randomized controlled trial. This study can merely generate a hypothesis because it was nonrandomized and included a significant selection bias. Infants were treated with LISA because a clinician had already decided that intubation and mechanical ventilation was not necessary. Despite the attempt to carefully match the control group, it is hard to overcome this.

LISA and MIST (minimally invasive surfactant treatment) are newer techniques in which the surfactant is instilled into the trachea using either a feeding tube or vascular catheter. Aside from requiring a great deal of skill and the fact that this technique is probably not amenable to use by trainees, I have a major concern about this treatment. Tracheal obstruction with bradycardia and hypoxia are not infrequent complications encountered during surfactant administration. Neither LISA nor MIST allows the operator to have control of the airway during surfactant administration, and this could create significant difficulty should this complication occur.

It may also be argued that although the airway itself is not technically instrumented, the procedure still requires laryngoscopy, which I would deem to still be invasive. It would be nice to do a proper randomized controlled trial and perhaps add measures of inflammation to address this point.

S. M. Donn, MD

Neurodevelopmental Outcomes of Very Low Birth Weight Preterm Infants Treated With Poractant Alfa versus Beractant for Respiratory Distress Syndrome
Eras Z, Dizdar EA, Kanmaz G, et al (Zekai Tahir Burak Maternity Teaching Hosp, Ankara, Turkey)
Am J Perinatol 31:463-468, 2014

Background.—Some controlled trials have shown significant differences in short-term clinical outcomes between poractant alfa and beractant in infants with respiratory distress syndrome (RDS). There is, however, no study showing the differences in long-term outcomes with these treatments.

Aim.—To determine and compare the neurodevelopmental outcomes of preterm infants with RDS treated with poractant alfa or beractant at 2 years of age.

Methods.—This was a prospective, longitudinal, single-center cohort study of infants born at ≤1,500 g and/or ≤32 weeks between 2008 and 2009 who received either poractant alfa ($n = 113$) or beractant ($n = 102$) for RDS. Neurological and developmental assessments were performed at a corrected age of 18 to 24 months.

Results.—About 33 of 113 infants (29.2%) in the poractant alfa group had neurodevelopmental impairment compared with 36 of 102 (35.2%) in the beractant group, and the results did not differ between the groups ($p = 0.339$). Similarly, no significant difference was found in the percentage of infants with cerebral palsy (11.5 vs. 16.7%, respectively; $p = 0.275$).

Conclusion.—Our findings suggest that poractant alfa and beractant are similar in terms of neurodevelopmental outcomes when used for the treatment of RDS in preterm infants.

▶ Surfactant administration improves survival of infants at risk for or with respiratory distress syndrome (RDS). Many trials and systematic reviews have compared commercially available surfactants, which differ in their origin, composition, and dosage.[1,2] However, until recently, only one such comparison trial published follow-up results beyond the neonatal period.[3]

Eras and collaborators reported follow-up at 18 to 24 months of a single-center original cohort of 260 infants of about 28.5 weeks of gestation and 1100-g birth weight with RDS treated with either poractant or beractant. Approximately 88% of survivors had a full developmental assessment using the Bayley Scale of Infant Development II at an average age of 21 months. Overall neurodevelopmental impairment (moderate to severe cerebral palsy [CP], bilateral hearing loss, blindness, or mental developmental index/physical developmental index < 70) occurred in about one-third, whereas CP was diagnosed in 11% to 16% of survivors. No differences between infants treated with either surfactant were identified. Abnormal neurologic outcomes in this study seem higher than follow-up reports from the United States and Europe,[4] which may reflect their relatively high incidence of sepsis and necrotizing enterocolitis, neonatal complications that can have an impact on long-term outcome.

The authors refer to their work as a prospective single-center cohort study conducted between January 2008 and January 2009 but subsequently describe randomization procedures and eligibility criteria in the methodology. These criteria are entirely different from the randomized trial comparing surfactants in the reference,[5] which was conducted in the same institution during an overlapping time period (July 2008 to June 2009). Thus, it is not clear whether infants in the follow-up study were originally part of the randomized trial conducted at the same institution. To add to the confusion, the 18- to 24-month follow-up was conducted between January 2010 and January 2012, at which time an infant born in January 2008 would already be 24 months, and those evaluated past February 2011 would have been past the eligibility window of 24 months. This notwithstanding, this study and that of Moya et al[3] demonstrate that the type of surfactant used during the neonatal period does not confer advantages in terms of neurodevelopment outcomes on follow-up.

F. Moya, MD

References

1. Singh N, Hawley KL, Viswanathan K. Efficacy of porcine versus bovine surfactants for preterm newborns with respiratory distress syndrome: systematic review and meta-analysis. *Pediatrics.* 2011;128:e1588-e1595.
2. Moya F, Maturana A. Animal-derived surfactants versus. past and current generation of synthetic surfactants: current status. *Clin Perinatol.* 2007;34:145-177.
3. Moya F, Sinha S, Gadzinowski J, et al. One-year follow up of very preterm infants who received lucinactant for prevention of respiratory distress syndrome: results from 2 multicenter randomized, controlled trials. *Pediatrics.* 2007;119: e1361-e1370.
4. Oskoui M, Coutinho F, Dykeman J, Jetté N, Pringsheim T. An update on the prevalence of cerebral palsy: a systematic review and meta-analysis. *Dev Med Child Neurol.* 2013;55:509-519.
5. Dizdar EA, Sari FN, Aydemir C, et al. A randomized, controlled trial of poractant alfa versus beractant in the treatment of preterm infants with respiratory distress syndrome. *Am J Perinatol.* 2012;29:95-100.

Bi-level CPAP does not improve gas exchange when compared with conventional CPAP for the treatment of neonates recovering from respiratory distress syndrome
Lampland AL, Plumm B, Worwa C, et al (Children's Hosps and Clinics of Minnesota, St Paul; et al)
Arch Dis Child Fetal Neonatal Ed 100:F31-F34, 2015

Aim.—We hypothesised that short-term application of bi-level nasal continuous positive airway pressure CPAP (SiPAP) compared with conventional nasal CPAP (nCPAP) at the same mean airway pressure in infants with persistent oxygen need recovering from respiratory distress syndrome would improve CO_2 removal with no change in oxygen requirement.

Design.—Non-blinded, randomised, observational four-period crossover study.

Setting/Population.—Level III NICU; low-birthweight infants requiring CPAP and oxygen while recovering from respiratory distress syndrome.

Methods.—Infants requiring nasal CPAP for >24 h prior to study enrolment, and fraction of inspired oxygen requirement (FiO_2) of 0.25–0.5, were randomised to either nCPAP or SiPAP. A crossover design with four 1 h treatment periods was used such that each infant received both treatments twice. Oxygen saturations (SaO_2), transcutaneous CO_2 ($tcCO_2$) and vital signs were monitored continuously. Polysomnographic recordings were analysed for apnoea, bradycardia and oxygen desaturation.

Results.—Twenty low-birthweight infants receiving 0.3 ± 0.04% supplemental oxygen on CPAP of 6 cm H_2O were studied at an average of

33 days of age (±23 days, SD). There were no differences in tcCO$_2$ or other physiological parameters except mean blood pressure, which was lower during nCPAP (52.3 ± 8.3 vs 54.4 ± 9.1 mm Hg; ±SD; $p < 0.01$). No differences in short or prolonged apnoea, bradycardia or significant desaturation events were observed.

Conclusions.—At similar mean airway pressures, SiPAP does not improve CO$_2$ removal, oxygenation or other studied physiological parameters with the exception of mean blood pressure, which was not clinically significant.

Trial Registration Number.—NCT01053455.

▶ As the pendulum continues to swing toward noninvasive respiratory support of preterm infants with respiratory distress syndrome, equipoise without evidence is a growing problem, often leading to the acceptance of different forms of continuous distending pressure without ascertaining scientific validity.

In this study, Lampland and colleagues compared bi-level continuous positive airway pressure (CPAP) to conventional CPAP using a crossover design in which infants received one or the other for four 1-hour periods, with infants receiving each method twice. Settings were selected to control mean airway pressure during each study period. Short-term outcome measures included evaluation of oxygenation by pulse oximetry, assessment of ventilation by transcutaneous PCO$_2$ tension, and the frequencies of apnea, bradycardia, and blood pressure. Only mean blood pressure showed a difference, being 2 mm Hg lower with CPAP, but this was hardly clinically significant. The investigators concluded that bi-level CPAP conferred no benefit in augmenting ventilation.

The authors acknowledged that synchronization of bi-level CPAP may have altered these results. Before we conclude that synchronization is the answer, we need more studies like this one to prove it.

S. M. Donn, MD

Changes in ventilator strategies and outcomes in preterm infants
Vendettuoli V, for the Italian Neonatal Network (Università degli Studi di Milano, Italy; et al)
Arch Dis Child Fetal Neonatal Ed 99:F321-F324, 2014

Background.—Although life-saving, intubation and mechanical ventilation can lead to complications including bronchopulmonary dysplasia (BPD). In order to reduce the incidence of BPD, non-invasive ventilation (NIV) is increasingly used.

Objective.—The aim of our study was to describe changes in ventilator strategies and outcomes between 2006 and 2010 in the Italian Neonatal Network (INN).

Design.—Multicentre cohort study.

Settings.—31 tertiary level neonatal units participating in INN in 2006 and 2010.

Patients.—2465 preterm infants 23–30 weeks gestational age (GA) without congenital anomalies.

Main Outcomes Measures.—Death, BPD and other variables defined according to Vermont Oxford Network. Logistic regressions, adjusting for confounders and clustering for hospitals, were used.

Results.—Similar numbers of infants were studied between 2006 and 2010 (1234 in 2006 and 1231 in 2010). The baseline risk of populations studied (GA, birth weight and Vermont Oxford Network Risk-Adjustment score) did not change. After adjusting for confounding variables, infants receiving invasive mechanical ventilation decreased (OR = 0.72, 95% CI 0.58 to 0.89) while NIV increased (OR = 1.75, 95% CI 1.39 to 2.21); intubation in delivery room decreased (OR = 0.64, 95% CI 0.51 to 0.79). Considering outcomes, there was a significant reduction in mortality (OR = 0.73, 95% CI 0.55 to 0.96) and in the combined outcome mortality or BPD (OR = 0.76, 95% CI 0.62 to 0.94).

Conclusions.—Despite a stable baseline risk, from 2006 to 2010, we observed a lower level of invasiveness, a reduction of mechanical ventilation and an increase of NIV use, and this was accompanied by a decrease in risk-adjusted mortality and BPD.

▶ Over the last 2 decades, the confluence of increasing concern about the role of barotrauma in development of chronic lung disease and availability of numerous new modes of and devices for supporting ventilation has led to widespread espousal of noninvasive ventilation strategies for neonates with respiratory insufficiency. This evolution in practice has come with shockingly sparse systematic evaluation of the indications for, efficacy of, or safety of these novel methods, creating uncertainty about the net effects of their extensive adoption. This report compares practices and outcomes in a consortium of neonatal units in Italy in 2006 and 2010, providing reassurance that those effects have at least not been negative. Although the abstract highlights the shift from invasive to noninvasive ventilation and reduction in delivery room intubation, there were also increases in use of high-frequency ventilation and surfactant during the initial resuscitation between 2006 and 2010. Modes of noninvasive ventilation included nasal intermittent mandatory ventilation, nasal continuous positive airway pressure, and high flow nasal cannula, each of which was used more frequently in the later era, so it would not be clear which approach(es) may have conferred any apparent advantage. These practice changes coincided with a significant decline in mortality, but it is not clear whether that resulted from fewer deaths due to respiratory failure or less mortality from other causes, or whether this might have resulted from other practice changes altogether. Although the abstract and text both note that increased use of noninvasive ventilation was accompanied by a decrease in mortality and bronchopulmonary dysplasia (BPD), it is important to note that this reflects the combined rate of those outcomes; there was no significant change in the rate of BPD, either with or without risk adjustment. These data do not permit a conclusion that changes in ventilator management caused, or were even temporally associated with, a reduction in respiratory deaths or morbidities. Nonetheless, the relatively robust sample sizes (1234 infants in the 2006 cohort and 1231 from 2010) provide sufficient power to indicate that increased use of noninvasive ventilation did not coincide with an increase in mortality (adjusted odds ratio [OR] 0.73, 95% confidence interval [CI] 0.55—0.96) or a large increase in BPD (adjusted OR 0.87, 95% CI 0.68—1.12). This reassurance should support equipoise about the safety of prospective trials of specific modes of noninvasive ventilation for specific varieties of respiratory failure, which are badly needed to guide informed application of these techniques.

W. E. Benitz, MD

Congenital chylothorax: a prospective nationwide epidemiological study in Germany
Bialkowski A, the Erhebungseinheit für seltene pädiatrische Erkrankungen in Deutschland Study Group (Univ of Tübingen, Germany; et al)
Arch Dis Child Fetal Neonatal Ed 100:F169-F172, 2015

Background.—Congenital chylothorax (CCT) is a rare disease of unknown aetiology. Treatment approaches vary; none has been evaluated prospectively.

Objective.—To prospectively determine incidence, treatment and outcome of infants with CCT born in Germany in 2012.

Design.—CCT was defined as non-traumatic chylous pleural effusion within 28 days after birth. As part of the Surveillance Unit for Rare Pediatric Conditions in Germany (Erhebungseinheit für seltene pädiatrische Erkrankungen in Deutschland), all paediatric departments (n = 432) received monthly reporting cards to notify the study centre of CCT cases, which were analysed based on anonymised questionnaires and discharge summaries. Data are shown as median (range) or n/N.

Results.—Of 37 cases reported, 28 met inclusion criteria. Questionnaires and/or discharge summaries were available for 27/28. Assuming complete reporting, the incidence of CCT was 1:24 000.

Nine infants suffered from proven or suspected syndromal anomalies, most frequently Noonan syndrome (5/9). Postnatally, 23 required mechanical ventilation, 3 continuous positive airway pressure; only 1 had no respiratory support. 17 infants were treated with inotropes/vasopressors, 25 required pleural drainage for 11 (1—36) days. In 13 infants, enteral feeds were withheld initially; 25 received medium-chain triglyceride diet at some time, 9 were treated with octreotide or somatostatin. 18 infants survived without, 6 with sequelae attributable to the underlying disorder; 3 infants died (median age at death 37 (2-144) days). Duration of hospital stay in survivors was 51 (20—127) days. Infants treated with octreotide or somatostatin had similar outcomes compared with those not treated.

Conclusions.—Based on this small observational study, CCT seems to have a favourable prognosis if not associated with genetic disorders.

▶ Although relatively rare, congenital chylothorax seems to be a more frequently encountered condition in perinatal centers, probably as a consequence of fetal surveillance and referral. As these authors note, there is a large variance in diagnosis and treatment. Thus, this prospective observation is a necessary first step to determine the epidemiology, incidence, and natural history of the disorder. As with any survey instrument, there may be a selection bias based on underreporting, and conclusions regarding the safety and efficacy of treatments can only generate a hypothesis to subject to a randomized clinical trial.

This study group determined a rate of 1 per 24 000 live births with a mortality approaching 11%. Infants who received octreotide or somatostatin had a longer duration of pleural drainage, a higher incidence of culture-proven sepsis, and more antithrombin administration, casting some doubt as to the efficacy and safety of these agents. Most important, the prognosis in this series was relatively favorable if the chylothorax was unassociated with a genetic disorder. These results should be addressed in the designs of subsequent treatment trials.

S. M. Donn, MD

Hospital Variation and Risk Factors for Bronchopulmonary Dysplasia in a Population-Based Cohort
Lapcharoensap W, Gage SC, Kan P, et al (Stanford Univ School of Medicine, CA; et al)
JAMA Pediatr 169:e143676, 2015

Importance.—Bronchopulmonary dysplasia (BPD) remains a serious morbidity in very low-birth-weight (VLBW) infants (<1500 g). Deregionalization of neonatal care has resulted in an increasing number of VLBW infants treated in community hospitals with unknown impact on the development of BPD.

Objective.—To identify individual risk factors for BPD development and hospital variation of BPD rates across all levels of neonatal intensive care units (NICUs) within the California Perinatal Quality Care Collaborative.

Design, Setting, and Participants.—Retrospective cohort study (January 2007 to December 2011) from the California Perinatal Quality Care Collaborative including more than 90% of California's NICUs. Eligible VLBW infants born between 22 to 29 weeks' gestational age.

Exposures.—Varying levels of intensive care.

Main Outcomes and Measures.—Bronchopulmonary dysplasia was defined as continuous supplemental oxygen use at 36 weeks' postmenstrual age. A combined outcome of BPD or mortality prior to 36 weeks was used. Multivariable logistic regression accounting for hospital as a random effect and gestational age as a risk factor was used to assess individual risk factors for BPD. This model was applied to determine risk-adjusted rates of BPD across hospitals and assess associations between levels of care and BPD rates.

Results.—The study cohort included 15 779 infants, of which 1534 infants died prior to 36 weeks' postmenstrual age. A total of 7081 infants, or 44.8%, met the primary outcome of BPD or death prior to 36 weeks. Combined BPD or death rates across 116 NICUs varied from 17.7% to

73.4% (interquartile range, 38.7%-54.1%). Compared with level IV NICUs, the risk for developing BPD was higher for level II NICUs (odds ratio, 1.23; 95% CI, 1.02-1.49) and similar for level III NICUs (odds ratio, 1.04; 95% CI, 0.95-1.14).

Conclusions and Relevance.—Bronchopulmonary dysplasia or death prior to 36 weeks' postmenstrual age affects approximately 45% of VLBW infants across California. The wide variability in BPD occurrence across hospitals could offer insights into potential risk or preventive factors. Additionally, our findings suggest that increased regionalization of NICU care may reduce BPD among VLBW infants.

▶ Bronchopulmonary dysplasia (BPD) is a serious cause of morbidity in preterm infants, and often results in impaired pulmonary function that may persist into adulthood. BPD affects approximately 40% of infants born at 28 weeks' gestation or less, with an increasing burden as gestational duration shortens. Prenatal factors such as chorioamnionitis and growth restriction, factors at birth such as male sex and low gestation, and postnatal factors such as ventilator support are associated with increased risk. Wide variation exists among centers for most neonatal morbidities, including BPD, and differences in many variables may contribute to center variation. In this population-based cohort in California over a recent 5-year period, Lapcharoensap used data from the California Perinatal Quality Care Collaborative (CPQCC) to examine the effect of the capabilities of newborn intensive care units (NICUs), reflected in their level of neonatal care using American Academy of Pediatrics designations, on BPD rates. Moderate-to-severe BPD was defined as use of supplemental oxygen at 36 weeks' postmenstrual age (PMA) or at hospital discharge if it occurred earlier, and transfers to another hospital were accounted for. Mortality before 36 weeks' PMA was included in the BPD definition because death is a competing outcome.

In this large sample, nearly 16 000 infants born between 22 and 29 weeks' gestational age and with birth weight between 401 and 1500 g were cared for in 116 CPQCC member hospitals that contributed at least 10 patients to the study population. Of these, the combined outcome of BPD or death affected 44.8%, 50.5% had no BPD, and the remainder had unknown outcome. Not unexpectedly, center rates of BPD or death varied widely, from 17.7% to 73.4%, a 4-fold difference. Level IV units had the least amount of center variation. Using a model that accounted for individual risk factors, rates of BPD or death were lower in level III (46.4%) or IV (47.8%) NICUs compared with level II (50.9%) NICUs (odds ratio, 1.23; 95% confidence interval, 1.02-1.49; level II compared with level IV).

This analysis confirmed several previously identified individual risk factors for BPD, such as male sex, lower gestational age, and maternal chorioamnionitis. The observation that lack of antenatal steroids is associated with increased BPD risk, in contrast to previous studies, may reflect a more contemporary population. The finding of lower rates of BPD or death for preterm infants cared for at level III and IV NICUs compared with level II NICUs supports the findings of others[1,2] that risk-appropriate care results in improved outcomes. Policy changes that support care settings appropriate for the level of illness may improve survival and reduce complications.

A. R. Stark, MD

References

1. Lasswell SM, Barfield WD, Rochat RW, Blackmon L. Perinatal regionalization for very low-birth-weight infants: a meta-analysis. *JAMA*. 2010;304:992-1000.
2. Lorch SA, Baiocchi M, Ahlberg CE, Small DS. The differential impact of delivery hospital on the outcomes of premature infants. *Pediatrics*. 2012;130:270-278.

Pulmonary Hypertension in Preterm Infants: Prevalence and Association with Bronchopulmonary Dysplasia
Mirza H, Ziegler J, Ford S, et al (Women & Infants Hosp/The Alpert Med School of Brown Univ, Providence, RI; Hasbro Children's Hosp/The Alpert Med School of Brown Univ, Providence, RI)
J Pediatr 165:909-914, 2014

Objective.—To determine whether early pulmonary hypertension (PH) at 10-14 days of life in preterm infants is associated with bronchopulmonary dysplasia (BPD) at 36 weeks' postmenstrual age (PMA).

Study Design.—This was a prospective observational cohort study of infants <28 weeks' gestation. Exclusion criteria were any major anomaly, genetic syndrome, or death before the initial echocardiogram. Echocardiograms were performed between 10 and 14 days of life and at 36 weeks' PMA to assess PH. BPD and its severity were determined at 36 weeks PMA by the National Institutes of Health workshop definition.

Results.—From March 2011 to April 2013, of 146 consecutively admitted infants <28 weeks, 120 were enrolled. One infant was excluded, 17 did not consent, and 8 died before undergoing a study echocardiogram. At 10-14 days of life, 10 infants had early PH (8%). Male sex (56% vs 40%), gestational age ($26^{+2} \pm 1^{+2}$ vs $25^{+6} \pm 1^{+4}$ weeks), birth weight (837 ± 205 g vs 763 ± 182 g), and small for gestational age (14% vs 20%) were not significantly different among infants with no PH and early PH, respectively. Infants with early PH required >0.3 fraction of inspired oxygen by day 10 of life (70% vs 27%, $P < .01$). Moderate/severe BPD or death was greater among infants with early PH (90%) compared with no PH (47%, relative risk 1.9, 95% CI 1.43-2.53).

Conclusion.—In this prospective, single-center cohort, early PH was associated with moderate/severe BPD or death at 36 weeks' PMA.

▶ This report of prospective monitoring for echocardiographic signs of pulmonary hypertension (PH) in 120 infants < 28 weeks' gestation at birth at a single regional center constitutes a microcosm of the challenges presented in sorting out the relationships among respiratory distress syndrome, bronchopulmonary dysplasia, and pulmonary hypertension. Of the infants who survived to have a screening echocardiogram at 10 to 14 days of age, 8% had signs of elevated pulmonary arterial pressure. Those infants were more likely to require an $FIO_2 > 0.3$ at day 10 after birth (70% vs 27%, $P = .0051$), intermittent positive pressure ventilation (IPPV) for >7 of the first 10 postnatal days (70% vs 28%, $P = .0065$), and more total days of IPPV (median of 26 vs 7 days, $P < .01$). It is not apparent, however, whether PH was a cause, consequence, or correlate of more severe respiratory failure. The role of persistent patency of the ductus arteriosus, which was also more common in infants with early PH (50% vs 10%, $P = .0004$), is also uncertain. Early PH did not predict PH at 36 weeks' postmenstrual age, however, because only 1 of the 10 infants with PH at 10 to 14 days (and 5 of the 118 infants evaluated at 36 weeks) had signs of PH at that age, despite a prevalence of bronchopulmonary dysplasia (BPD) of $>50\%$ (61 of 120) in this cohort. These data not only suggest that PH may be a less common complication of BPD than suggested by prior studies but also demonstrate that the timing of screening is a critical determinant of ascertainment of affected babies and that early PH is likely to resolve even in infants who develop a prolonged requirement for supplemental oxygen. The implications of these observations are concisely summarized in the final paragraph of this article: "Some experts have recommended universal screening for PH in extremely premature infants with severe respiratory disease or infants with moderate or severe BPD; however, the optimal timing for this screening has not been determined. Furthermore, whether early recognition and intervention to treat PH in extremely premature infants can decrease the incidence of adverse outcomes, including BPD, is unknown. Further research is needed to determine the optimal time for PH screening and to assess potential benefits of treating early PH in extremely premature infants." It will be wise to await the results of such research before implementing protocols for identification and treatment of PH in convalescent extremely low birth weight infants.

W. E. Benitz, MD

Noninvasive Inhaled Nitric Oxide Does Not Prevent Bronchopulmonary Dysplasia in Premature Newborns

Kinsella JP, Cutter GR, Steinhorn RH, et al (Univ of Colorado School of Medicine/Children's Hosp, Aurora; Univ of Alabama at Birmingham School of Public Health; Univ of California—Davis Children's Hosp, Sacramento; et al)
J Pediatr 165:1104-1108, 2014

Objective.—To assess the efficacy and safety of early, noninvasive inhaled nitric oxide (iNO) therapy in premature newborns who do not require mechanical ventilation.

Study Design.—We performed a multicenter randomized trial including 124 premature newborns who required noninvasive supplemental oxygen within the first 72 hours after birth. Newborns were stratified into 3 different groups by birth weight (500-749, 750-999, 1000-1250 g) prior to randomization to iNO (10 ppm) or placebo gas (controls) until 30 weeks postmenstrual age. The primary outcome was a composite of death or bronchopulmonary dysplasia (BPD) at 36 weeks postmenstrual age.

Secondary outcomes included the need for and duration of mechanical ventilation, severity of BPD, and safety outcomes.

Results.—There was no difference in the incidence of death or BPD in the iNO and placebo groups (42% vs 40%, $P = .86$, relative risk $= 1.06$, 0.7-1.6). BPD severity was not different between the treatment groups. There were no differences between the groups in the need for mechanical ventilation (22% vs 23%; $P = .89$), duration of mechanical ventilation (9.7 vs 8.4 days; $P = .27$), or safety outcomes including severe intracranial hemorrhage (3.4% vs 6.2%, $P = .68$).

Conclusions.—We found that iNO delivered noninvasively to premature infants who have not progressed to early respiratory failure is a safe treatment, but does not decrease the incidence or severity of BPD, reduce the need for mechanical ventilation, or alter the clinical course.

▶ Emergence of the construct of a "new bronchopulmonary dysplasia (BPD)" characterized primarily by arrest of alveolar septation rather than bronchiolar desquamation and obstruction ("old BPD") was followed by several reports of amelioration of that pathology in animal models by administration of exogenous inhaled nitric oxide. Those observations led to clinical trials in human infants, which have been generally disappointing but produced in turn, several hypotheses about subgroups of preterm infants who might benefit from this therapy. One such subgroup was infants with less severe respiratory distress syndrome, as reflected in their pretreatment oxygenation indices. The trial reported here is the second published report of effects of inhaled nitric oxide in infant with relatively mild respiratory failure—in this case, preterm infants weighing 500 to 1250 g whose disease had not progressed to the point of requiring invasive ventilation. The trial design included early initiation (before 72 hours of age), administration of test gas (placebo or nitric oxide) for a minimum of 2 weeks, and a dose of 10 ppm, obviating potential criticisms that treatment was started too late, stopped too soon, or given in an insufficient amount. Much the same as the EUNO and NEWNO investigators in similar trials,[1,2] these investigators demonstrated no effects on any primary or secondary outcome. Collectively, these trials should lay to rest the hypothesis that inhaled nitric oxide improves outcomes of preterm infants with mild-to-moderate respiratory disease. The lesson that apparently promising subgroup analyses demand confirmation in prospective controlled trials must also be extended to other hypotheses generated from previous trials. Until such data are available, use of inhaled nitric oxide in preterm infants with particular characteristics—African Americans, exposure to oligohydramnios, echocardiographic evidence of pulmonary hypertension, and the like—should be viewed as an unproven therapy.

W. E. Benitz, MD

References

1. Mercier JC, Hummler H, Durrmeyer X, et al. Inhaled nitric oxide for prevention of bronchopulmonary dysplasia in premature babies (EUNO): a randomised controlled trial. *Lancet.* 2010;376:346-354.

2. Yoder BA. *Inhaled NO for Prevention of BPD: Update on the NEWNO Trial.* Washington, DC: Hot Topics in Neonatology; 2013.

Inhaled nitric oxide in preterm infants with prolonged preterm rupture of the membranes: a case series
Semberova J, O'Donnell SM, Franta J, et al (Coombe Women and Infants Univ Hosp, Dublin, Ireland; et al)
J Perinatol 35:304-306, 2015

The available evidence does not support the routine use of inhaled nitric oxide (iNO) in the care of premature infants. We present a case series of 22 preterm infants born after prolonged preterm premature rupture of membranes and oligohydramnios with respiratory failure. Oxygenation index decreased significantly after commencement of iNO.

▶ Despite consensus statements in 2011 and again in 2014 that noted a lack of evidence for benefit from administration of inhaled nitric oxide (iNO) to preterm infants with respiratory failure and recommended against such treatment, use of iNO in this population is not infrequent and may be increasing.[1] One reason for this apparently inconsistent behavior may be the 9 previous small case series that suggest beneficial effects of iNO in preterm infants born after prolonged rupture of membranes associated with oligohydramnios, lung hypoplasia, and pulmonary hypertension. These reports include a total of 63 infants treated with iNO for whom immediate physiological responses could be characterized. Treatment with iNO appeared to be associated with improved oxygenation and reduced mean airway pressures.

This report adds to that collective experience and reaches similar conclusions. In this group of 22 preterm (<32 weeks' gestation) infants born after preterm premature rupture of membranes ≥7 days, the oxygenation index decreased from 29.7 ± 15.2 before to 9.2 ± 5.7 1 hour after initiation of iNO ($P < .0001$), mean airway pressure decreased from 11.8 ± 2.1 cm H_2O before to 8.6 ± 1.8 cm H_2O 24 hours after initiation of iNO ($P < .0001$), and arterial oxygen tension increased from 44 ± 19 mm Hg before to 94 ± 83 mm Hg 1 hour after initiation of iNO. These prompt responses are impressive, and it seems intuitive that ultimate outcomes were correspondingly improved. Although comparison of outcomes with iNO treatment with other experiences with similar infants suggests that may be so, this has certainly not been established; only 1 of the existing reports (a post hoc analysis) describe data from a randomized clinical trial.[2] While noting that "larger randomized trials are desirable," these authors "advocate iNO treatment in this particular population." Others have expressed doubts about the feasibility of randomized trials, on the basis of an estimated incidence of only 0.03% of all births[3] (ie, about 1200 affected infants per year in the United States). If the efficacy of iNO in such cases is sufficient to reduce mortality by 50% to the approximately 15% observed in this cohort, however, enrollment of only 240 infants in a randomized trial would be sufficient to resolve this question. In pursuit of that goal, advocates of iNO use in this high-risk subgroup should be encouraged to develop a trial, and others should enroll their eligible patients.

W. E. Benitz, MD

References

1. Ellsworth MA, Harris MN, Carey WA, et al. Off-label use of inhaled nitric oxide after release of NIH Consensus Statement. *Pediatrics*. 2015;135:643-648.
2. Chock VY, Van Meurs KP, Hintz SR, et al. Inhaled nitric oxide for preterm premature rupture of membranes, oligohydramnios, and pulmonary hypoplasia. *Am J Perinatol*. 2009;26:317-322.
3. Ball MK, Steinhorn RH. Inhaled nitric oxide for preterm infants: a Marksman's approach. *J Pediatr*. 2012;161:379-380.

An Update on the Impact of Postnatal Systemic Corticosteroids on Mortality and Cerebral Palsy in Preterm Infants: Effect Modification by Risk of Bronchopulmonary Dysplasia
Doyle LW, Halliday HL, Ehrenkranz RA, et al (Univ of Melbourne, Australia; Queen's Univ, Belfast, Northern Ireland; Yale Univ School of Medicine, New Haven, CT; et al)
J Pediatr 165:1258-1260, 2014

Infants at higher risk of bronchopulmonary dysplasia had increased rates of survival free of cerebral palsy after postnatal corticosteroid treatment in a previous metaregression of data from 14 randomized controlled trials. The relationship persists and is stronger in an updated analysis with data from 20 randomized controlled trials.

▶ Bronchopulmonary dysplasia (BPD) represents a common morbidity in infants born preterm. Despite 20 randomized controlled trials over 30 years, systemic corticosteroids remain a controversial therapy to prevent BPD. Corticosteroids effectively reduce the duration of mechanical ventilation and the incidence of BPD; however, corticosteroids may have direct neurotoxic effects in the developing brain. Because both BPD and corticosteroids demonstrate an association with cerebral palsy, considering the risk/benefit relationship in the context of underlying risk of BPD allows clinicians to contextualize the results of these trials for application to individual clinical scenarios. In 2005, Doyle and colleagues reported a weighted meta-regression analysis of 14 randomized controlled trials of corticosteroid therapy in preterm infants at risk for BPD. When the risk of BPD was below 35%, corticosteroid treatment significantly increased the risk of cerebral palsy or death. When the risk of BPD exceeded 65%, treatment reduced combined risk. In this update, the authors considered 6 additional trials as well as further follow-up data from the 14 original trials published since 2005. Additional data slightly narrowed the confidence intervals but otherwise had little effect on the regression line (lower confidence interval for harm at 33% and upper confidence interval for benefit at 60%). Combining the data above with predictive algorithms for the risk of BPD (https://neonatal.rti.org/index.cfm?fuseaction=BPDCalculator.start), clinicians have the ability to consider this controversial therapy with nuance and counsel families accurately on risk and benefit.

C. McPherson

Detection of Bloodstream Infections and Prediction of Bronchopulmonary Dysplasia in Preterm Neonates with an Electronic Nose

Rogosch T, Herrmann N, Maier RF, et al (Philipps-Univ Marburg, Germany; et al)
J Pediatr 165:622-624, 2014

We show that smellprints of volatile organic components measured with an electronic nose (Cyranose 320; Smiths Detection Group Ltd, Watford, United Kingdom) differ between tracheal aspirates from preterm neonates with or without laboratory-confirmed bloodstream infections and with or without subsequent development of bronchopulmonary dysplasia. Tracheal aspirate smellprints could be useful noninvasive diagnostic markers for preterm neonates.

▶ The nose knows. Many animals have a better sense of smell than humans; for example, canines have been used to detect a variety of medical conditions (among other things, such as illicit drugs or explosives) without knowing exactly what volatile molecules their nose might be detecting. The study by Rogosch et al describes application of an "electronic nose" for a similar purpose, using the Cyranose 320 detector to identify "smellprints " (like fingerprints) of organic volatile compounds from tracheal aspirates associated with bronchopulmonary dysplasia (BPD). Even though the numbers are small, the linear discriminant analysis of smellprints measured with the electronic nose was able to distinguish smell prints of neonates with and without BPD. Even storage of the samples did not affect the smellprints. This pattern-recognition approach may be less than satisfying for the basic scientist who might wish to know more about the particular volatile organic compounds emanating from the tracheal aspirates. Nonetheless, the technique is sufficient for clinical application in the same way biomarkers may be useful for diagnosis or prediction of various medical conditions. That is, diagnosis and prediction can be based on association and not necessarily causal relationships. Nonetheless, such biomarker pattern identification could lead to a better understanding of causal pathways as well, depending on what is actually being detected.

The notion of using trace volatile components of breath for diagnostic or prediction purposes is not new. Also, what we would consider to be volatile might vary depending on the vapor pressure of the substance and what can be detected. As detectors have improved over the years, the potential for identifying many low-level volatile constituents in breath or in other substances such as tracheal aspirates has increased, making this measurement approach more practical. Although a tracheal aspirate is used in this study, it is not inconceivable that simply taking a smell print of the breath of an infant might provide similar information. For example, carbon monoxide (CO), which typically is used as an index of bilirubin production, can also reflect lipid peroxidation in the lung in the context of mechanical ventilation and oxygen exposure. Of course, there are many more substances that might be assayed in breath and provide information about local lung injury or endogenous metabolism.

Another feature of breath sampling that is attractive is that if excretion rates can be estimated, metabolic rates can be estimated. This would allow prediction of a syndrome before the syndrome manifests clinically, such as estimating ammonia production and identifying an elevated production rate because of a urea cycle deficit before ammonia has accumulated to a level in circulation that it might affect neurologic function or cause injury. Such an approach has already been used to estimate bilirubin production, indexed by CO production, identifying individuals with hemolysis before the pigment accumulates to a high level in circulation, thus making prevention of hyperbilirubinemia a possibility rather than correction of the abnormal state ex post facto—a riskier proposition.

D. K. Stevenson, MD

The Effect of the National Shortage of Vitamin A on Death or Chronic Lung Disease in Extremely Low-Birth-Weight Infants

Tolia VN, Murthy K, McKinley PS, et al (Baylor Health Care System, Dallas, TX; Northwestern Univ, Chicago, IL; Clear Lake Regional Med Ctr, Webster, TX; et al)

JAMA Pediatr 168:1039-1044, 2014

Importance.—Prophylactic vitamin A supplementation has been shown to reduce the incidence of chronic lung disease or death in extremely low-birth-weight infants. Beginning in 2010, a national shortage reduced the supply of vitamin A available.

Objective.—To estimate the association between vitamin A supplementation and death or chronic lung disease in the context of the recent drug shortage. Intercenter variability in vitamin A use was assessed secondarily.

Design, Setting, and Participants.—Retrospective cohort study of 7925 infants with birth weights between 401 and 1000 g who were cared for in US neonatal intensive care units managed by the Pediatrix Medical Group. Infants were discharged between January 1, 2010, and June 30, 2012, and data were collected from the Pediatrix Clinical Data Warehouse. Infants who had major congenital anomalies, died during the first 3 days of life, or had missing data were excluded from the analysis.

Exposures.—Vitamin A supplementation.

Main Outcomes and Measures.—The primary outcome was either death before hospital discharge or chronic lung disease, defined as receiving any respiratory support at 36 weeks' corrected gestational age.

Results.—Of the 6210 eligible infants, 3011 (48.5%) experienced the primary outcome. Those who received vitamin A were more immature and more likely to receive mechanical ventilation during the first 3 days of life. During the study period, vitamin A supplementation significantly decreased (27.2% to 2.1%); however, the primary outcome was similar (48.4% to 49.5%; $P=.40$). Vitamin A was unrelated to death or chronic lung disease in unadjusted or multivariable analyses (relative risk [RR], 0.97; 95% CI, 0.91-1.03; $P=.32$) when demographic and clinical information were considered. After classifying centers by vitamin A use, the center of birth was significantly associated with the outcome, with birth in low- and medium-use centers related to a reduced likelihood of death or chronic lung disease.

Conclusions and Relevance.—The occurrence of death or chronic lung disease appears unaffected by the recent shortage of vitamin A. However, the center of birth appears to be an important risk factor for these infants' outcomes.

▶ In 1999, the Neonatal Research Network of the Eunice Kennedy Shriver National Institute of Child Health and Human Development published what is still the largest clinical trial of vitamin A supplementation for prevention of bronchopulmonary dysplasia.[1] The trial enrolled subjects with birth weights 401 to 1000 g in 1996 and 1997. That trial demonstrated modest, but significant, reductions in rates of the combined outcome of death or oxygen requirement at 36 weeks' postmenstrual age (55% vs 62%; number needed to treat = 14.5) and of oxygen use at 36 weeks' postmenstrual age (47 vs 56%; number needed to treat = 11.8). There were no differences in neurodevelopmental outcomes or respiratory morbidities in these subjects at 18 to 22 months of age, however.[2] Perhaps because of these mixed results, only a small fraction of neonatology services adopted routine vitamin A supplementation. The low penetration of this practice is reflected in the small proportion of potentially eligible infants (approximately 30%) who received vitamin A supplements in the baseline period described in this report of a "natural experiment" that developed when vitamin A preparations suitable for intramuscular injection became commercially unavailable in late 2010. Because of that shortage, vitamin A administration to extremely low birth weight babies at the centers contributing to this cohort virtually ceased (Fig in the original article). The rate of bronchopulmonary dysplasia did not increase, as would be expected with elimination of an effective therapy, however. These authors go to considerable lengths to develop statistical models that might explain that unexpected observation. Adjustment for gestational age, being small for gestational age, sex, race, severity of illness, and center demonstrated no relationship between vitamin A supplementation, and death or chronic lung disease (relative risk [RR], 0.97; 95% confidence interval [CI]: 0.91–1.03). Stratification of centers by extent of vitamin use among eligible infants revealed lower rates of death or bronchopulmonary dysplasia in centers where use of vitamin A was low (< 25%; adjusted RR 0.90, 95% CI: 0.82–0.98) or moderate (25%–50%; adjusted RR 0.88, CI: 0.78–0.98), but not in those at which vitamin A use was more prevalent (50%–75% or >75%; adjusted RR 0.97 and 1.01, 95% CI: 0.89–1.07 and 0.94–1.09, respectively), where an effect of supplementation should have been greater. These data cast doubt on the applicability of the now-old Neonatal Research Network results in the current era and merit careful thought as centers contemplate resumption of routine intramuscular vitamin A injections for these tiny infants now that appropriate formulations are once again commercially available. Although the benefits remain uncertain, the pain of multiple injections is much less so.

W. E. Benitz, MD

References

1. Tyson JE, Wright LL, Oh W, et al. Vitamin A supplementation for extremely-low-birth-weight infants. National Institute of Child Health and Human Development Neonatal Research Network. *N Engl J Med.* 1999;340:1962-1968.
2. Ambalavanan N, Tyson JE, Kennedy KA, et al. Vitamin A supplementation for extremely low birth weight infants: outcome at 18 to 22 months. *Pediatrics.* 2005;115:e249-e254.

Cardiovascular function in children who had chronic lung disease of prematurity
Joshi S, Wilson DG, Kotecha S, et al (Cardiff Univ, UK; Univ Hosp of Wales, Cardiff, UK)
Arch Dis Child Fetal Neonatal Ed 99:F373-F379, 2014

Objectives.—Although increased pulmonary arterial pressure is common in infancy in preterm infants who develop chronic lung disease of prematurity (CLD), it is unknown if the increase persists into childhood. We, therefore, assessed if 8–12-year-old children with documented CLD in infancy had evidence of right ventricular dysfunction or pulmonary arterial hypertension at rest or in response to acute hypoxia when compared to preterm and term-born controls.

Methods.—We studied 90 children: 60 born at ≤32 weeks of gestation (28 with CLD and 32 preterm controls), and 30 term-born controls. All had echocardiography including myocardial velocity imaging, at rest and while breathing 15% oxygen and 12% oxygen for 20 min each.

Results.—Baseline oxygen saturation, heart rate, blood pressure and echocardiographic markers of left and right ventricular function were similar in all three groups. While breathing 12% oxygen, the oxygen saturation decreased to 81.9% in the CLD group compared to 85.1% ($p < 0.05$) and 84.7% ($p < 0.01$) in the preterm and term controls, respectively. In response to hypoxia, all three groups showed increases in velocity of tricuspid regurgitation, end-diastolic velocity of pulmonary regurgitation, and right ventricular relaxation time; and decreases in pulmonary arterial acceleration time and the ratio of right ventricular acceleration time to ejection time. However, there were no differences between groups.

Conclusions.—Childhood survivors of CLD have comparable left and right ventricular function at 8—12 years of age to preterm and term-born children, and no evidence of increased pulmonary arterial pressure even after hypoxic exposure.

▶ Not long after bronchopulmonary dysplasia (BPD) was first recognized in 1967, it became apparent that both hypercarbia and electrocardiographic signs of cor pulmonale portend dismal outcomes. Over the decades, both the nature of the disease and the tools available for diagnosis of pulmonary hypertension have evolved. With more frequent echocardiographic assessment of right heart function in infants with BPD, retrospective reviews have indicated that as many as 25% of preterm infants with BPD have signs of pulmonary hypertension (PH).[1] Other studies have suggested that PH, especially if severe, is associated with high mortality rates. Those observations have led to recommendations for echocardiographic screening of infants who continue to require supplemental oxygen at 36 weeks' postmenstrual age, and sometimes for further evaluation by cardiac catheterization or computed tomographic angiography and treatment with a growing assortment of medications. There is scant evidence to guide those practices, however. In general, infants with BPD (including those discharged home with supplemental oxygen) gradually improve and have favorable long-term outcomes. Three-quarters of infants with BPD and signs of PH at 2 months of age had documented improvement after a median interval of approximately 3 months.[1] Now this report provides information about the status of PH at age 8 to 12 years in infants who met criteria for BPD at 36 weeks' postmenstrual age. Remarkably, evaluations while breathing 21%, 15%, and 12% oxygen revealed no differences in an array of echocardiographic measures of left and right ventricular function and pulmonary arterial pressures between children who had chronic lung disease (CLD) of prematurity, former preterm infants who did not have CLD, and those born at term. The authors concluded that "asymptomatic survivors of CLD have normal resting cardiovascular function in childhood, and that there are no late cardiovascular consequences of CLD." These divergent observations are not easy to reconcile. One possibility is that the latter observations reflect survivor bias, such that only those infants with the least severe BPD survived to have those late follow-up evaluations. Another possibility is that PH eventually resolved in even more severe cases, as appears to be the general case for PH in infants with BPD.[1] A much more complete understanding of the natural history of this complication of BPD will be required to distinguish these possibilities. Until there is evidence that guides identification of infants with BPD who are destined to have poor outcomes from progressive pulmonary vascular disease and that treatments targeted to acutely lower pulmonary artery pressure in those high-risk babies prevents those outcomes, it may be wise to take a restrained approach to the use of invasive diagnostic procedures and unproven therapies in these infants.

W. E. Benitz, MD

Reference

1. An HS, Bae EJ, Kim GB, et al. Pulmonary hypertension in preterm infants with bronchopulmonary dysplasia. *Korean Circ J*. 2010;40:131-136.

8 Central Nervous System and Special Senses

Neonatal encephalopathy and the association to asphyxia in labor
Jonsson M, Ågren J, Nordén-Lindeberg S, et al (Uppsala Univ, Sweden; et al)
Am J Obstet Gynecol 211:667.e1-667.e8, 2014

Objective.—In cases with moderate and severe neonatal encephalopathy, we aimed to determine the proportion that was attributable to asphyxia during labor and to investigate the association between cardiotocographic (CTG) patterns and neonatal outcome.

Study Design.—In a study population of 71,189 births from 2 Swedish university hospitals, 80 cases of neonatal encephalopathy were identified. Cases were categorized by admission CTG patterns (normal or abnormal) and by the presence of asphyxia (cord pH, <7.00; base deficit, ≥12 mmol/L). Cases with normal admission CTG patterns and asphyxia at birth were considered to experience asphyxia related to labor. CTG patterns were assessed for the 2 hours preceding delivery.

Results.—Admission CTG patterns were normal in 51 cases (64%) and abnormal in 29 cases (36%). The rate of cases attributable to asphyxia (ie, hypoxic ischemic encephalopathy) was 48 of 80 cases (60%), most of which evolved during labor (43/80 cases; 54%). Both severe neonatal encephalopathy and neonatal death were more frequent with an abnormal, rather than with a normal, admission CTG pattern (13 [45%] vs 11 [22%]; $P=.03$), and (6 [21%] vs 3 [6%]; $P=.04$), respectively. Comparison of cases with an abnormal and a normal admission CTG pattern also revealed more frequently observed decreased variability (12 [60%] and 8 [22%], respectively) and more late decelerations (8 [40%] and 1 [3%], respectively).

Conclusion.—Moderate and severe encephalopathy is attributable to asphyxia in 60% of cases, most of which evolve during labor. An abnormal admission CTG pattern indicates a poorer neonatal outcome and more often is associated with pathologic CTG patterns preceding delivery.

▶ In this observational study, investigators attempted to determine whether there was a difference in early and later brain MRI findings in infants undergoing hypothermia for hypoxic-ischemic encephalopathy. Forty-three infants were selected in this 7-year cohort study because they had undergone both an early MRI examination during hypothermic treatment and a later scan after therapy had been completed. There was a strong concordance between studies in infants who developed structural brain injury; early abnormal studies had 100% specificity and sensitivity at predicting later abnormalities.

Aside from the obvious selection bias—severely affected infants were more likely to have been examined early—interpretation of the results is a "glass half-full, glass half-empty" scenario. Early MRI may have utility in a research setting, but if the results do not differ from later MRI, why subject a critically ill infant to the risks of transport and the procedure? In fact, I would argue that even in this population, routine posthypothermia is an unnecessary procedure. Our group has shown that only seizures and the inability to feed orally are correlated to positive MRI findings.[1] Less may be more.

S. M. Donn, MD

Reference

1. Sarkar S, Donn SM, Bapuraj JR, Bhagat I, Dechert RE, Barks JD. Does clinical evaluation one week after therapeutic hypothermia predict brain MRI abnormalities? *J Perinatol*. 2013;33:538-542.

Diagnostic Accuracy of Fetal Heart Rate Monitoring in the Identification of Neonatal Encephalopathy

Graham EM, Adami RR, McKenney SL, et al (Bloomberg School of Public Health, MD; Johns Hopkins Univ School of Medicine, Baltimore, MD)
Obstet Gynecol 124:507-513, 2014

Objective.—To estimate the diagnostic accuracy of electronic fetal heart rate abnormalities in the identification of neonates with encephalopathy treated with whole-body hypothermia.

Methods.—Between January 1, 2007, and July 1, 2013, there were 39 neonates born at two hospitals within our system treated with whole-body hypothermia within 6 hours of birth. Neurologically normal control neonates were matched to each case by gestational age and mode of delivery in a two-to-one fashion. The last hour of electronic fetal heart rate monitoring before delivery was evaluated by three obstetricians blinded to outcome.

Results.—The differences in tracing category were not significantly different (neonates in the case group 10.3% I, 76.9% II, 12.8% III; neonates in the control group 9.0% I, 89.7% II, 1.3% III; $P=.18$). Bivariate analysis showed neonates in the case group had significantly increased late decelerations, total deceleration area 30 (debt 30) and 60 minutes (debt 60) before delivery and were more likely to be nonreactive. Multivariable logistic regression showed neonates in the case group had a significant decrease in early decelerations ($P=.03$) and a significant increase in debt 30 (.01) and debt 60 ($P = .005$). The area under the receiver operating characteristic curve, sensitivity, and specificity were 0.72, 23.1%, and 94.9% for early decelerations; 0.66, 33.3%, and 87.2% for debt 30, and 0.68, 35.9%, and 89.7% for debt 60, respectively.

Conclusion.—Abnormalities during the last hour of fetal heart rate monitoring before delivery are poorly predictive of neonatal hypoxic—ischemic encephalopathy qualifying for whole-body hypothermia treatment within 6 hours of birth.

Level of Evidence.—II.

▶ This study attempted to correlate abnormalities in electronic heart rate monitoring with neonatal encephalopathy. The authors analyzed the last hour of monitoring in 39 newborns who qualified for whole body hypothermia and compared them to a control group that was neurologically normal and matched for mode of delivery and gestational age. Little correlation was found, and the authors concluded that abnormal tracings in this setting are poorly predictive of hypoxic-ischemic encephalopathy and qualifying for hypothermic neuroprotection.

We should not be surprised by these findings. One of the hypotheses that have plagued all of the cooling trials is the a priori assumption that brain injury occurred within a 6-hour window of birth, and affected infants would display the requisite neonatal neurologic syndrome and concurrent disturbances in physiology and acid—base balance. Unfortunately, probably many of these infants were injured earlier in labor or prenatally. Thus, we face a "chicken and egg" scenario. Is the tracing abnormal because the brain is displaying an abnormal tolerance of labor, or is there truly a hypoxic state that the tracings reflect?

A parallel to the early days of extracorporeal membrane oxygenation may exist. We defined the treatment rather than the underlying condition that led to its implementation. In addition to ambiguity about timing, differences in the pathophysiology must be accounted. Was it prolonged, partial asphyxia, or was it near total? Did it result from altered uteroplacental function, cord compression, diminished oxygen carrying capacity, or inflammation/infection? Hypothermia is not the disease, it's the treatment, and the electronic fetal monitoring is perhaps not the "smoking gun."

S. M. Donn, MD

Heart rate variability in hypoxic ischemic encephalopathy: correlation with EEG grade and 2-y neurodevelopmental outcome
Goulding RM, Stevenson NJ, Murray DM, et al (Irish Centre for Fetal and Neonatal Translational Res, Cork, Ireland)
Pediatr Res 77:681-687, 2015

Background.—The study aims to describe heart rate variability (HRV) in neonatal hypoxic ischemic encephalopathy (HIE) and correlate HRV with electroencephalographic (EEG) grade of HIE and neurodevelopmental outcome.

Methods.—Multichannel EEG and electrocardiography (ECG) were assessed at 12—48 h after birth in healthy and encephalopathic full-term neonates. EEGs were graded (normal, mild, moderate, and severe). Neurodevelopmental outcome was assessed at 2 y of age. Seven HRV features were calculated using normalized-RR (NN) interval. The correlation of these features with EEG grade and outcome were measured using Spearman's correlation coefficient.

Results.—HRV was significantly associated with HIE severity ($P < 0.05$): standard deviation of NN interval (SDNN) ($r = -0.62$), triangular interpolation of NN interval histogram (TINN) ($r = -0.65$), mean NN interval ($r = -0.48$), and the very low frequency (VLF) ($r = -0.60$), low frequency (LF) ($r = -0.67$) and high frequency (HF) components of the NN interval ($r = -0.60$). SDNN at 24 and 48 h were significantly associated ($P < 0.05$) with neurodevelopmental outcome ($r = -0.41$ and -0.54, respectively).

Conclusion.—HRV is associated with EEG grade of HIE and neurodevelopmental outcome. HRV has potential as a prognostic tool to complement EEG.

▶ Therapeutic hypothermia has remarkably improved outcomes for increasing numbers of infants affected by the scourge of hypoxic-ischemic encephalopathy (HIE). Nevertheless, accurately predicting outcomes for infants with HIE remains challenging. Advances in electroencephalography (EEG) and neuroimaging have shed a good deal more predictive light than might have been offered in times past. In their current publication, Goulding and colleagues might well have added another predictor to our HIE toolkit: heart rate variability (HRV). The investigators evaluated parameters of HRV at 12 to 48 hours of postnatal age in relationship to EEG and neurodevelopmental (ND) outcome at 2 years and found an association with each outcome. Decreases in HRV parameters were associated with more severely abnormal EEG findings and adverse ND outcomes at age 2. When Griffin and Moorman first cited heart rate analysis as a predictor of neonatal sepsis,[1] the observation seemed implausible. Not only have their findings been validated, but currently heart rate analyses have been shown to be predictive for other disorders, such as impending myocardial infarction. Goulding and colleagues' current findings seem a logical extension of the observed link between decreased fetal heart rate variability and its association with fetal distress. Hopefully, sophisticated analyses of this most basic vital sign will be automated and/or incorporated into standard monitoring software for bedside use.

L. J. Van Marter, MD, MPH

Reference

1. Griffin M, Moorman JR. Toward the early diagnosis of neonatal sepsis and sepsis-like illness using novel heart rate analysis. *J Pediatrics.* 2001;107:97-104.

Brain Temperature in Neonates with Hypoxic-Ischemic Encephalopathy during Therapeutic Hypothermia

Wu T-W, McLean C, Friedlich P, et al (Univ of Southern California, Los Angeles)
J Pediatr 165:1129-1134, 2014

Objective.—To noninvasively determine brain temperature of neonates with hypoxic-ischemic encephalopathy (HIE) during and after therapeutic hypothermia.

Study Design.—Using a phantom, we derived a calibration curve to calculate brain temperature based on chemical shift differences in magnetic resonance spectroscopy. We enrolled infants admitted for therapeutic hypothermia and assigned them to a moderate HIE (M-HIE) or severe HIE (S-HIE) group based on Sarnat staging. Rectal (core) temperature and magnetic resonance spectroscopy data used to derive regional brain temperatures (basal ganglia, thalamus, and cortical gray matter) were acquired concomitantly during and after therapeutic hypothermia. We compared brain and rectal temperature in the M-HIE and S-HIE groups during and after therapeutic hypothermia using 2-tailed *t*-tests.

Results.—Eighteen patients (14 with M-HIE and 4 with S-HIE) were enrolled. As expected, both brain and rectal temperatures were lower during therapeutic hypothermia than after therapeutic hypothermia. Brain temperature in patients with S-HIE was higher than in those with M-HIE both during (35.1 ± 1.3°C vs 33.7 ± 1.2°C; $P < .01$) and after therapeutic hypothermia (38.1 ± 1.5°C vs 36.8 ± 1.3°C; $P < .01$). The brain–rectal temperature gradient was also greater in the S-HIE group both during and after therapeutic hypothermia.

Conclusion.—For this analysis of a small number of patients, brain temperature and brain–rectal temperature gradient were higher in neonates with S-HIE than in those with M-HIE during and after therapeutic hypothermia. Further studies are needed to determine whether further decreasing brain temperature in neonates with S-HIE is safe and effective in improving outcome.

▶ Rectal or esophageal temperatures are used to guide the treatment of neonatal hypoxic/ischemic encephalopathy (HIE) with therapeutic hypothermia. Invasive measurement of brain temperature in adults with acute brain injury indicates that brain temperature frequently exceeds systemic temperature.[1,2] In the above observational study the investigators used magnetic resonance thermometry to evaluate the reliability of rectal temperature as a surrogate measure of brain temperature in infants undergoing therapeutic hypothermia for neonatal HIE.

Magnetic resonance studies were done to assess brain temperature during and after therapeutic hypothermia. The mean ages at the time of the first and second studies were 57 ± 10 hours and 6.3 ± 2.8 days, respectively. As expected, overall brain temperature during therapeutic hypothermia was higher than target core temperature. Of note, brain temperature and brain-recta gradient during and after therapeutic hypothermia were significantly higher in infants with severe HIE than in those with moderate HIE. These observations suggest that for infants with severe HIE, therapeutic hypothermia at the current target temperature might be less effective in lowering brain temperature and indicate that rectal temperature may not be a reliable surrogate measure of brain temperature. The authors speculate that these findings may partially explain the diminished neuroprotective effect of therapeutic hypothermia in infants with severe HIE compared with those with moderate HIE.

L. A. Papile, MD

References

1. Rumana CS, Gopinath SP, Uzura M, Valadka AB, Robertson CS. Brain temperature exceeds systemic temperature in head-injured patients. *Crit Care Med.* 1998;26:562-567.
2. Childs C, Vail A, Protheroe R, King AT, Dark PM. Differences between brain and rectal temperatures during routine critical care of patients with severe traumatic brain injury. *Anaesthesia.* 2005;60:759-765.

Cognitive Outcomes After Neonatal Encephalopathy

Pappas A, for the Hypothermia Extended Follow-up Subcommittee of the *Eunice Kennedy Shriver* NICHD Neonatal Research Network (Wayne State Univ, Detroit, MI; et al)
Pediatrics 135:e624-e634, 2015

Objectives.—To describe the spectrum of cognitive outcomes of children with and without cerebral palsy (CP) after neonatal encephalopathy, evaluate the prognostic value of early developmental testing and report on school services and additional therapies.

Methods.—The participants of this study are the school-aged survivors of the National Institute of Child Health and Human Development Neonatal Research Network randomized controlled trial of whole-body hypothermia. Children underwent neurologic examinations and neurodevelopmental and cognitive testing with the Bayley Scales of Infant Development—II at 18 to 22 months and the Wechsler intelligence scales and the Neuropsychological Assessment—Developmental Neuropsychological Assessment at 6 to 7 years. Parents were interviewed about functional status and receipt of school and support services. We explored predictors of cognitive outcome by using multiple regression models.

Results.—Subnormal IQ scores were identified in more than a quarter of the children: 96% of survivors with CP had an IQ <70, 9% of children without CP had an IQ <70, and 31% had an IQ of 70 to 84. Children with a mental developmental index, <70 at 18 months had, on average, an adjusted IQ at 6 to 7 years that was 42 points lower than that of those with a mental developmental index >84 (95% confidence interval, −49.3 to −35.0; $P < .001$). Twenty percent of children with normal IQ and 28% of those with IQ scores of 70 to 84 received special educational support services or were held back ≥1 grade level.

Conclusions.—Cognitive impairment remains an important concern for all children with neonatal encephalopathy.

▶ This study is a secondary analysis of prospectively collected data from the National Institute of Child Health and Human Development Neonatal Research Network multicenter trial of whole-body hypothermia that recruted participants between 2000 and 2003. The primary outcome of the trial, death or neurodevelopmental disability at 18 months of age, did not differ for the hypothermia-treated cohort and the control group. Longitudinal follow-up at 7 years of age again found no difference in death or neurodevelopmental disability between the 2 groups.

Formal neuropsychological assessment at 6 to 7 years of age occurred in 78% (110 of 140) of surviving study children. Of the 31 surviving children with IQ scores less than 70 at 7 years of age, 74% had cerebral palsy, whereas 96% of the 23 children with cerebral palsy had an IQ less than 70. The authors state in the discussion that "this is the largest study to date to address an unfortunate tenet of mythology regarding the lack of association between cognitive impairment and neonatal encephalopathy among survivors without cerebral palsy." The statement is misleading in that it implies that hypoxic-ischemic encephalopathy (HIE) sufficiently severe to result in mental retardation will not affect neuromotor systems. HIE is a cause-specific subset of neonatal encephalopathy and its presence does not exclude additional causes of mental retardation.

L. A. Papile, MD

Cognitive Outcomes of Preterm Infants Randomized to Darbepoetin, Erythropoietin, or Placebo

Ohls RK, Kamath-Rayne BD, Christensen RD, et al (Univ of New Mexico, Albuquerque; Cincinnati Children's Hosp, OH; Intermountain Health Care, Salt Lake City, UT; et al)
Pediatrics 133:1023-1030, 2014

Background.—We previously reported decreased transfusions and donor exposures in preterm infants randomized to Darbepoetin (Darbe) or erythropoietin (Epo) compared with placebo. As these erythropoiesis-stimulating agents (ESAs) have shown promise as neuroprotective agents, we hypothesized improved neurodevelopmental outcomes at 18 to 22 months among infants randomized to receive ESAs.

Methods.—We performed a randomized, masked, multicenter study comparing Darbe (10 µg/kg, 1×/week subcutaneously), Epo (400 U/kg, 3×/week subcutaneously), and placebo (sham dosing 3×/week) given through 35 weeks' postconceptual age, with transfusions administered according to a standardized protocol. Surviving infants were evaluated at 18 to 22 months' corrected age using the Bayley Scales of Infant Development III. The primary outcome was composite cognitive score.

TABLE 4.—Neurodevelopmental Outcomes

	Darbe $n=27$	Epo $n=29$	P*	ESA[a] $n=56$	Placebo $n=24$	Unadjusted Odds Ratio (95% CI)	P*	Adjusted for Gender, Maternal Education Odds Ratio (95% CI)	P*
Cognitive score <85	0 (0)	3 (10.3)	0.12	3 (5.4)	6 (25.0)	0.17 (0.04–0.75)	0.02	0.18 (0.04–0.82)	0.03
Cognitive score <80	0 (0)	3 (10.3)	0.12	3 (5.4)	5 (20.8)	0.22 (0.05–0.99)	0.05	0.24 (0.05–1.13)	0.07
Cognitive score <70	0 (0)	1 (3.5)	0.50	1 (1.8)	2 (8.3)	0.20 (0.02–2.32)	0.20	0.24 (0.02–2.93)	0.26
NDI,[b] N (%)	3 (11.1)	4 (13.8)	0.88	7 (12.5)	10 (41.7)	0.20 (0.06–0.62)	0.005	0.21 (0.07–0.68)	0.009
CP;[c]	0 (0)	0 (0)	1.00	0 (0)	5 (20.8)	N/A	0.002	N/A	<0.001
Visual deficit	2 (7.4)	0 (0)	0.27	2 (3.6)	1 (4.2)	0.85 (0.07–9.87)	0.91	0.72 (0.06–8.74)	0.80
Hearing deficit	0 (0)	1 (3.5)	0.50	1 (1.8)	1 (4.2)	0.42 (0.03–6.98)	0.54	0.48 (0.03–8.59)	0.62
NDI or death, N (%)	4/28 (14.3)	5/30 (16.7)	0.92	9/58 (15.5)	13/27 (48.2)	0.20 (0.07–0.56)	0.002	0.22 (0.07–0.70)	0.01
Moderate NDI,[d] N (%)	3 (11.1)	2 (6.9)	0.45	5 (8.9)	9 (37.5)	0.16 (0.05–0.56)	0.004	0.18 (0.05–0.63)	0.008
Moderate NDI or death, N (%)	4/28 (14.3)	3/30 (10.0)	0.48	7/58 (12.1)	12/27 (44.4)	0.17 (0.06–0.51)	0.002	0.20 (0.06–0.67)	0.009

* P values for comparisons between Darbe and Epo were computed using 2 methods depending on characteristics of the data. For the NDI measures, P values were computed using logistic regression with gender and maternal education as covariates. For the remaining measures, P values were computed using ANCOVA with only gender as a covariate. Percentages for NDI or death include deaths during initial hospitalization. CI, confidence interval. N/A, not applicable.
[a]Treated groups are combined.
[b]NDI is defined as having either CP, visual deficit, hearing deficit, or a cognitive score <85.
[c]Given the absence of CP cases in the ESA treatment group, odds ratios cannot be accurately estimated. P values given for CP were computed using Fisher's exact tests for the unadjusted P value and using ANCOVA with gender as the only covariate for the remaining P values.
[d]Moderate NDI is defined as having either CP, visual deficit, hearing deficit, or a cognitive score <70.
Reproduced with permission from Pediatrics. Ohls RK, Kamath-Rayne BD, Christensen RD, et al. Cognitive Outcomes of Preterm Infants Randomized to Darbepoetin, Erythropoietin, or Placebo. Pediatrics. 2014;133:1023-1030. Copyright © 2014, by the American Academy of Pediatrics.

Assessments of object permanence, anthropometrics, cerebral palsy, vision, and hearing were performed.

Results.—Of the original 102 infants (946 ± 196 g, 27.7 ± 1.8 weeks' gestation), 80 (29 Epo, 27 Darbe, 24 placebo) returned for follow-up. The 3 groups were comparable for age at testing, birth weight, and gestational age. After adjustment for gender, analysis of covariance revealed significantly higher cognitive scores among Darbe (96.2 ± 7.3; mean ± SD) and Epo recipients (97.9 ± 14.3) compared with placebo recipients (88.7 ± 13.5; $P = .01$ vs ESA recipients) as was object permanence ($P = .05$). No ESA recipients had cerebral palsy, compared with 5 in the placebo group ($P < .001$). No differences among groups were found in visual or hearing impairment.

Conclusions.—Infants randomized to receive ESAs had better cognitive outcomes, compared with placebo recipients, at 18 to 22 months. Darbe and Epo may prove beneficial in improving long-term cognitive outcomes of preterm infants (Table 4).

▶ Retrospective reviews and posthoc analyses of randomized trials have suggested that early treatment with erythropoietin may improve long-term neurodevelopmental outcomes of extremely low birth weight preterm infants. Until this report, this hypothesis had not been tested in randomized, controlled trials in which neurodevelopmental outcome was a prospective primary outcome. Although the numbers are small, this comparison of erythropoietin (Epo), darbepoetin (Darbe), and placebo provides the first demonstration of improved neurodevelopment associated with this class of drugs. Compared with placebo recipients, infants treated with either erythropoietic agent had significantly higher composite cognitive scores and object permanence measures on the Bayley Scales of Infant Development at 18 to 22 months of age, as summarized in the abstract of the article. In addition, several other measures of neurodevelopmental outcome were significantly better in the treatment group, as shown in the following table (adapted from Table 4 of the article).

NDI is defined as having cerebral palsy, visual deficit, hearing deficit, or a cognitive score < 85; moderate NDI is similarly defined but with cognitive score < 70. These results were not substantially different after adjustment for infant sex and maternal education.

Are these impressive results sufficient to support widespread adoption of this treatment? Although both the magnitude and statistical significance of the observed differences are robust, only 80 subjects (24 in the placebo group) completed the trial. Because encouraging results from small initial trials are often followed by negative results of larger ones, it seems wise to await the results of other larger trials. The Swiss EPO Neuroprotection Trial has completed enrollment, but the primary outcome of neurodevelopmental status at 24 months of age has not been reported. The Preterm Erythropoietin Neuroprotection Trial, the largest to date, continues to enroll subjects. The status of 2 additional trials in China is uncertain. Enthusiasm for this intervention should be restrained until those studies can more fully inform practice.

W. E. Benitz, MD

Effects of Hypothermia for Perinatal Asphyxia on Childhood Outcomes
Azzopardi D, for the TOBY Study Group (King's College London, UK; et al)
N Engl J Med 371:140-149, 2014

Background.—In the Total Body Hypothermia for Neonatal Encephalopathy Trial (TOBY), newborns with asphyxial encephalopathy who received hypothermic therapy had improved neurologic outcomes at 18 months of age, but it is uncertain whether such therapy results in longer-term neurocognitive benefits.

Methods.—We randomly assigned 325 newborns with asphyxial encephalopathy who were born at a gestational age of 36 weeks or more to receive standard care alone (control) or standard care with hypothermia to a rectal temperature of 33 to 34°C for 72 hours within 6 hours after birth. We evaluated the neurocognitive function of these children at 6 to 7 years of age. The primary outcome of this analysis was the frequency of survival with an IQ score of 85 or higher.

Results.—A total of 75 of 145 children (52%) in the hypothermia group versus 52 of 132 (39%) in the control group survived with an IQ score of 85 or more (relative risk, 1.31; $P = 0.04$). The proportions of children who died were similar in the hypothermia group and the control group (29% and 30%, respectively). More children in the hypothermia group than in the control group survived without neurologic abnormalities (65 of 145 [45%] vs. 37 of 132 [28%]; relative risk, 1.60; 95% confidence interval, 1.15 to 2.22). Among survivors, children in the hypothermia group, as compared with those in the control group, had significant reductions in the risk of cerebral palsy (21% vs. 36%, $P = 0.03$) and the risk of moderate or severe disability (22% vs. 37%, $P = 0.03$); they also had significantly better motor-function scores. There was no significant between-group difference in parental assessments of children's health status and in results on 10 of 11 psychometric tests.

Conclusions.—Moderate hypothermia after perinatal asphyxia resulted in improved neurocognitive outcomes in middle childhood. (Funded by the United Kingdom Medical Research Council and others; TOBY ClinicalTrials.gov number, NCT01092637.)

▶ Most neonatal clinical trials have been limited to relatively short-term outcomes. This can be especially misleading when neurodevelopmental status is the primary outcome measure. The investigators of the TOBY whole-body cooling trial are to be commended for publishing 6- to 7-year follow-up of infants enrolled in the original clinical trial conducted between 2002 and 2006. In the interim, multiple international trials have established hypothermia as the standard of care for infants sustaining a presumed intrapartum asphyxial insult. This study by Azzopardi et al is reassuring for several reasons. First and foremost, neurocognitive outcomes were better in infants undergoing cooling, and second, hypothermic treatment did not appear to result in an increase in morbid survival. The study design also accounted for those lost to follow-up, reducing the risk of selection bias.

There should no longer be any hesitation to offer treatment to babies who meet criteria used in the major trials.

S. M. Donn, MD

Maternal allopurinol administration during suspected fetal hypoxia: a novel neuroprotective intervention? A multicentre randomised placebo controlled trial
Kaandorp JJ, Benders MJNL, Schuit E, et al (Univ Med Ctr, Utrecht, The Netherlands; et al)
Arch Dis Child Fetal Neonatal Ed 100:F216-F223, 2015

Objective.—To determine whether maternal allopurinol treatment during suspected fetal hypoxia would reduce the release of biomarkers associated with neonatal brain damage.

Design.—A randomised double-blind placebo controlled multicentre trial.

Patients.—We studied women in labour at term with clinical indices of fetal hypoxia, prompting immediate delivery.

Setting.—Delivery rooms of 11 Dutch hospitals.

Intervention.—When immediate delivery was foreseen based on suspected fetal hypoxia, women were allocated to receive allopurinol 500 mg intravenous (ALLO) or placebo intravenous (CONT).

Main Outcome Measures.—Primary endpoint was the difference in cord S100ß, a tissue-specific biomarker for brain damage.

Results.—222 women were randomised to receive allopurinol (ALLO, n = 111) or placebo (CONT, n = 111). Cord S100ß was not significantly different between the two groups: 44.5 pg/mL (IQR 20.2–71.4) in the ALLO group versus 54.9 pg/mL (IQR 26.8–94.7) in the CONT group (difference in median −7.69 (95% CI −24.9 to 9.52)). Post hoc subgroup analysis showed a potential treatment effect of allopurinol on the proportion of infants with a cord S100ß value above the 75th percentile in girls (ALLO n = 5 (12%) vs CONT n = 10 (31%); risk ratio (RR) 0.37 (95% CI 0.14 to 0.99)) but not in boys (ALLO n = 18 (32%) vs CONT n = 15 (25%); RR 1.4 (95% CI 0.84 to 2.3)). Also, cord neuroketal levels were significantly lower in girls treated with allopurinol as compared with placebo treated girls: 18.0 pg/mL (95% CI 12.1 to 26.9) in the ALLO group versus 32.2 pg/mL (95% CI 22.7 to 45.7) in the CONT group (geometric mean difference −16.4 (95% CI −24.6 to −1.64)).

Conclusions.—Maternal treatment with allopurinol during fetal hypoxia did not significantly lower neuronal damage markers in cord blood. Post hoc analysis revealed a potential beneficial treatment effect in girls.

Trial Registration Number.—NCT00189007, Dutch Trial Register NTR1383.

▶ This study sought to determine whether administration of intravenous allopurinol to laboring mothers experiencing a presumed episode of fetal hypoxia could reduce the concentrations of biomarkers associated with neonatal brain injury. It was a masked, placebo-controlled trial in which 222 women were randomized to receive drug or placebo. An abnormal fetal heart rate monitoring pattern was used as a surrogate for fetal hypoxia, and if a decision to terminate labor by immediate delivery was made, allopurinol or placebo was administered to the mother intravenously. Severity of hypoxia was assessed after the fact by measurement of venous lactate and arterial pH on cord blood samples obtained following delivery.

Allopurinol treatment had no effect on reducing biomarkers of brain injury, although a posthoc analysis suggests that it may have an effect on female fetuses. However, it appears that this treatment population was probably not significantly affected to show any clinically significant impact of treatment. Mean cord pH in both groups was 7.19, Apgar scores were equivalent, base excess was the same, and there were no differences in the incidence of hypoglycemia. No infant developed seizures or hypoxic-ischemic encephalopathy.

Before we label allopurinol a novel neuroprotective drug, it needs to be tested on a population of fetuses that needs neuroprotection.

S. M. Donn, MD

Melatonin use for neuroprotection in perinatal asphyxia: a randomized controlled pilot study
Aly H, Elmahdy H, El-Dib M, et al (George Washington Univ and Children's Natl Med Ctr, DC; Tanta Univ, Egypt)
J Perinatol 35:186-191, 2015

Objective.—Melatonin has been shown to be neuroprotective in animal models. The objective of this study is to examine the effect of melatonin on clinical, biochemical, neurophysiological and radiological outcomes of neonates with hypoxic–ischemic encephalopathy (HIE).

Study Design.—We conducted a prospective trial on 45 newborns, 30 with HIE and 15 healthy controls. HIE infants were randomized into: hypothermia group ($N = 15$; received 72-h whole-body cooling) and melatonin/hypothermia group ($N = 15$; received hypothermia and five daily enteral doses of melatonin 10 mg kg^{-1}). Serum melatonin, plasma superoxide dismutase (SOD) and serum nitric oxide (NO) were measured at enrollment for all infants ($N = 45$) and at 5 days for the HIE groups ($N = 30$). In addition to electroencephalography (EEG) at enrollment, all surviving HIE infants were studied with brain magnetic resonance imaging (MRI) and repeated EEG at 2 weeks of life. Neurologic evaluations and Denver Developmental Screening Test II were performed at 6 months.

Result.—Compared with healthy neonates, the two HIE groups had increased melatonin, SOD and NO. At enrollment, the two HIE groups did not differ in clinical, laboratory or EEG findings. At 5 days, the melatonin/hypothermia group had greater increase in melatonin ($P < 0.001$) and decline in NO ($P < 0.001$), but less decline in SOD ($P = 0.004$). The melatonin/hypothermia group had fewer seizures on follow-up EEG and less white matter abnormalities on MRI. At 6 months, the melatonin/hypothermia group had improved survival without neurological or developmental abnormalities ($P < 0.001$).

Conclusion.—Early administration of melatonin to asphyxiated term neonates is feasible and may ameliorate brain injury.

▶ Multiple randomized clinical trials have convincingly demonstrated that induced hypothermia initiated within 6 hours of birth is an effective and safe therapy for moderate to severe neonatal hypoxic-ischemic encephalopathy (HIE). However, because 40% to 50% of infants with HIE who are treated with hypothermia will either die or have severe neurodevelopmental impairment, there is an abiding interest in exploring potential adjuvant therapies.

In this study, the investigators sought to study the feasibility and efficacy of administering melatonin to infants with neonatal HIE who were undergoing hypothermia. The rationale for choosing melatonin relates to its demonstrated antioxidant, antiinflammatory, and antiapoptotic properties in animal models subjected to oxidative stress and the fact that it freely crosses the blood—brain barrier.[1] In contrast to previously published clinical studies in infants, melatonin was given enterally, not intravenously, and it would appear that the product used was not of medical grade but rather an over-the-counter preparation.[2,3] Both of these factors could potentially affect the pharmacokinetics of melatonin. Furthermore, there were twice as many infants in the hypothermia-alone cohort who had severe HIE compared with the melatonin/ hypothermia group, potentially leading to bias regarding developmental outcome. In view of these limitations, it is difficult to ascribe the beneficial changes noted to melatonin therapy.

L. A. Papile, MD

References

1. Gitto E, Marseglia L, Manti S, et al. Protective role of melatonin in neonatal disease. *Oxid Med Cell Longev.* 2013;2013:980374.
2. Gitto E, Reiter RJ, Cordaro SP, et al. Oxidative and inflammatory parameters in respiratory distress syndrome of the preterm infant: beneficial effects of melatonin. *Am J Perinatal.* 2004;21:209-216.
3. Gitto E, Romeo C, Reiter RJ, et al. Melatonin reduces oxidative stress in surgical neonates. *J Pediatr Surg.* 2004;39:184-189.

Effect of Depth and Duration of Cooling on Deaths in the NICU Among Neonates With Hypoxic Ischemic Encephalopathy: A Randomized Clinical Trial

Shankaran S, for the Eunice Kennedy Shriver National Institute of Child Health and Human Development Neonatal Research Network (Wayne State Univ, Detroit, MI; et al)
JAMA 312:2629-2639, 2014

Importance.—Hypothermia at 33.5°C for 72 hours for neonatal hypoxic ischemic encephalopathy reduces death or disability to 44% to

55%; longer cooling and deeper cooling are neuroprotective in animal models.

Objective.—To determine if longer duration cooling (120 hours), deeper cooling (32.0°C), or both are superior to cooling at 33.5°C for 72 hours in neonates who are full-term with moderate or severe hypoxic ischemic encephalopathy.

Design, Setting, and Participants.—A randomized, 2 × 2 factorial design clinical trial performed in 18 US centers in the Eunice Kennedy Shriver National Institute of Child Health and Human Development (NICHD) Neonatal Research Network between October 2010 and November 2013.

Interventions.—Neonates were assigned to 4 hypothermia groups; 33.5°C for 72 hours, 32.0°C for 72 hours, 33.5°C for 120 hours, and 32.0°C for 120 hours.

Main Outcomes and Measures.—The primary outcome of death or disability at 18 to 22 months is ongoing. The independent data and safety monitoring committee paused the trial to evaluate safety (cardiac arrhythmia, persistent acidosis, major vessel thrombosis and bleeding, and death in the neonatal intensive care unit [NICU]) after the first 50 neonates were enrolled, then after every subsequent 25 neonates. The trial was closed for emerging safety profile and futility analysis after the eighth review with 364 neonates enrolled (of 726 planned). This report focuses on safety and NICU deaths by marginal comparisons of 72 hours' vs 120 hours' duration and 33.5°C depth vs 32.0°C depth (predefined secondary outcomes).

Results.—The NICU death rates were 7 of 95 neonates (7%) for the 33.5°C for 72 hours group, 13 of 90 neonates (14%) for the 32.0°C for 72 hours group, 15 of 96 neonates (16%) for the 33.5°C for 120 hours group, and 14 of 83 neonates (17%) for the 32.0°C for 120 hours group. The adjusted risk ratio (RR) for NICU deaths for the 120 hours group vs 72 hours group was 1.37 (95% CI, 0.92-2.04) and for the 32.0°C group vs 33.5°C group was 1.24 (95% CI, 0.69-2.25). Safety outcomes were similar between the 120 hours group vs 72 hours group and the 32.0°C group vs 33.5°C group, except major bleeding occurred among 1% in the 120 hours group vs 3% in the 72 hours group (RR, 0.25 [95% CI, 0.07-0.91]). Futility analysis determined that the probability of detecting a statistically significant benefit for longer cooling, deeper cooling, or both for NICU death was less than 2%.

Conclusions and Relevance.—Among neonates who were full-term with moderate or severe hypoxic ischemic encephalopathy, longer cooling, deeper cooling, or both compared with hypothermia at 33.5°C for 72 hours did not reduce NICU death. These results have implications for patient care and design of future trials.

Trial Registration.—clinicaltrials.gov Identifier: NCT01192776.

▶ More is not always better. Since 1999, 5 randomized controlled trials have demonstrated improved outcomes among infants with acute hypoxic-ischemic neonatal encephalopathy who were treated with reduction in body or head temperature to 33°C to 34°C for 72 hours, yet approximately half of such infants still have significant permanent neurodevelopmental deficits. In search of alternatives that might reduce that disease burden, Shankaran and the Eunice Kennedy Shriver National Institute of Child Health and Human Development Neonatal Research Network asked whether longer or deeper cooling (or both) might be more effective. Because serial interim safety analyses revealed a small probability (<2%) that further enrollment would lead to identification of a s gnificant difference in mortality among treatment groups, the trial was closed after 364 of the planned 726 subjects. Although neither reached statistical significance, the odds ratios for mortality suggested that mortality may be increased by deeper (32°C) or longer (120 hours) hypothermia. Although predefined safety event rates did not differ among treatment groups, infants in the prolonged (120 hours) cooling group had more arrhythmias (7% vs 1%; $P = 0.02$), more anuria (9% vs 3%; $P = 0.01$), and longer hospital stays (mean 26.4 vs 21.6 days; $P = .002$), and those in the deeper cooling (32°C) group more frequently required nitric ode (34% vs 24%; $P = 0.03$) or extracorporeal membrane oxygenation (9% vs 4%; $P = .005$) and more days of supplemental oxygen (mean 8.8 vs 8.0; $P = 0.02$). These data raise substantial concerns that deeper or longer cooling regimens may result in worse, rather than better, outcomes, potentially including higher mortality rates. Happily for the many babies who have benefited from this treatment over the past decade and a half, the initial choice of temperature and duration for hypothermic treatment appears to have been at least very close to optimal.

W. E. Benitz, MD

Effect of Depth and Duration of Cooling on Deaths in the NICU Among Neonates With Hypoxic Ischemic Encephalopathy: A Randomized Clinical Trial

Shankaran S, for the Eunice Kennedy Shriver National Institute of Child Health and Human Development Neonatal Research Network (Wayne State Univ, Detroit, MI; et al)
JAMA 312:2629-2639, 2014

Importance.—Hypothermia at 33.5°C for 72 hours for neonatal hypoxic ischemic encephalopathy reduces death or disability to 44% to 55%; longer cooling and deeper cooling are neuroprotective in animal models.

Objective.—To determine if longer duration cooling (120 hours), deeper cooling (32.0°C), or both are superior to cooling at 33.5°C for 72 hours in neonates who are full-term with moderate or severe hypoxic ischemic encephalopathy.

Design, Setting, and Participants.—A randomized, 2 × 2 factorial design clinical trial performed in 18 US centers in the Eunice Kennedy Shriver National Institute of Child Health and Human Development (NICHD) Neonatal Research Network between October 2010 and November 2013.

Interventions.—Neonates were assigned to 4 hypothermia groups; 33.5°C for 72 hours, 32.0°C for 72 hours, 33.5°C for 120 hours, and 32.0°C for 120 hours.

Main Outcomes and Measures.—The primary outcome of death or disability at 18 to 22 months is ongoing. The independent data and safety monitoring committee paused the trial to evaluate safety (cardiac arrhythmia, persistent acidosis, major vessel thrombosis and bleeding, and death in the neonatal intensive care unit [NICU]) after the first 50 neonates were enrolled, then after every subsequent 25 neonates. The trial was closed for emerging safety profile and futility analysis after the eighth review with 364 neonates enrolled (of 726 planned). This report focuses on safety and NICU deaths by marginal comparisons of 72 hours' vs 120 hours' duration and 33.5°C depth vs 32.0°C depth (predefined secondary outcomes).

Results.—The NICU death rates were 7 of 95 neonates (7%) for the 33.5°C for 72 hours group, 13 of 90 neonates (14%) for the 32.0°C for 72 hours group, 15 of 96 neonates (16%) for the 33.5°C for 120 hours group, and 14 of 83 neonates (17%) for the 32.0°C for 120 hours group. The adjusted risk ratio (RR) for NICU deaths for the 120 hours group vs 72 hours group was 1.37 (95% CI, 0.92-2.04) and for the 32.0°C group vs 33.5°C group was 1.24 (95% CI, 0.69-2.25). Safety outcomes were similar between the 120 hours group vs 72 hours group and the 32.0°C group vs 33.5°C group, except major bleeding occurred among 1% in the 120 hours group vs 3% in the 72 hours group (RR, 0.25 [95% CI, 0.07-0.91]). Futility analysis determined that the probability of detecting a statistically significant benefit for longer cooling, deeper cooling, or both for NICU death was less than 2%.

Conclusions and Relevance.—Among neonates who were full-term with moderate or severe hypoxic ischemic encephalopathy, longer cooling, deeper cooling, or both compared with hypothermia at 33.5°C for 72 hours did not reduce NICU death. These results have implications for patient care and design of future trials.

Trial Registration.—clinicaltrials.gov Identifier: NCT01192776.

▶ It is now standard clinical practice to cool term infants with moderate to severe hypoxic-ischemic encephalopathy (HIE) to 33°C to 34°C for 72 hours. However, the choice of both the depth and duration of cooling used is based on best estimates from data derived in the course of preclinical studies. In fact, additional preclinical data suggest that both deeper and longer cooling may lead to a more beneficial outcome. In this randomized clinical trial, both strategies were incorporated in a factorial design. It should be noted that data collection pertaining to the primary outcome of the trial, death or moderate to severe neurodevelopmental disability at 18 to 22 months of age, has not yet been completed. However, the Eunice Kennedy Shriver National Institute of Child Health and Human Development Neonatal Research Network steering committee of principal investigators opted to report short-term secondary outcomes before the primary outcome of the trial was known to inform clinicians and other investigators of the apparent futility and potential harm of deeper cooling or longer duration of cooling compared with hypothermia at 33.5° for 72 hours.

L. A. Papile, MD

Association Between Early Administration of High-Dose Erythropoietin in Preterm Infants and Brain MRI Abnormality at Term-Equivalent Age

Leuchter RH-V, Gui L, Poncet A, et al (Univ Hosp of Geneva, Switzerland; et al)
JAMA 312:817-824, 2014

Importance.—Premature infants are at risk of developing encephalopathy of prematurity, which is associated with long-term neurodevelopmental delay. Erythropoietin was shown to be neuroprotective in experimental and retrospective clinical studies.

Objective.—To determine if there is an association between early high-dose recombinant human erythropoietin treatment in preterm infants and biomarkers of encephalopathy of prematurity on magnetic resonance imaging (MRI) at term-equivalent age.

Design, Setting, and Participants.—A total of 495 infants were included in a randomized, double-blind, placebo-controlled study conducted in Switzerland between 2005 and 2012. In a nonrandomized subset of 165 infants (n = 77 erythropoietin; n = 88 placebo), brain abnormalities were evaluated on MRI acquired at term-equivalent age.

Interventions.—Participants were randomly assigned to receive recombinant human erythropoietin (3000 IU/kg; n = 256) or placebo (n = 239) intravenously before 3 hours, at 12 to 18 hours, and at 36 to 42 hours after birth.

Main Outcomes and Measures.—The primary outcome of the trial, neurodevelopment at 24 months, has not yet been assessed. The secondary outcome, white matter disease of the preterm infant, was semiquantitatively assessed from MRI at term-equivalent age based on an established scoring method. The resulting white matter injury and gray matter injury scores were categorized as normal or abnormal according to thresholds established in the literature by correlation with neurodevelopmental outcome.

Results.—At term-equivalent age, compared with untreated controls, fewer infants treated with recombinant human erythropoietin had abnormal scores for white matter injury, white matter signal intensity, periventricular white matter loss, and gray matter injury.

Outcomes	No. (%) With Abnormal Score		Birth Weight–Adjusted Risk Ratio (95% CI)
	Erythropoietin Group (n = 77)	Placebo Group (n = 88)	
White matter injury	17 (22)	32 (36)	0.58 (0.35-0.96)
White matter signal intensity	2 (3)	10 (11)	0.20 (0.05-0.90)
Periventricular white matter loss	14 (18)	29 (33)	0.53 (0.30-0.92)
Gray matter injury	5 (7)	17 (19)	0.34 (0.13-0.89)

Reprinted from Leuchter RH-V, Gui L, Poncet A, et al. Association Between Early Administration of High-Dose Erythropoietin in Preterm Infants and Brain MRI Abnormality at Term-Equivalent Age. JAMA. 2014;312:817-824, Copyright 2014, American Medical Association. All rights reserved.

Conclusions and Relevance.—In an analysis of secondary outcomes of a randomized clinical trial of preterm infants, high-dose erythropoietin treatment within 42 hours after birth was associated with a reduced risk of brain injury on MRI. These findings require assessment in a randomized trial designed primarily to assess this outcome as well as investigation of the association with neurodevelopmental outcomes.

Trial Registration.—clinicaltrials.gov Identifier: NCT00413946.

▶ This is the initial report from the largest randomized controlled trial of erythropoietin for neuroprotection in extremely preterm infants completed to date, in which infants ≥26 and <32 weeks' gestation at birth were treated with 3 doses of erythropoietin (3000 IU) at <3 hours, 12 to 18 hours, and 36 to 48 hours after birth. It provides a description of neuroimaging results at term-equivalent age in convenience samples of subjects in each arm of the trial. Infants in the erythropoietin group were significantly less likely to have evidence of both white and gray matter injury, as assessed using a multicomponent scoring tool that is predictive of later neurodevelopmental outcomes, including cognitive delay, motor delay, and cerebral palsy.[1] Imaging data are available for only 165 of the 461 subjects in the trial (77 of 236 erythropoietin-treated subjects and 88 of 225 controls); others were excluded because of lack of access to magnetic resonance imaging at 3 of the 5 participating centers, lack of parent consent, or poor-quality images. This selection process has potential for introduction of bias with respect to imaging outcomes. Although the rates of abnormalities in imaging findings are lower in the treatment group, it remains uncertain whether their magnitude is sufficient to result in long-term impairments. The sample size may not be sufficient to detect differences in less common injury manifestations, and the short course of therapy may prove insufficient for achievement of long-term benefits. Data on neurodevelopmental outcomes from this trial are not yet available, but these preliminary data also provide further evidence of safety of this treatment. Mortality rates (12 of 236 vs 12 of 225, respectively) did not differ between treatment groups, and rates of major complications of prematurity (retinopathy of prematurity, sepsis, requirement for respiratory support) were similar in the 2 groups of infants in the imaging subset. Although these results are promising, it will be important to await results of comprehensive neurodevelopmental assessments before adoption of this treatment into clinical practice.

W. E. Benitz, MD

Reference

1. Woodward LJ, Anderson PJ, Austin NC, et al. Neonatal MRI to predict neurodevelopmental outcomes in preterm infants. *N Engl J Med.* 2006;355:685-694.

Association Between Early Administration of High-Dose Erythropoietin in Preterm Infants and Brain MRI Abnormality at Term-Equivalent Age

Leuchter RH-V, Gui L, Poncet A, et al (Univ Hosp of Geneva, Switzerland; et al)
JAMA 312:817-824, 2014

Importance.—Premature infants are at risk of developing encephalopathy of prematurity, which is associated with long-term neurodevelopmental delay. Erythropoietin was shown to be neuroprotective in experimental and retrospective clinical studies.

Objective.—To determine if there is an association between early high-dose recombinant human erythropoietin treatment in preterm infants and biomarkers of encephalopathy of prematurity on magnetic resonance imaging (MRI) at term-equivalent age.

Design, Setting, and Participants.—A total of 495 infants were included in a randomized, double-blind, placebo-controlled study conducted in Switzerland between 2005 and 2012. In a nonrandomized subset of 165 infants (n = 77 erythropoietin; n = 88 placebo), brain abnormalities were evaluated on MRI acquired at term-equivalent age.

Interventions.—Participants were randomly assigned to receive recombinant human erythropoietin (3000 IU/kg; n = 256) or placebo (n = 239) intravenously before 3 hours, at 12 to 18 hours, and at 36 to 42 hours after birth.

Main Outcomes and Measures.—The primary outcome of the trial, neurodevelopment at 24 months, has not yet been assessed. The secondary outcome, white matter disease of the preterm infant, was semiquantitatively assessed from MRI at term-equivalent age based on an established scoring method. The resulting white matter injury and gray matter injury scores were categorized as normal or abnormal according to thresholds established in the literature by correlation with neurodevelopmental outcome.

Results.—At term-equivalent age, compared with untreated controls, fewer infants treated with recombinant human erythropoietin had abnormal scores for white matter injury, white matter signal intensity, periventricular white matter loss, and gray matter injury.

Outcomes	No. (%) With Abnormal Score		Birth Weight–Adjusted Risk Ratio (95% CI)
	Erythropoietin Group (n = 77)	Placebo Group (n = 88)	
White matter injury	17 (22)	32 (36)	0.58 (0.35-0.96)
White matter signal intensity	2 (3)	10 (11)	0.20 (0.05-0.90)
Periventricular white matter loss	14 (18)	29 (33)	0.53 (0.30-0.92)
Gray matter injury	5 (7)	17 (19)	0.34 (0.13-0.89)

Reprinted from Leuchter RH-V, Gui L, Poncet A, et al. Association Between Early Administration of High-Dose Erythropoietin in Preterm Infants and Brain MRI Abnormality at Term-Equivalent Age. JAMA. 2014;312:817-824, Copyright 2014, American Medical Association. All rights reserved.

Conclusions and Relevance.—In an analysis of secondary outcomes of a randomized clinical trial of preterm infants, high-dose erythropoietin treatment within 42 hours after birth was associated with a reduced risk of brain injury on MRI. These findings require assessment in a randomized trial designed primarily to assess this outcome as well as investigation of the association with neurodevelopmental outcomes.

Trial Registration.—clinicaltrials.gov Identifier: NCT00413946.

▶ Major neurodevelopmental delays, such as learning and attention deficits during school age, cognitive delays, and cerebral palsy (CP), are common outcomes for extremely low birth weight (ELBW) infants, and successful neuroprotective interventions have yet to be developed. Erythropoiesis-stimulating agents (ESAs), such as erythropoietin (Epo) and darbepoetin (Darbe), have antiapoptotic, antiinflammatory, and trophic effects on neurons and oligodendrocytes and have the potential to mitigate injury during this critical window of development. Recent studies in animals and humans evaluating the nonhematopoietic effects of ESAs suggest a strong potential for neuroprotection via the above mechanisms.

Juan-Claude Fauchere and colleagues devised a randomized controlled trial of high-dose Epo administered within the first 48 hours of life, with a plan to evaluate developmental outcomes at 2 years. Although 2-year developmental testing has not been completed, Leuchter and colleagues published magnetic resonance imaging (MRI) data on a subset (77 of 229 Epo-treated and 88 of 219 placebo-treated) of Fauchere's high-dose Epo study infants who underwent MRI at term-equivalent age. Fewer Epo-treated infants had abnormal white matter or gray matter injury scores, and fewer had evidence of periventricular white matter loss. Although there were no significant differences between groups in any grade head ultrasound identified intracranial hemorrhage (ICH) in the original population (JC Fauchere, personal communication), it is unclear what percentage of those infants with ICH underwent MRI at term.

MRI performed at term-equivalent age has been proposed as a means of predicting neurodevelopmental outcomes; it remains to be seen if the subset of infants with MRI abnormalities also have cognitive delays. More importantly, the much anticipated developmental outcomes of the high-dose Epo study will add significantly to the current evidence that ESAs are neuroprotective in premature infants.

R. Ohls, MD

Brain Magnetic Resonance Imaging in Infants with Surgical Necrotizing Enterocolitis or Spontaneous Intestinal Perforation versus Medical Necrotizing Enterocolitis
Merhar SL, Ramos Y, Meinzen-Derr J, et al (Cincinnati Children's Hosp Med Ctr, OH)
J Pediatr 164:410-412, 2014

Magnetic resonance imaging of the brain was performed in 26 preterm infants with necrotizing enterocolitis (NEC) or spontaneous intestinal perforation at term equivalent age. Infants with surgical NEC or spontaneous intestinal perforation had significantly more brain injury on magnetic resonance imaging compared with infants with medical NEC, even after adjustment for confounders.

▶ This study of 26 preterm infants with necrotizing enterocolitis (NEC) or spontaneous intestinal perforation (SIP) substantiates previous studies (referenced in the article) that show differences in neurodevelopmental outcome in these infants (especially the ones requiring surgery) compared with infants who did not develop NEC.

As stated by the authors, this is small study, without control infants who did not have medical or surgical NEC as a comparison group. Thus it is not surprising that the medical NEC infants actually had better scores (lower injury) than the group containing all the infants. The diagnosis of medical NEC may not be as trivial as many think, and it is common that disagreements occur in the evaluation of radiographs by neonatologists and/or radiologists. Thus, whether the infants with medical NEC (Stage 2) were correctly diagnosed is a question, as is whether this actually represents necrosis or inflammation of the intestine. If not, then there would be no surprise that these infants had minimal if any MRI signs of central nervous system (CNS) injury. Is this valuable information? Probably so, because the need to follow infants closely with medical NEC in terms of neurodevelopmental outcomes would not be as great as the surgical infants.

In terms of the pathogenesis of the MRI findings, the authors discuss various theories, but it is possible that the same inciting stimulus that caused the infant to necessitate surgery for NEC/SIP may also be at the root of the abnormal MRI findings and might have caused CNS damage even without the episode of surgical NEC/SIP. Trying to dissect this experimentally will be a challenge but is worth further investigation.

J. Neu, MD

Prenatal unilateral cerebellar hypoplasia in a series of 26 cases: significance and implications for prenatal diagnosis
Massoud M, Cagneaux M, Garel C, et al (Université Claude Bernard Lyon I, France; Lyon et Hôpital Armand Trousseau, Paris, France; et al)
Ultrasound Obstet Gynecol 44:447-454, 2014

Objective.—To define imaging patterns of unilateral cerebellar hypoplasia (UCH), discuss possible pathophysiological mechanisms and underline the etiology and prognosis associated with these lesions.

Methods.—In this retrospective study we reviewed the charts of 26 fetuses diagnosed between 2003 and 2011 with UCH, defined by asymmetrical cerebellar hemispheres with or without decreased transverse cerebellar diameter. The review included analysis of the anatomy of the cerebellar hemispheres, including foliation, borders and parenchymal echogenicity, and of the severity of the hypoplasia. Data from clinical and biological work-up and follow-up were obtained.

Results.—Our series could be divided into two groups according to whether imaging features changed progressively or remained constant during follow-up. In Group 1 ($n = 8$), the progression of imaging features, echogenic cerebellar changes and/or hyposignal in T2*-weighted MR images were highly suggestive of ischemic/hemorrhagic insult. In Group 2 ($n = 18$), imaging features remained constant during follow-up; UCH was associated with abnormal foliation in three proven cases of clastic lesions, a cystic lesion was noted in three cases of PHACE (posterior fossa anomalies, hemangioma, arterial anomalies, cardiac abnormalities/aortic coarctation, eye abnormalities) syndrome and, in the remaining cases, UCH remained unchanged, with no imaging pattern typical of hemorrhage. In 24 cases the infant was liveborn and follow-up was continued in 23, for a mean period of 3 years. Among these, neurological complications were identified in seven (in one of seven (at a mean of 46 months) in Group 1 and in six of 16 (at a mean of 35 months) in Group 2). The surface loss of cerebellar hemisphere was >50% in 19/24 fetuses and the vermis was clearly normal in appearance in 19/24. Predisposing factors for fetal vascular insult were identified in eight cases: these included maternal alcohol addiction, diabetes mellitus, congenital cytomegalovirus infection and pathological placenta with thrombotic vasculopathy and infarctions.

Conclusion.—UCH is defined as a focal lesion of the cerebellum that may be secondary to hemorrhage and/or ischemic insult, suggesting a clastic origin, particularly when imaging follow-up reveals changes over time. UCH may also be a clue for the prenatal diagnosis of PHACE syndrome. The amount of surface loss of cerebellar hemisphere does not correlate with poor prognosis. UCH with normal vermis is often associated with normal outcome.

▶ This represents an interesting collection of cases over a long period of time with a number of take home messages. Advances in neuroimaging and genetic testing have greatly improved clinical diagnosis, counseling, and prognostic information for a variety of conditions including cerebellar hypoplasia.

Cerebellar hypoplasia (CH) refers to a cerebellum with a reduced volume and is a common, but nonspecific, neuroimaging finding. The etiological spectrum of CH is wide and includes both primary (malformative) and secondary (disruptive) conditions. The series described in this article fit well into this broad classification with progressive lesions due to vascular disruptions and a larger group with static lesions. There is an extensive differential diagnosis for cerebellar hypoplasia with an excellent review by Poretti et al.[1]

Cerebellar hypoplasia may be seen with chromosomal aberrations (eg, trisomy 13 and 18), metabolic disorders (eg, Smith-Lemli-Opitz syndrome, and adenylosuccinase deficiency), genetic syndromes (eg, CHARGE syndrome), and brain malformations (primary posterior fossa malformations, eg, Dandy-Walker malformation, pontine tegmental cap dysplasia, or global brain malformations such as tubulopathies and α-dystroglycanopathies). Secondary (disruptive) conditions include prenatal infections (eg, cytomegalovirus), exposure to teratogens, and extreme prematurity. Neuroimaging provides key information to categorize CH based on the pattern of involvement: unilateral CH, CH with mainly vermis involvement, global CH with involvement of both vermis and hemispheres, and pontocerebellar hypoplasia.

In this series, vascular disruptions were common, and diabetes, alcohol, and congenital infections played a role. The distinction between malformations and disruptions is important for counseling. Prognosis was better if the vermis was intact.

Overall, I was pleasantly surprised by the relatively good neurodevelopmental outcome, which speaks to the plasticity of the neonatal brain.

A. A. Fanaroff, MBBCh, FRCPE

Reference

1. Poretti A, Boltshauser E, Doherty D. Cerebellar hypoplasia: differential diagnosis and diagnostic approach. *Am J Med Genet C Semin Med Genet*. 2014;166C: 211-226.

Eye disorders in newborn infants (excluding retinopathy of prematurity)
Wan MJ, VanderVeen DK (Boston Children's Hosp, Boston, MA)
Arch Dis Child Fetal Neonatal Ed 100:F264-F269, 2015

A screening eye examination is an essential part of the newborn assessment. The detection of many ocular disorders in newborn infants can be achieved through careful observation of the infant's visual behaviour and the use of a direct ophthalmoscope to assess the ocular structures and check the red reflex. Early diagnosis and subspecialty referral can have a critical impact on the prognosis for many ocular conditions, including potentially blinding but treatable conditions such as congenital cataracts, life-threatening malignancies such as retinoblastoma and harbingers of disease elsewhere such as sporadic aniridia and its association with the development of Wilms tumour.

▶ This was an excellent review of ocular disorders of the newborn, complete with excellent color photographs of conditions such as leukocoria, corneal opacification, coloboma of the iris and eyelid, Horner's syndrome, and epiblepharon. The authors reinforce the importance of the screening eye examination and its importance in diagnosing treatable conditions to preserve visual function and avoid life-threatening conditions such as malignancies and systemic diseases. I strongly encourage neonatologists and pediatricians to read this review and keep a copy of it handy.

S. M. Donn, MD

The Pediatric Cataract Register (PECARE): analysis of age at detection of congenital cataract
Haargaard B, Nyström A, Rosensvärd A, et al (Glostrup Univ Hosp, Copenhagen, Denmark; Univ of Gothenburg, Sweden; St. Erik Eye Hosp, Stockholm, Sweden; et al)
Acta Ophthalmol 93:24-26, 2015

Purpose.—To analyse and discuss screening for the detection of congenital cataract in two Nordic countries, Denmark and Sweden.

Methods.—Until 2011, in Denmark, no guideline concerning screening for congenital cataract existed. Since 2011, Danish guidelines regarding eye examination include examination with a pencil light at age 5 weeks, whereas newborn red reflex examination using a handheld ophthalmoscope is routine protocol in Swedish maternity wards. Data regarding age of referral were derived from the Pediatric Cataract Register (PECARE). All children operated on before 1 year of age between January 2008 and December 2012 were included. Statistical comparison of the different screening strategies was made.

Results.—The number of children undergoing surgery for congenital cataract before 1 year of age was 31 (17 bilateral cases) in Denmark and 92 (38 bilateral cases) in Sweden. The proportion was 14 per 100.000 children in Denmark and 16 in Sweden ($p < 0.05$). There was a statistically significant difference between Denmark and Sweden in the percentage of children referred within 42 days of birth ($p < 0.0001$) and within 100 days ($p < 0.001$).

Conclusion.—Due to the screening procedure with red reflex examination, congenital cataract in Swedish children is detected significantly earlier than in Danish children (Fig 1).

▶ In this era of electronic monitoring, sophisticated automated screening for hearing deficits and heart disease, electronic recordkeeping, "-omics," "big data," and reliance on expert systems, it has become easy to lose sight of the importance of basic tools for patient assessment—and perhaps even fashionable to question their utility on the grounds that they have not been systematically

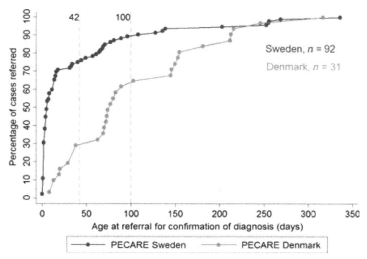

FIGURE 1.—The percentage of paediatric cataract cases referred to an ophthalmologist in relation to age at referral during the time period 2008—2012. (Reprinted from Haargaard B, Nyström A, Rosensvärd A, et al. The pediatric cataract register (PECARE): analysis of age at detection of congenital cataract. *Acta Ophthalmol.* 2015;93:24-26, Copyright 2015, Acta Ophthalmologica Scandinavica Foundation.)

evaluated and are therefore not "evidence based." Now and then, an opportunity arises to address that criticism, and this is a report of just such an opening. These authors have been able to evaluate the utility of evaluation of the pupillary red reflex as a standard component of the predischarge newborn examination by comparing referral patterns for infants with congenital cataracts in demographically similar Scandinavian countries that used disparate approaches to screening. In Sweden, assessment of the red reflex using a handheld ophthalmoscope has been a long-standing recommendation, with reported compliance in 90% of maternity wards.[1] In Denmark, no screening was recommended until adoption of examination with a small flashlight in 2011. The latter practice did not alter the age at referral compared with not screening at all. Ophthalmoscopic red reflex assessment was associated with much earlier referral for ophthalmological evaluation. In Sweden, nearly 70% of the cases were identified in the first 3 weeks after birth, compared with fewer than 20% in Denmark, where referrals predominantly occurred after well baby examinations at 2 and 4 months of age (Fig 1). This report does not include data on the timing of cataract surgery or long-term rates of amblyopia, which await further follow-up and analysis of patients in this binational registry. These data are compelling evidence of the utility of the old-fashioned physical examination in comprehensive screening of newborn infants for medical conditions, from cataracts to anal patency, and many things in between.

W. E. Benitz, MD

Reference

1. Magnusson G, Bizjajeva S, Haargaard B, Lundström M, Nyström A, Tornqvist K. Congenital cataract screening in maternity wards is effective: evaluation of the Paediatric Cataract Register of Sweden. *Acta Paediatr.* 2013;102:263-267.

Late Reconstruction of Brachial Plexus Birth Palsy
Sibbel SE, Bauer AS, James MA (Shriners Hosp for Children Northern California, Sacramento)
J Pediatr Orthop 34:S57-S62, 2014

Brachial plexus birth palsy (BPBP) presents to the physician on a clinical spectrum, and may substantially impair the child. Potential interventions to improve function for the child with BPBP include physical therapy, microsurgical nerve reconstruction and nerve transfers, soft-tissue balancing and reconstruction with musculotendinous transfers, and osteotomies. Some interventions, such as nerve reconstruction, are best performed in infancy; others, such as muscle transfers and osteotomies, are performed to treat manifestations of this condition that appear later in childhood. Although controversy continues to exist regarding the natural history and surgical management of these patients, recent literature has improved our understanding of surgical indications, anticipated outcomes, and potential complications. On the basis of current evidence, we present here the recommendations for surgical intervention in the upper extremity of children with BPBP, and encourage early referral to a brachial plexus specialist to establish care.

▶ Supination deformity of the forearm is an undesirable sequela of neonatal brachial plexus palsy (NBPP). Although surgical treatment of NBPP via nerve reconstruction experienced a lively revival in the 1990s, infants with more extensive or severe injury to the nerves of the brachial plexus (extending from spinal nerve roots C5-T1) during the perinatal period continue to suffer chronic muscular weakness/imbalance.[1-3] For example, weakness of the biceps brachii (innervated by nerve roots C5,6) and/or supinator muscle (C6,7) results in the inability to rotate the radius to turn the palm up which leads to consequent pronation posture and contractures. Similarly, weakness of the pronator teres (C6,7) and pronator quadratus (C7,8) results in the inability to turn the palm down, which leads to consequent supination posture and chronic deformity. Because forearm supination and pronation are complementary movements that allow humans to flip the palm up or down, the lack of either or both of these movements significantly affects activities of daily living and of normal childhood development (eg, feeding, biking, keyboarding).

Supination deformity typically begins as a "dynamic" deformity before progressing to a "fixed" disablement. Initially, the supination deformity is at a "dynamic" stage, during which the patients maintain passive supination range of motion (ROM) without significant active ROM; conservative treatment such as physical therapy or splinting is recommended at this stage to strengthen the agonist muscles or to loosen/weaken the antagonists.[4,5] However, chronic loss of passive supination ROM results in shortening of the interosseous membrane and in subsequent bony deformities comprising the "fixed" stage.[6,7] The appearance of dynamic or fixed forearm deformities has both physical and psychosocial ramifications. Decline in a developing child's self-confidence and decrease in the ability to participate in sporting or social events can lead to further chronic disablements. In both dynamic and fixed deformities, surgical intervention can ameliorate the lack of function and improve aesthetics. Common surgical treatments for supination deformity include forearm osteotomies, biceps rerouting, interosseous membrane release, tendon transfer, and combinations of these treatments. However, the indications for surgery, timing of surgery, type of procedure, recurrence rates, and especially the outcomes of surgery remain controversial.

In an attempt to provide treatment suggestions for supination deformity associated with NBPP, Metsaars et al conducted a timely systematic review and meta-analysis to evaluate the outcomes for patients with NBPP who underwent surgery for supination deformity.[8] However, the lack of randomized trials or comparable large cohort studies precluded an extensive analysis, consequently limiting the authors to a mere summary of the published data. Only 13 studies with primary outcomes on 238 patients (157 osteotomies and 71 biceps rerouting) were included in the review. Even with limited case series/report data, surgery resulted in significant improvements in the position of the forearm, with approximately 70 to 80% gains in pronation despite the complications of hardware failure, biceps rupture, and recurrence.

With regard to patient selection, patients with more severe deformities achieved better outcomes, but this statement should be considered within the context of the heterogeneity of preoperative descriptions of the patients within the included studies. However, this does make sense intuitively because patients with more severe deformity have more that they are capable of gaining through surgical intervention. This is not to say that patients with more severe deformity had better functional outcomes but rather that such patients achieved a higher degree of correction toward pronation. The authors suggest a supination deformity at rest of ≥60 degrees as a primary indication for surgery; additionally, they indicate that different degrees of passive ROM serve as the determinants for the specific type of procedure (osteotomy vs muscle rerouting), consistent with other reports. Although passive range of motion is important in determining the optimal surgical procedure, it should not be considered when deciding whether to surgically intervene. The decision to operate should be made solely on the basis of the degree of supination deformity at rest. Importantly, patients should be advised that the goal for surgery is to better position the forearm but not to increase active pronation, because the latter is not supported by published reports despite the type of procedure. With regard to the age of intervention, the authors were unable to provide any literature-supported guidelines. The suggestion of surgical intervention at 6 to 8 years is based solely on expert opinion when considering the functional needs of children starting school (consider that a supination deformity would preclude keyboard use), the compliance of the patient/family with postoperative therapy, and the stage (dynamic or fixed) of the supination deformity. With regard to adverse effects related to the type of procedure, the authors present a significant 20% to 40% recurrence rate in the osteotomy group but none in the biceps rerouting group. This may be because muscle growth/normal development could contribute to recurrence of deformity for younger children even after osteotomy procedure. This concept supports the addition of biceps rerouting to the forearm osteotomy for patients less than 6 years.

Finally, the assessment of outcomes after surgery for supination deformity deserves further exploration. The authors note the heterogeneity of the included studies and in the reporting of outcomes that may weaken the primary conclusion regarding the positive outcomes of surgical intervention for supination deformity. Little agreement exists among practitioners regarding the use of NBPP evaluation instruments in the current literature.[9] Valid and reliable evaluation instruments developed specifically for the NBPP population are significantly lacking, manifesting difficulties in evaluating the overall impact/effectiveness of clinical treatments in a consistent and comparative manner. Most, if not all, of the outcomes data reside within the International Classification of Function—Body Function and Structure domain, rather in the Activity and Participation domain.[10] Accordingly, the main outcome reported in the included articles is degree of deformity correction. There is little in the way of outcomes reporting with regard to functional use of the affected limb. It may be that using such outcomes would provide a more complete picture as to whether surgical intervention is beneficial. Nonetheless, previous studies have reported an improvement in wrist/finger extension and Raimondi score when the forearm is corrected into a more functionally pronated position.[2,11] Therefore, true outcomes after surgical intervention for supination deformity should consider all International Classification of Functioning domains, and future studies should comprise consideration of spontaneous (not practitioner-elicited) use of the affected arm in activities of daily living with attention to the psychosocial impact of the disablement.

Supination deformity in children with NBPP affects their daily activities, participation, and overall development. Any advances in understanding the indications for treatment, timing of intervention, and type of procedure leading to a positive outcome are welcomed by practitioners trying to prescribe treatment in a field with few guidelines. This study by Metsaars et al takes a significant step in this direction. Finally, a commentary regarding the primary condition underlying the supination deformity would be incomplete without mentioning the international variability in its name. Metsaars et al refer to this condition as "obstetric brachial plexus injury." This nomenclature implies an obstetrical causation/fault, although none may have occurred during the perinatal period. In fact, a recent survey of US-based practitioners demonstrated a strong (94%) preference for alternative terms, such as NBPP.[12]

K. W-C. Chang, MA
T. J. Wilson, MD
L. J-S. Yang, MD, PhD

References

1. Yang LJS, Chung KC, McGillicuddy JE, eds. Practical Management of Pediatric and Adult Brachial Plexus Palsies. 1st ed. London, United Kingdom: Elsevier Saunders; 2012.
2. Yam A, Fullilove S, Sinisi M, Fox M. The supination deformity and associated deformities of the upper limb in severe birth lesions of the brachial plexus. *J Bone Joint Surg Br.* 2009;91:511-516.
3. Yang LJ. Neonatal brachial plexus palsy—management and prognostic factors. *Semin Perinatol.* 2014;38:222-234.
4. Rasmussen L, Justice D, Chang KW, Nelson VS, Yang LJ. Home exercise DVD promotes exercise accuracy by caregivers of children and adolescents with brachial plexus palsy. *PM R.* 2013;5:924-930.
5. Wang AA, Hutchinson DT, Coleman DA. One-bone forearm fusion for pediatric supination contracture due to neurologic deficit. *J Hand Surg Am.* 2001;26:611-616.
6. Gilbert A, Brockman R, Carlioz H. Surgical treatment of brachial plexus birth palsy. *Clin Orthop Relat Res.* 1991:39-47.
7. Kozin SH. Treatment of the supination deformity in the pediatric brachial plexus patient. *Tech Hand Up Extrem Surg.* 2006;10:87-95.
8. Metsaars WP, Nagels J, Pijils BG, Langenhoff JM, Nelissen RG. Treatment of supination deformity for obstetric brachial plexus injury: a systematic review and meta-analysis. *J Hand Surg Am.* 2014;39:1948-1958.e2.
9. Chang KW, Justice D, Chung KC, Yang LJ. A systematic review of evaluation methods for neonatal brachial plexus palsy. *J Neurosurg Pediatr.* 2013 [Epub ahead of print].
10. World Health Organization. *International Classification of Functioning, Disability and Health: ICF.* Geneva, Switzerland: WHO; 2001.
11. Allende CA, Gilbert A. Forearm supination deformity after obstetric paralysis. *Clin Orthop Relat Res.* 2004:206-211.
12. Phua PD, Al-Samkari HT, Borschel GH. Is the term "obstetrical brachial plexus palsy" obsolete? an international survey to assess consensus among peripheral nerve surgeons. *J Plast Reconstr Aesthet Surg.* 2012;65:1227-1232.

9 Gastrointestinal Health and Nutrition

Intestinal Microbiota Development in Preterm Neonates and Effect of Perinatal Antibiotics
Arboleya S, Sánchez B, Milani C, et al (Instituto de Productos Lácteos de Asturias (IPLA), Villaviciosa, Asturias, Spain; Univ of Parma, Italy; et al)
J Pediatr 166:538-544, 2015

Objectives.—To assess the establishment of the intestinal microbiota in very low birthweight preterm infants and to evaluate the impact of perinatal factors, such as delivery mode and perinatal antibiotics.

Study Design.—We used 16S ribosomal RNA gene sequence-based microbiota analysis and quantitative polymerase chain reaction to evaluate the establishment of the intestinal microbiota. We also evaluated factors affecting the microbiota, during the first 3 months of life in preterm infants (n = 27) compared with full-term babies (n = 13).

Results.—Immaturity affects the microbiota as indicated by a reduced percentage of the family *Bacteroidaceae* during the first months of life and by a higher initial percentage of *Lactobacillaceae* in preterm infants compared with full term infants. Perinatal antibiotics, including intrapartum antimicrobial prophylaxis, affects the gut microbiota, as indicated by increased *Enterobacteriaceae* family organisms in the infants.

Conclusions.—Prematurity and perinatal antibiotic administration strongly affect the initial establishment of microbiota with potential consequences for later health.

▶ A majority of preterm very low birth weight infants are exposed to antibiotics, either before or shortly after birth or both.[1] Surveys in the United States show that the rate of culture-proven bacteremia in these infants is only between 1% and 2%.[1] Hence, a large number of preterm infants are being subjected to a course of antibiotics that may be of questionable value and even harmful.

The use of routine antibiotic prophylaxis during pregnancy to avoid adverse maternal and neonatal outcomes is also widespread despite a lack of evidence for efficacy.[2] Although the monetary cost of this preemptive and unproven measure is high, the cost in terms of antibiotic-induced harm has only recently been questioned. In the preterm neonate, the rationale often provided for this widespread use of antibiotics includes the immature immune system of these infants, the possibility that preterm delivery may have been caused by infection in the mother, and that the respiratory distress these infants undergo most often simply due to immaturity cannot be readily distinguished from pneumonia. The average length of treatment of this "standard of care" practice is between 5 and 7 days.[3] The rationale for such widespread antibiotic use is also partially based on opinions that use of intravenous antibiotics is safe or at the very least outweighs the benefits of not providing them. This is proving to be incorrect. Recent studies have shown an association between duration of early antibiotic use with increased odds of developing necrotizing enterocolitis,[3,4] a disease with extremely high mortality and morbidity.[5]

This study is highly pertinent to the foregoing concerns in that it compares the intestinal microbiota development in term versus preterm infants and compares the development of the intestinal microbiota over time in preterm infants exposed or not exposed to antibiotics. There are obvious differences in the taxa of microbes in term infants not exposed to antibiotics compared with the preterm infants. Within the preterm infant groups not exposed versus exposed to antibiotics, interesting differences are found at 10, 30, and 90 days showing that early antibiotics usage may result in long-term effects on the microbes present in the intestines of these infants.

There are several caveats to this study. The numbers of subjects (n) were very low. It is also difficult to control for the numerous potentially confounding factors such as feeding type, feeding amount, and delivery mode. Differences in gestational age (25 vs 32 weeks) may also result in variation between microbial colonization over time.

Nevertheless, the differences seen associated with antibiotic usage underline the fact that more studies are needed to determine the long-term effects on the host that may result from perturbations in the infant intestinal microbiota due to early antibiotic usage.

J. Neu, MD

References

1. Clark RH, Bloom BT, Spitzer AR, Gerstmann DR. Reported medication use in the neonatal intensive care unit: data from a large national data set. *Pediatrics.* 2006; 117:1979-1987.
2. Thinkhamrop J, Hofmeyr GJ, Adetoro O, Lumbiganon P, Ota E. Antibiotic prophylaxis during the second and third trimester to reduce adverse pregnancy outcomes and morbidity. *Cochrane Database Syst Rev.* 2015:CD002250.
3. Cotten CM, Taylor S, Stoll B, et al. Prolonged duration of initial empirical antibiotic treatment is associated with increased rates of necrotizing enterocolitis and death for extremely low birth weight infants. *Pediatrics.* 2009;123:58-66.
4. Alexander VN, Northrup V, Bizzarro MJ. Antibiotic exposure in the newborn intensive care unit and the risk of necrotizing enterocolitis. *J Pediatr.* 2011;159: 392-397.
5. Neu J, Walker WA. Necrotizing enterocolitis. *N Engl J Med.* 2011;364:255-264.

Bacteriological, Biochemical, and Immunological Properties of Colostrum and Mature Milk From Mothers of Extremely Preterm Infants

Moles L, Manzano S, Fernández L, et al (Universidad Complutense de Madrid, Spain; Probisearch, Tres Cantos, Spain; et al)
J Pediatr Gastroenterol Nutr 60:120-126, 2015

Objectives.—The objective of this work was to elucidate the influence of extremely premature birth (gestational age 24–27 weeks) on the microbiological, biochemical, and immunological composition of colostrum and mature milk.

Methods.—A total of 17 colostrum and 34 mature milk samples were provided by the 22 mothers of extremely preterms who participated in this study. Bacterial diversity was assessed by culture-based methods, whereas the concentration of lactose, glucose, and *myo*-inositol was determined by a gas chromatography procedure. Finally, the concentrations of a wide spectrum of cytokines, chemokines, growth factors, and immunoglobulins were measured using a multiplex system.

Results.—Bacteria were present in a small percentage of the colostrum and milk samples. Staphylococci, streptococci, and lactobacilli were the main bacterial groups isolated from colostrum, and they could be also isolated, together with enterococci and enterobacteria, from some mature milk samples. The colostrum concentrations of lactose and glucose were significantly lower than those found in mature milk, whereas the contrary was observed in relation to *myo*-inositol. The concentrations of most cytokines and immunoglobulins in colostrum were higher than in mature milk, and the differences were significant for immunoglobulin G3, immunoglobulin G4, interleukin (IL)-6, interferon-γ, interleukin-4 (IL-4), IL-13, IL-17, macrophage-monocyte chemoattractant protein-1 and macrophage inflammatory protein-1β.

Conclusions.—The bacteriological, biochemical, and immunological content of colostrum and mature milk from mothers of extremely preterm infants is particularly valuable for such infants. Efforts have to be made to try that preterm neonates receive milk from their own mothers or from donors matching, as much as possible, the gestational age of the preterm.

▶ We are progressing into an era of personalized medicine. In fact, a "Precision Medicine Coalition" (http://www.personalizedmedicinecoalition.org/) plans to allocate significant research funds for research related to this area. This is germane to the practice of neonatal intensive care in that we are increasingly beginning to recognize special qualities of human milk especially when derived from the infant's own mother at times that are synchronized with the infant.

This article nicely describes a comparative analysis of colostrum and mature milk derived from mothers of babies who delivered extremely preterm. The investigators were careful to avoid differentiation between foremilk and hindmilk by taking a representative aliquot of the entire feeding (2 mL). Several covariates were considered that included type of delivery, antibiotic and corticosteroid use, chorioamnionitis, and mother's age. Differences were found using culture-based techniques to identify the microbiota of the colostrum and mature milk samples. *Staphylococcus* species were borderline higher in colostrum, but *Lactobacillus*, *Enterococcus*, and *Enterobacteria* were higher in mature milk samples. The differences in microbes are of interest and may be germane to differential stimulation of the intestinal immune response at different stages of lactation and infant development.

Lactose and glucose were slightly higher in mature milk, the relevance of which is difficult to speculate. However, myoinositol was significantly higher in colostrum. Whether this teleologically may play a protective role in prevention of pathology such as lung disease or retinopathy is speculative. Various cytokines, chemokines, and hematopoietic stimuli differed significantly between colostrum and mature milk. Again, these differences are intriguing as well as hypothesis generating.

When we provide donor milk to infants in the neonatal intensive care unit, the microbes are largely removed, as are the live cellular elements and much of the enzymatic activity. Donor milk usually also is derived from mature milk rather than colostrum, hence has considerably different properties than colostrum. This needs to be kept in mind when we wait for long periods to enterally feed preterm infants and then use mature milk rather than colostrum. This study begs that we pay more attention to the maturity level of the milk that we provide to preterms, as well as do more investigation to better develop a more "personalized" approach to caring for these infants.

J. Neu, MD

Breast milk, microbiota, and intestinal immune homeostasis
Walker WA, Iyengar RS (MassGeneral Hosp for Children, Boston, MA)
Pediatr Res 77:220-228, 2015

Newborns adjust to the extrauterine environment by developing intestinal immune homeostasis. Appropriate initial bacterial colonization is necessary for adequate intestinal immune development. An environmental determinant of adequate colonization is breast milk. Although the full-term infant is developmentally capable of mounting an immune response, the effector immune component requires bacterial stimulation. Breast milk stimulates the proliferation of a well-balanced and diverse microbiota, which initially influences a switch from an intrauterine TH2 predominant to a TH1/TH2 balanced response and with activation of T-regulatory cells by breast milk–stimulated specific organisms (*Bifidobacteria, Lactobacillus*, and *Bacteroides*). As an example of its effect, oligosaccharides in breast milk are fermented by colonic bacteria producing an acid milieu for bacterial proliferation. In addition, short-chain fatty acids in breast milk activate receptors on T-reg cells and bacterial genes, which preferentially mediate intestinal tight junction expression and anti-inflammation. Other components of breast milk (defensins, lactoferrin, etc.) inhibit pathogens and further contribute to microbiota composition. The breast milk influence on initial intestinal microbiota also prevents expression of immune-mediated diseases (asthma, inflammatory bowel disease, type 1 diabetes) later in life through a balanced initial immune response, underscoring the necessity of breastfeeding as the first source of nutrition.

▶ This superb review article beautifully describes the evolution of intestinal immunity and the important role played by components of breast milk at every step in the process. It is a must-read for all who care for newborns.

L. J. Van Marter, MD, MPH

Bioactive peptides released from *in vitro* digestion of human milk with or without pasteurization
Wada Y, Lönnerdal B (Univ of California, Davis; et al)
Pediatr Res 77:546-553, 2015

Background.—Pasteurized donor human milk (HM) serves as the best alternative for breast-feeding when availability of mother's milk is limited. Pasteurization is also applied to mother's own milk for very low birth weight infants, who are vulnerable to microbial infection. Whether pasteurization affects protein digestibility and therefore modulates the profile of bioactive peptides released from HM proteins by gastrointestinal digestion, has not been examined to date.

Methods.—HM with and without pasteurization (62.5°C for 30 min) were subjected to *in vitro* gastrointestinal digestion, followed by peptidomic analysis to compare the formation of bioactive peptides.

Results.—Some of the bioactive peptides, such as caseinophosphopeptide homologues, a possible opioid peptide (or propeptide), and an antibacterial peptide, were present in undigested HM and showed resistance to *in vitro* digestion, suggesting that these peptides are likely to exert their bioactivities in the gastrointestinal lumen, or be stably transported to target organs. *In vitro* digestion of HM released a large variety of bioactive peptides such as angiotensin I-converting enzyme-inhibitory, antioxidative, and immunomodulatory peptides. Bioactive peptides were released largely in the same manner with and without pasteurization.

Conclusion.—Provision of pasteurized HM may be as beneficial as breast-feeding in terms of milk protein-derived bioactive peptides.

▶ Human milk, with its attendant beneficial properties is increasingly being used in the United States neonatal intensive care units (NICUs) for very low birth weight preterm infants. With recent American Academy of Pediatrics recommendations, donor milk is being recommended as a surrogate if infant's own mother's milk is not available. However, this donor milk is pasteurized, usually at 62.5°C for 30 minutes, to avoid potential milk-transmitted infections. This process is also used by some NICUs for infant's own mother's milk. Despite getting rid of certain bacteria and viruses, this treatment also is known to have effects on live cells (kills them), enzymes, immunomodulatory proteins, and hormones such as insulin.

This study evaluated the effects of pasteurization on human milk protein with and without *in vitro* digestion (acidic conditions, pH = 4 and enzymatic hydrolysis with porcine pepsin and pancreatin). The peptides were measured by liquid chromatography coupled with tandem mass spectrometry. Resulting peptides were searched for "bioactivities" using established databases.

The results showed that some of the proteins showed resistance to the digestion process. These proteins likely would also resist digestion in the upper GI tract and exert their effects in the intestinal lumen, on the intestinal surface or beyond. A large number of digestive products were found (more than double the amount of original proteins) that would be considered "bioactive" compared with primary structures on known databases. Caseins, lactalbumin, and lactoferrin and osteopontin were the major parent proteins evaluated. Many of the peptides measured were short peptide fragments. Those between 2 and 4 amino acid chain lengths were not evaluated.

The most important finding in this study is that peptides were released from digestion in the same manner with and without pasteurization. It is still unclear, however, what pasteurization does to the secondary, tertiary, and quaternary structure of these peptides and proteins, thus potentially negating their "bioactivity" so that simply finding the same amino acid sequence in a database may not correspond directly to the actual function of the protein or peptide. As the authors state in their conclusion, in vivo investigations are warranted to substantiate whether these peptides and proteins may actually exert their activities in an optimal manner after the pasteurization process.

J. Neu, MD

Human milk microRNA and total RNA differ depending on milk fractionation
Alsaweed M, Hepworth AR, Lefèvre C, et al (Univ of Western Australia, Crawley; Deakin Univ, Victoria, Australia; et al)
J Cell Biochem, 2015 [Epub ahead of print]

MicroRNA have been recently discovered in human milk signifying potentially important functions for both the lactating breast and the infant. Whilst human milk microRNA have started to be explored, little data exist on the evaluation of sample processing and analysis to ensure that a full spectrum of microRNA can be obtained. Human milk comprises three main fractions: cells, skim milk and lipids. Typically, the skim milk fraction has been measured in isolation despite evidence that the lipid fraction may contain more microRNA. This study aimed to standardize isolation of microRNA and total RNA from all three fractions of human milk to determine the most appropriate sampling and analysis procedure for future studies. Three different methods from eight commercially available kits were tested for their efficacy in extracting total RNA and microRNA from the lipid, skim and cell fractions of human milk. Each fraction yielded different concentrations of RNA and microRNA, with the highest quantities found in the cell and lipid fractions, and the lowest in skim milk. The column-based phenol-free method was the most efficient extraction method for all three milk fractions. Two microRNAs were expressed and validated in the three milk fractions by qPCR using the three recommended extraction kits for each fraction. High expression levels were identified in the skim and lipid milk factions for these microRNAs. These results suggest that careful consideration of both the human milk sample preparation and extraction protocols should be made prior to embarking upon research in this area.

▶ MicroRNAs (miRNAs) comprise approximately 22 nucleotide bases that are thought to play important roles in regulation of gene expression. They do this by targeting mRNAs by repression or cleavage. miRNAs have been found to be present in high abundance in milks of many species, including humans. At this juncture, we know little about the functional importance of these compounds in milk, but we do know that these are relatively stable molecules that appear to resist acid digestion at pH levels found in the stomach and appear to be small enough to be passively transported through the intestinal barrier.[1] The precise function of these molecules in breast milk is not known, but preliminary evidence suggests that they may play a role in increasing regulatory T cells, inducing B-cell differentiation, and thus may play a role in immunologic conditions such as allergy, atopy, and asthma.[1]

This article, although more of a methods development study, indicates that miRNAs in human milk are found primarily within cells or fat globules or other vesicles such as exosomes. The lipid fraction appears to be particularly rich in these compounds. The article also describes several aspects of analysis that need to be considered.

I consider this to be an exciting new area of human milk research. Is it possible that these molecules reflect the individual mother's diet and other environmental exposures that may offer special benefits primarily to her own infant? Are these compounds found in donor milk or formula? How do they differ from individual mothers' fresh milk samples? Does colostrum differ from the mature milk? What effects might these mRNAs have on the infant intestinal tract? The next few years of research into this area may yield interesting and highly practical results.

J. Neu, MD

Reference

1. Kosaka N, Izumi H, Sekine K, Ochiya T. microRNA as a new immune-regulatory agent in breast milk. *Silence*. 2010;1:7.

Enteral Granulocyte-Colony Stimulating Factor and Erythropoietin Early in Life Improves Feeding Tolerance in Preterm Infants: A Randomized Controlled Trial
El-Ganzoury MM, Awad HA, El-Farrash RA, et al (Ain Shams Univ, Cairo, Egypt)
J Pediatr 165:1140-1145, 2014

Objective.—To evaluate the efficacy and safety of enteral recombinant human granulocyte colony-stimulating factor (rhG-CSF) and recombinant human erythropoietin (rhEPO) in preventing feeding intolerance.

Study Design.—An interventional randomized control trial was conducted in 90 preterm infants born at ≤33 weeks gestational age. The neonates were assigned to 4 groups; 20 received rhG-CSF, 20 received rhEPO, 20 received both, and 30 received distilled water (placebo control). The test solution was given at the beginning of enteral feeding and was discontinued when enteral intake reached 100 mL/kg/day or after a maximum of 7 days, whichever came first. Feeding tolerance and adverse effects of treatment were assessed. Serum granulocyte colony-stimulating factor and erythropoietin levels were measured on days 0 and 7 of treatment.

Results.—All neonates tolerated the treatment without side effects. Neonates who received rhG-CSF and/or rhEPO had better feeding tolerance, as reflected by earlier achievement of 75 mL/kg/day, 100 mL/kg/day, and full enteral feeding of 150 mL/kg/day with earlier weight gain and a shorter hospital stay ($P < .05$). The risk of necrotizing enterocolitis was reduced from 10% to 0% in all treatment groups ($P < .05$). There was a shorter duration of withholding of feeding secondary to feeding intolerance among neonates receiving both rhG-CSF and rhEPO compared with those receiving placebo ($P < .05$). Serum levels of granulocyte colony-stimulating factor and erythropoietin at 0 and 7 days did not differ across the treatment groups.

Conclusions.—Enteral administration of rhG-CSF and/or rhEPO improves feeding outcome and decreases the risk of necrotizing enterocolitis in preterm neonates. The mechanism may involve the prevention of villous atrophy.

▶ Traditionally, when thinking about granulocyte colony-stimulating factor (GCSF) administration to preterm infants, you would be considering sepsis and neutropenia in which it has been shown to lower mortality.[1] Erythropoietin (EPO), in contrast, has been used successfully to reduce the need for blood transfusions and is being investigated as an adjuvant therapy for severe hypoxic ischemic encephalopathy.[2] These cytokines have diverse functions including maintenance of gut integrity and stimulation of growth of the intestinal villi when administered orally. Both these factors are present in amniotic fluid, which the fetus drinks in huge quantities, and human milk. The integrity and impermeability of the intestinal tract is maintained by tight junctions (TJs) formed between adjacent intestinal epithelial cells. Disruption of TJs and loss of barrier function is one of the mechanisms that are associated with a number of gastrointestinal diseases, including neonatal necrotizing enterocolitis (NEC).[3] As noted by the authors, human milk is protective against NEC, and the human milk factor EPO is protective of both endothelial cell-to-cell and blood–brain barriers. Shiou et al[4] demonstrated that EPO protects enterocyte barrier function by supporting expression of the TJ protein ZO-1.

This well-designed, if small, randomized controlled study from Egypt, supports these concepts of gut protection with a combination of GCSF and EPO. It was reassuring to see no side effects and many beneficial effects including shorter times to full feeds and shorter hospital stay. It was disappointing to learn how few of these babies received human milk. The study population is too small to get too excited about the absence of NEC in all the subjects, including the control population. However, this approach is worth pursuing. Indeed, the authors have begun pursuing this approach with a more complex product composed of a simulated amniotic fluid containing 115 mEq/L sodium chloride, 17 mEq/L sodium acetate 4 mEq/L potassium chloride, 225 ng/mL rhG-CSF, 4400 mU/mL rhEPO, and human serum albumin with a final concentration of 0.05%.

A. A. Fanaroff, MBBCh, FRCPE

References

1. Chaudhuri J, Mitra S, Mukhopadhyay D, Chakraborty S, Chatterjee S. Granulocyte colony-stimulating factor for preterms with sepsis and neutropenia: a randomized controlled trial. *J Clin Neonatol.* 2012;1:202-206.
2. Rangarajan V, Juul SE. Erythropoietin: emerging role of erythropoietin in neonatal neuroprotection. *Pediatr Neurol.* 2014;51:481-488.
3. Rogers EE, Bonifacio SL, Glass HC, et al. Erythropoietin and hypothermia for hypoxic-ischemic encephalopathy. *Pediatr Neurol.* 2014;51:657-662.
4. Shiou SR, Yu Y, Chen S, et al. Erythropoietin protects intestinal epithelial barrier function and lowers the incidence of experimental neonatal necrotizing enterocolitis. *J Biol Chem.* 2011;286:12123-12132.

Enteral Granulocyte-Colony Stimulating Factor and Erythropoietin Early in Life Improves Feeding Tolerance in Preterm Infants: A Randomized Controlled Trial
El-Ganzoury MM, Awad HA, El-Farrash RA, et al (Ain Shams Univ, Cairo, Egypt)
J Pediatr 165:1140-1145, 2014

Objective.—To evaluate the efficacy and safety of enteral recombinant human granulocyte colony-stimulating factor (rhG-CSF) and recombinant human erythropoietin (rhEPO) in preventing feeding intolerance.

Study Design.—An interventional randomized control trial was conducted in 90 preterm infants born at ≤33 weeks gestational age. The neonates were assigned to 4 groups; 20 received rhG-CSF, 20 received rhEPO, 20 received both, and 30 received distilled water (placebo control). The test solution was given at the beginning of enteral feeding and was discontinued when enteral intake reached 100 mL/kg/day or after a maximum of 7 days, whichever came first. Feeding tolerance and adverse effects of treatment were assessed. Serum granulocyte colony-stimulating factor and erythropoietin levels were measured on days 0 and 7 of treatment.

Results.—All neonates tolerated the treatment without side effects. Neonates who received rhG-CSF and/or rhEPO had better feeding tolerance, as reflected by earlier achievement of 75 mL/kg/day, 100 mL/kg/day, and full enteral feeding of 150 mL/kg/day with earlier weight gain and a shorter hospital stay ($P < .05$). The risk of necrotizing enterocolitis was reduced from 10% to 0% in all treatment groups ($P < .05$). There was a shorter duration of withholding of feeding secondary to feeding intolerance among neonates receiving both rhG-CSF and rhEPO compared with those receiving placebo ($P < .05$). Serum levels of granulocyte colony-stimulating factor and erythropoietin at 0 and 7 days did not differ across the treatment groups.

Conclusions.—Enteral administration of rhG-CSF and/or rhEPO improves feeding outcome and decreases the risk of necrotizing enterocolitis in preterm neonates. The mechanism may involve the prevention of villous atrophy.

▶ Despite ongoing advances in understanding of the underlying pathophysiology and clinical epidemiology of necrotizing enterocolitis (NEC), supplemented by occasional reports correlating particular practice changes with reduced rates of NEC in high-risk populations, reductions in attack rates have proven difficult to sustain. On the contrary, a recent report from a large clinical trials consortium suggests that mortality rates attributable to NEC may have increased over the last decade.[1] This small but well-designed and carefully executed randomized trial provides hope for changing this frustrating circumstance. The most important results are described in the abstract reproduced here, but a few additional details deserve attention. The infants in the 4 arms of the trial did not differ in gestational age (overall mean 30.5 weeks), birth weight (1.29 kg), age at initiation of feeding (2.0 days), or proportion fed only proprietary formula (37% overall; only 1 infant was fed human milk exclusively). The authors highlight the observed reduction in the rate of NEC from 10% (3 of 30) in the placebo group to 0% (0 of 20) in each of the 3 treatment groups; intergroup comparisons are statistically significant only after pooling data from the 3 treatment groups (0 of 60; $P = .013$ vs placebo); this does not appear to have been an a priori hypothesis and should therefore be viewed with some caution. Ancillary results suggest that this important result may be reproducible in larger trials, however. Comparing all treatment groups to the placebo group, the mean time to achievement of full feeding was reduced by 3.5 days (P values for group comparisons vs placebo 0.005, 0.032, and 0.006), number of days on which feedings were withheld by 4.9 days ($P = .05$, .59, and .037), and length of hospital stay by 14 days ($P < .001$ for all groups vs placebo). The authors report that serum levels of granulocyte colony-stimulating factor (G-CSF) and erythropoietin (EPO) on days 0 and 7 did not vary among treatment groups, but only data for the G-CSF and EPO + G-CSF groups are presented; a detailed comparison with the placebo group is not provided. No adverse effects of treatment were identified. These results may not generalize to facilities where exclusive use of human milk (maternal or donor) is the predominant practice. These observations encourage further investigation of this treatment, but general adoption should await results of adequately powered trials.

W. E. Benitz, MD

Reference

1. Patel RM, Kandefer S, Walsh MC, et al. Causes and timing of death in extremely premature infants from 2000 through 2011. *N Engl J Med.* 2015;372:331-340.

Influences of Breast Milk Composition on Gastric Emptying in Preterm Infants

Perrella SL, Hepworth AR, Simmer KN, et al (Univ of Western Australia, Crawley)
J Pediatr Gastroenterol Nutr 60:264-271, 2015

Objectives.—The aim of the present study was to determine whether specific biochemical and energy concentrations influence gastric emptying of unfortified and fortified mother's own milk (MOM) in stable preterm infants, and whether gastric emptying differs between feeds of unfortified MOM and feeds fortified with S-26 or FM 85 human milk fortifier (HMF) when infants are fed the same volume under similar conditions. Influences of infant gestation, age, and weight, and feed characteristics were also explored.

Methods.—Stomach volumes of 25 paired unfortified and fortified MOM feeds were monitored prefeed and postfeed delivery and at 30-minute intervals thereafter. For each feed, MOM samples were analyzed to determine concentrations of total protein, casein, whey, carbohydrate, lactose, fat, and energy. Fortified feed compositions were calculated by adding fortifier biochemical and energy concentrations to unfortified MOM concentrations. Ultrasound images were used to calculate infant stomach volumes. Statistical comparisons were made of paired stomach volume measurements.

Results.—Higher feed concentrations of casein were associated with faster gastric emptying during feed delivery ($P = 0.007$). When compared with unfortified MOM, S-26 fortified feeds emptied similarly, whereas FM 85 fortified feeds emptied more slowly both during feed delivery and during the postprandial period ($P = 0.002$, <0.001, respectively). Gastric emptying was slower for 2-hourly feeds compared with that for 3-hourly feeds ($P = 0.003$) and in supine position compared with that in prone ($P = 0.001$).

Conclusions.—Breast milk composition influences gastric emptying in stable preterm infants, with feeds of higher casein concentration emptying faster during feeding than otherwise equivalent feeds, and FM 85 fortified MOM emptying more slowly than unfortified MOM.

▶ Measurement of gastric volumes, critical to the determination of gastric emptying, has for a long time presented a challenge to clinicians. Availability of bedside ultrasound has potentially solved this dilemma and offers the means to study the factors that influence gastric emptying in the preterm infant. Perrella et al from Australia reported that for preterm infants serial gastric volumes are repeatable (within 2 mL) and ratings of intragastric echogenicity and curding are moderately consistent when fed milk of the same volume and composition.[1,2] In a series of reports, they concluded that gastric emptying during feed delivery is influenced with infant positioning, fortification of breast milk, and feeding frequency.[2,3] They concluded that breast milk composition influences gastric emptying in stable preterm infants, with feeds of higher casein concentration emptying faster during feeding than otherwise equivalent feeds, and the FM 85 human milk fortifier, fortified mother's own milk (MOM), emptying more slowly than unfortified MOM.

The study abstracted here was designed to determine the specific effects of components of MOM compared with fortified milk on gastric emptying. Gastric emptying was slower for 2-hourly feeds compared with that for 3-hourly feeds and in supine position compared with that in prone. The amount of casein in the feed was also influential on gastric emptying.

Motility of the gastrointestinal tract or lack thereof in preterm infants has long been a thorny issue. Having the ability to minimally invasively monitor gastric emptying together with the knowledge of the factors that influence gastric emptying should facilitate management of this problem. We are indebted to this team from Western Australia for this excellent series of studies.

A. A. Fanaroff, MBBCh, FRCPE

References

1. Perrella SL, Hepworth AR, Simmer KN, Hartmann PE, Geddes DT. Repeatability of gastric volume measurements and intragastric content using ultrasound in preterm infants. *J Pediatr Gastroenterol Nutr.* 2014;59:254-263.
2. Perrella SL, Hepworth AR, Simmer KN, Geddes DT. Validation of ultrasound methods to monitor gastric volume changes in preterm infants. *J Pediatr Gastroenterol Nutr.* 2013;57:741-749.
3. Perrella SL, Hepworth AR, Gridneva Z, Simmer KN, Hartmann PE, Geddes DT. Gastric emptying and curding of pasteurized donor human milk and mother's own milk in preterm infants. *J Pediatr Gastroenterol Nutr.* 2015 [Epub ahead of print].

Influences of Breast Milk Composition on Gastric Emptying in Preterm Infants
Perrella SL, Hepworth AR, Simmer KN, et al (Univ of Western Australia, Crawley)
J Pediatr Gastroenterol Nutr 60:264-271, 2015

Objectives.—The aim of the present study was to determine whether specific biochemical and energy concentrations influence gastric emptying of unfortified and fortified mother's own milk (MOM) in stable preterm infants, and whether gastric emptying differs between feeds of unfortified MOM and feeds fortified with S-26 or FM 85 human milk fortifier (HMF) when infants are fed the same volume under similar conditions. Influences of infant gestation, age, and weight, and feed characteristics were also explored.

Methods.—Stomach volumes of 25 paired unfortified and fortified MOM feeds were monitored prefeed and postfeed delivery and at 30-minute intervals thereafter. For each feed, MOM samples were analyzed to determine concentrations of total protein, casein, whey, carbohydrate, lactose, fat, and energy. Fortified feed compositions were calculated by adding fortifier biochemical and energy concentrations to unfortified MOM concentrations. Ultrasound images were used to calculate infant stomach volumes. Statistical comparisons were made of paired stomach volume measurements.

Results.—Higher feed concentrations of casein were associated with faster gastric emptying during feed delivery ($P = 0.007$). When compared with unfortified MOM, S-26 fortified feeds emptied similarly, whereas FM 85 fortified feeds emptied more slowly both during feed delivery and during the postprandial period ($P = 0.002, <0.001$, respectively). Gastric emptying was slower for 2-hourly feeds compared with that for 3-hourly feeds ($P = 0.003$) and in supine position compared with that in prone ($P = 0.001$).

Conclusions.—Breast milk composition influences gastric emptying in stable preterm infants, with feeds of higher casein concentration emptying faster during feeding than otherwise equivalent feeds, and FM 85 fortified MOM emptying more slowly than unfortified MOM.

▶ One of the most vexing problems in caring for low birth weight preterm infants in the neonatal intensive care unit (NICU) is the baby who presents with feeding intolerance. We often resort to pharmacologic therapy without giving much thought about relatively simple adjustments such as positioning, timing of feedings, and composition of feedings. Although many NICUs are attempting to feed these infants their own mother's milk or donor milk, the protein and mineral composition is inadequate to meet the requirements for these rapidly growing infants, thus they often are supplemented by fortifiers. Each infant's own mother's milk may also differ over time and from other mothers' milk.

The intestine at different developmental stages may respond quite differently to the composition of feedings. This study evaluated the effects of various compositional differences on gastric emptying using an ultrasound-based equation that evaluated residual gastric volume. A higher concentration of casein was associated with faster gastric emptying. A fortifier that utilized extensively hydrolyzed whey resulted in more rapid emptying than a 40:60 casein whey mixture. Every 2-hour feedings compared with 3-hour feedings resulted in more gastric contents remaining in the stomach (13.4% higher). The supine position resulted in slower emptying than the prone. Not surprising, continuous positive airway pressure resulted in a 36% greater gastric volume retained compared with those not receiving respiratory support. Unfortified feeds resulted in faster gastric emptying of almost 2 times that of one of the fortified preparations. This could have been due to higher osmolality of this feeding preparation.

The effects seen in this study should provide us with considerations for simple alterations that may improve feeding tolerance.

J. Neu, MD

A randomised trial of re-feeding gastric residuals in preterm infants

Salas AA, Cuna A, Bhat R, et al (Univ of Pennsylvania, Philadelphia; Univ of Missouri-Kansas City; Univ of Maryland, Baltimore; et al)
Arch Dis Child Fetal Neonatal Ed 100:F224-F228, 2015

Objective.—To determine whether re-feeding of gastric residual volumes reduces the time needed to achieve full enteral feeding in preterm infants.

Design.—Parallel-group randomised controlled trial with a 1:1 allocation ratio.
Setting.—Regional referral neonatal intensive care unit.
Patients.—72 infants of gestational age $23^{0/7}$ to $28^{6/7}$ weeks receiving minimal enteral nutrition (<24 mL/kg/day) during the first week after birth.
Interventions.—Infants were randomised to either be re-fed with gastric residual volumes (Re-feeding group) or receive fresh formula/human milk (Fresh-feeding group) whenever large gastric residual volumes were noted.
Main Outcome Measure.—The primary efficacy end point was time to achieve full enteral feeding (≥ 120 mL/kg/day) after randomisation.
Results.—The mean time to full enteral feeding was 10.0 days in the Re-feeding group and 11.3 days in the Fresh-feeding group (mean difference favouring re-feeding: -1.3 days; 95% CI -2.9 to 0.3; $p = 0.11$). The composite safety end point of spontaneous intestinal perforation, surgical necrotising enterocolitis, or death occurred in 6 of 36 infants (17%) in the Re-feeding group versus 10 of 36 infants (28%) in the Fresh-feeding group ($p = 0.26$).
Conclusions.—Re-feeding gastric residual volumes in extremely preterm infants does not reduce time to achieve full enteral feeding. This trial suggests that re-feeding might be as safe as fresh feeding, but further research is needed, due to lack of sufficient statistical power in this study for safety analysis.
Trial Registration Number.—NCT01420263NCT01420263.

▶ Neonatal intensive care has long concentrated on the lung, the heart, the brain, and prevention of infection. Despite nutrition playing a critical role in brain development, the attitude toward enteral nutrition has been rather casual and perhaps even indifferent with the thought that parenteral nutrition will tide them over the critical period. During the past decade, there has been intense focus on establishing enteral nutrition with human milk and starting minimal gut stimulation as soon as possible after birth.

Nonetheless, feeding intolerance or gastric immotility, defined as the inability to digest enteral feedings associated with increased gastric residuals (GR), abdominal distension, and/or emesis, is commonplace in preterm infants. This results in discontinuation of feeds and reevaluation of the feeding protocol. Concerns for necrotizing enterocolitis make what is most commonly a benign condition a cause of major concern. Which brings us to the question at hand: What to do with gastric residuals? Should we even be measuring gastric residuals? Well, we move from the art of feeding to the science of feeding. New data, however, generated in these randomized trials, will help to move these questions to the evidence-based side of neonatal care.

Li, working with my editorial colleague Josef Neu,[1] in their review point out that "It is routine practice in most neonatal intensive care units to measure the volume and color of gastric residuals (GRs) prior to enteral bolus feedings in preterm very low birth weight infants. However, there is paucity of evidence supporting the routine use of this technique. Moreover, owing to the lack of uniform standards in the management of GRs, wide variations exist as to what constitutes significant GR volume, the importance of GR color and frequency of GR evaluation, and the color or volume standards that dictate discarding or returning GRs. The presence of large GR volumes or green-colored residuals prior to feeding often prompts subsequent feedings to be withheld or reduced because of possible necrotizing enterocolitis resulting in delays in enteral feeding." The alternative is to abandon the practice of GR evaluation, a practice for which there is little evidence.

Salas's report indicates that refeeding old GR or fresh human milk did not affect time to full enteral feeds. They of course call for more randomized trials. By aspirating gastric contents, Chen[2] showed that prone position resulted in more rapid clearing of GRs. Unfortunately, the evidence remains skimpy, and feeding will continue to be an art, not a science.[3] My bias is that it is unnecessary to measure residuals in the absence of spitting or distension, but it is just a gut feeling.

A. A. Fanaroff, MBBCh, FRCPE

References

1. Li YF, Lin HC, Torrazza RM, Parker L, Talaga E, Neu J. Gastric residual evaluation in preterm neonates: a useful monitoring technique or a hindrance? *Pediatr Neonatol.* 2014;55:335-340.
2. Chen SS, Tzeng YL, Gau BS, Kuo PC, Chen JY. Effects of prone and supine positioning on gastric residuals in preterm infants: a time series with cross-over study. *Int J Nurs Stud.* 2013;50:1459-1467.
3. Su BH, Lin HY, Huang FK, Tsai ML. Gastric residuals, feeding intolerance, and necrotizing enterocolitis in preterm infants. *Pediatr Neonatol.* 2015;56:136-137.

Abdominal Circumference or Gastric Residual Volume as Measure of Feed Intolerance in VLBW Infants
Kaur A, Kler N, Saluja S, et al (Sir Ganga Ram Hosp, New Delhi, India)
J Pediatr Gastroenterol Nutr 60:259-263, 2015

Background.—The aim of the study was to compare prefeed abdominal circumference (AC) and gastric residual volume (GRV) as a measure of feed intolerance in very-low-birth-weight infants (VLBW).

Methods.—Eighty VLBW infants were randomized to 2 groups; feed intolerance was monitored by measuring either GRV group or prefeed AC group. The primary outcome was time to full enteral feeds (180 mL·kg^{-1}·day^{-1}). Other main outcome measures were feed interruption days, duration of parenteral nutrition, incidence of culture positive sepsis, necrotizing enterocolitis, mortality, and duration of hospital stay.

Results.—The median (interquartile range) time to achieve full feeds was 10 (9–13) versus 14 (12–17.5) days in AC and GRV groups, respectively ($P < 0.001$). Infants in AC group had fewer feed interruption days (0 [0–2] vs 2.0 [1, 5], $P < 0.001$) and shorter duration of parenteral nutrition ($P < 0.001$). The incidence of culture-positive sepsis in AC and GRV groups was 17.5% and 30%, respectively ($P = 0.18$). Duration of hospital stay and mortality were comparable in both the groups.

Conclusions.—Prefeed AC as a measure of feed intolerance in VLBW infants may shorten the time taken to achieve full feeds.

▶ Measurement of gastric residual volumes just before gavage feedings of very low birth weight (VLBW) infants is deeply ingrained in the culture of neonatal intensive care. Increased gastric residuals are commonly believed to be a sign of feeding intolerance and are often cited as an early warning sign of impending necrotizing enterocolitis (NEC). The origins of these beliefs are obscure, and there is surprisingly little evidence to support them. More than a decade ago, Mihatsch et al found that gastric residual volumes were not predictive of the volume of enteric feedings achieved at 14 days of age[1] and suggested that a more tolerant stance toward gastric residuals might be warranted. Now this randomized trial confirms that reliance on abdominal circumference measurements rather than gastric residuals for assessment of feeding tolerance in VLBW infants results in more rapid achievement of full enteral feeding volumes, fewer days of parenteral nutrition, and fewer episodes of and days of feeding interruption because of perceived feeding intolerance. The sample size was not adequate to assess effects on rates of NEC, sepsis, or mortality, but there was no suggestion that the risk of these outcomes might be increased. Although the stated objective of this trial was to assess the utility of abdominal circumference as a tool for assessment of feeding tolerance, no data relating changes in those measurements to predict feeding problems or to correlate them with the risk of other adverse outcomes is provided, so those measurements may actually have been simply uninformative. Indeed, data from a similar but smaller trial of elimination of gastric residual measurements[2] suggests that the differences observed in this trial may reflect inadequacies of gastric residual measurements more than efficacy of abdominal circumference measurements. Although the numbers of subjects in these trials is small, they are sufficient to establish that gastric residual measurements fail to meet one of the prime requirements for a screening test: a low false-positive rate. Because large gastric residuals are nonspecific, they lead to unnecessary interruptions of and delays in advancement of feedings in VLBW infants. Until well-designed trials establish thresholds for concern and demonstrate utility in management of VLBW infants, our patients are likely to be better off without performance of routine gastric residual measurements.

W. E. Benitz, MD

References

1. Mihatsch WA, von Schoenaich P, Fahnenstich H, et al. The significance of gastric residuals in the early enteral feeding advancement of extremely low birth weight infants. *Pediatrics*. 2002;109:457-459.
2. Torrazza RM, Parker LA, Li Y, Talaga E, Shuster J, Neu J. The value of routine evaluation of gastric residuals in very low birth weight infants. *J Perinatol*. 2015;35:57-60.

Breast-Feeding Improves Gut Maturation Compared With Formula Feeding in Preterm Babies

Reisinger KW, de Vaan L, Kramer BW, et al (Maastricht Univ Med Ctr, The Netherlands)
J Pediatr Gastroenterol Nutr 59:720-724, 2014

Objective.—The incidence of necrotizing enterocolitis (NEC) is higher in formula-fed babies than in breast-fed babies, which may be caused by breastfeeding− induced gut maturation. The effect of breast-feeding on gut maturation has been widely studied in animal models. This study aimed to assess the effects of breast-feeding on intestinal maturation in prematurely born babies by evaluating postnatal changes in urinary intestinal fatty acid binding protein (I-FABP) levels, a specific enterocyte marker.

Methods.—Gut maturation in 40 premature babies (<37 weeks of gestation) without gastrointestinal morbidity was studied, of whom 21 were exclusively breast-fed and 19 were formula-fed infants. Urinary I-FABP levels as the measure of gut maturation were measured at 5, 12, 19, and 26 days after birth.

Results.—In breast-fed infants, there was a significant increase in median urinary I-FABP levels between 5 and 12 days after birth (104 [78−340] pg/ mL to 408 [173−1028] pg/mL, $P = 0.002$), whereas I-FABP concentration in formula-fed infants increased between 12 and 19 days after birth (105 [44−557] pg/mL, 723 [103−1670] pg/mL, $P = 0.004$). Breast-fed babies had significantly higher median urinary I-FABP levels at postnatal day 12 ($P = 0.01$).

Conclusions.—The time course of the postnatal increase in urinary I-FABP levels reflecting gut maturation was significantly delayed in formula-fed babies, suggesting a delayed physiological response in formula-fed compared with breast-fed infants.

▶ The gastrointestinal (GI) tract is a multipurpose organ with a prime function for digestion and absorption of nutrients, but it also serves as a major bacterial repository—the GI biome, and performs major endocrine, neural, and immunologic functions. For example, Rehfeld pointed out that "Gastrointestinal hormones are peptides released from endocrine cells and neurons in the digestive tract. More than 30 hormone genes are currently known to be expressed in the gastrointestinal tract, which makes the gut the largest hormone producing organ in the body."[1] The maturity of the GI tract determines whether the nutritional needs of the preterm infant can be accomplished enterally or require additional parenteral nutrition with its attendant risks. Enteral nutrition is of major importance for the growth and development of the GI tract, which depends on the amount and composition of feeds. We also remain acutely aware that the brain of very low birth weight infants is particularly vulnerable to under nutrition. Any discussion on the immature GI tract inevitably turns to necrotizing enterocolitis. This article is no exception, and the benefits of human milk are highlighted.

The high prevalence worldwide of enteric diseases and dysfunction in neonates has led to much interest in understanding the role of nutrients and food components, especially human milk, in the maintenance and functioning of the GI tract. Despite the major limitations of a single-center study with significant loss of the cohort by 19 days such that statistical significance at this time cannot be determined, I found the concepts expressed to be intriguing. The article introduced me to the role of intestinal fatty acid-binding protein (I-FABP) as an indicator of gut maturity.[2] I-FABP is a small cytosolic protein, exclusively present in mature enterocytes of the small intestine and colon. It is released into the circulation when enterocytes detach from villi at the end of their life span and pass the glomerular filter so they can be measured in the urine. Human milk, rich in I-FABP when compared with formula, accelerates gut maturation, which occurs at least a week earlier than in formula-fed infants. No doubt more studies exploring the ways and means of maturing the gastrointestinal tract and modifying the biome will be forthcoming, and multiple factors will be found to play roles. Putting together the pieces of the puzzle will enable enhanced nutrition and better outcomes for all infants.

A. A. Fanaroff, MBBCh, FRCPE

References

1. Rehfeld JF. Gastrointestinal hormones and their targets. *Adv Exp Med Biol.* 2014; 817:157-175.
2. Reisinger KW, Elst M, Derikx JP, et al. Intestinal fatty acid-binding protein: a possible marker for gut maturation. *Pediatr Res.* 2014;76:261-268.

Randomized Trial of Human Milk Cream as a Supplement to Standard Fortification of an Exclusive Human Milk-Based Diet in Infants 750-1250 g Birth Weight

Hair AB, Blanco CL, Moreira AG, et al (Texas Children's Hosp, Houston; Univ of Texas Health Science Ctr, San Antonio; et al)

J Pediatr 165:915-920, 2014

Objective.—To evaluate whether premature infants who received an exclusive human milk (HM)-based diet and a HM-derived cream supplement (cream) would have weight gain (g/kg/d) at least as good as infants receiving a standard feeding regimen (control).

Study Design.—In a prospective noninferiority, randomized, unmasked study, infants with a birth weight 750-1250 g were randomly assigned to the control or cream group. The control group received mother's own milk or donor HM with donor HM-derived fortifier. The cream group received a HM-derived cream supplement if the energy density of the HM tested <20 kcal/oz using a near infrared HM analyzer. Infants were continued on the protocol until 36 weeks postmenstrual age. Primary outcomes included growth velocities and amount of donor HM-derived fortifier used. The hypothesis of noninferiority was established if the lower bound of the one-sided 95% CI for the difference in weight velocities exceeded -3 g/kg/day.

Results.—There were no differences between groups in baseline demographics for the 78 infants studied except racial distribution (P =.02). The cream group (n = 39) had superior weight (14.0 ± 2.5 vs 12.4 ± 3.0 g/kg/d, P =.03) and length (1.03 ± 0.33 vs 0.83 ± 0.41 cm/wk, P =.02) velocity compared with the control group (n = 39). There were no significant differences in amount of fortifier used between study groups. The 1-sided 95% lower bound of the CI for the difference in mean velocity (cream-control) was 0.38 g/kg/d.

Conclusions.—Premature infants who received HM-derived cream to fortified HM had improved weight and length velocity compared with the control group. HM-derived cream should be considered an adjunctive supplement to an exclusive HM-based diet to improve growth rates in premature infants.

▶ This study, a Randomized Trial of Human Milk Cream as a Supplement to Standard Fortification of an Exclusive Human Milk-Based Diet in Infants 750-1250 g Birth Weight, evaluated the use of a human milk-derived cream (standardized to 25% lipids with 2.5 kcal/mL, mean 12.5 calories/kg). The cream group received the same standard feeding regimen but with the addition of the donor human milk-derived cream supplement. The study used human milk analyses once fortified feeds were tolerated using the human milk-derived fortifier. A near-infrared analyzer was used to determine the caloric content of a daily 24-hour batch sample, but the information was not available to the investigators at the study sites.[1] They found an increase in weight velocity of 1.6 g/k/d and length gain velocity of 0.17 cm/wk associated with the addition of the cream.[1]

Infants in this study received either their own mother's milk or donor human milk. There are a number of studies that suggest there is tremendous variability among macronutrient composition among the milks of mothers of premature infants, and donor milk may be especially low in protein and fat. The high variability in nutrient content makes meeting nutrient recommendations inherently inaccurate. Milk composition varies with volume of milk expressed, the type of milk obtained (foremilk or hind milk), and the stage of lactation. For example, 2-fold to 3-fold differences in protein, fat, and hence energy have been demonstrated.[2,3] Additionally, the milk from a woman delivering prematurely has a decreasing protein content with the duration of lactation. We found among 85 samples of preterm human milk at varying stages of lactation that 31% of the samples were below 18 calories per ounce and 14% were below 16 calories per ounce.[3] However, is this the answer—to routinely add energy to promote growth? What about considerations of body composition? When you add energy alone, you decrease the protein/energy ratio, which influences body leanness or adiposity.

Fortification strategies include standard fixed dosage or blind fortification, adjustable based on blood urea nitrogen (BUN) as a surrogate for protein nutriture and targeted or individualized, customized fortification. Protein is limiting for growth, and it is essential for optimal neurodevelopment.[4] Adequate protein fortification of human milk is therefore critical. Did the infants in either group of this study receive enough protein?

Standardized fortification assumes an average composition of breast milk that is being fortified and then adding a fixed dosage of fortifier. The variability in content of milk is not taken into account, and inadequate protein intake is typical, as is less than optimal energy.[5] The changing protein content of preterm milk over lactation makes fortification challenging without analyses or another strategy. Fortifiers make an assumption that the protein concentration of the milk will be approximately 1.4 g/dL to be able to label the product as to the ultimate protein concentration achieved by addition of the fortifier. Donor milk is not nearly as variable but provides a much lower protein intake (0.9-1.0 g/dL). Therefore, it is difficult if not impossible to meet the protein requirements with standard fortification.

Adjustable fortification using BUN as a surrogate for protein nutriture uses metabolic response to feeding.[6] Serial determinations of BUN allow the provision of additional protein to the standard fortification regimen, analogous to the study reviewed in this review except that additional protein is provided based on metabolic response rather than blindly. In the adjustable fortification study, weight gain velocity was 4 g/k/d greater and head circumference velocity was 0.7 cm/week greater.[6]

The third strategy is targeted with analyses of human milk to guide supplementation. We have shown the possibilities of such an approach by demonstrating how this technique could be used on a number of samples of milk from our pool of preterm milk samples from mothers and a donor pool.[5] A recent study showed excellent growth among both routinely fortified very low-birth-weight infants and those whose milk was adjusted with all 3 macronutrients based on a 12-hour daily batch human milk analyses. The milk samples were obtained on 10 study infants and 20 matched fortified controls who did not receive any supplement.[6] There were 650 pooled samples of human milk, and all of them required at least 1 macronutrient adjustment to meet European Society for Paediatric Gastroenterology Hepatology and Nutrition requirements for the macronutrients as the goal for supplementation.[6]

In an editorial, Bill Hay asked the question, "Would an additional 1 g/k/d of protein be too much for these infants in whom the mother has good protein content?"[5] He concluded this was not likely, that many measurements of human milk protein consistently show levels of protein in mothers' milk for preterm infants to be below 2 g/dL.[3] Adding a 1 g/k/d of protein to such milk would produce 3 g/dL and an intake of 4.5 g/k/d at 150 ml/k/d. The protein provided this way would decrease as the protein of the mothers' milk decrease as lactation progresses.

Now we have the consideration that an adjunctive supplemental human milk cream at 12.5 calories per kilogram per day. Of course, to date there is no protein supplement made from human milk to maintain exclusive human milk-fed diet if on the human-derived fortifier.

Does it seem like we need a different fortifier? Perhaps one with more protein and energy that maintains a protein/energy ratio that promotes lean body mass? The answer to these proposed strategies must begin to take into account the effects on body composition and then the long-term implications through larger studies relating prematurity, postnatal growth, and body composition on adult outcomes.

D. H. Adamkin, MD

References

1. Radmacher PG, Lewis SL, Adamkin DH. Individualizing fortification of human milk using real time human milk analysis. *J Neonatal Perinatal Med*. 2013;6:319-323.

2. Adamkin DH, Radmacher PG. Fortification of human milk in very low birth weight infants (VLBW <1500 g birth weight). *Clin Perinatol.* 2014;41:405-421.
3. Hay WW. Optimizing protein intake in preterm infants. *J Perinatol.* 2009;29(7): 455-466.
4. Arslanaglu S, Moro G, Ziegler E, the Working Group on Nutrition. Optimization of human milk fortification for preterm infants: new concepts and recommendations. *J Perinat Med.* 2010;38:233-238.
5. Rochow N, Fusch G, Choi A, et al. Target fortification of breast milk with fat, protein, and carbohydrates for preterm infants. *J Pediatr.* 2013;163:1001-1007.
6. Polberger S, Axelsson I, Raiha N. Growth of the very low birth weight infants on varying amounts of human milk protein. *Pediatr Res.* 1989;25:414-419.

Glycerin Enemas and Suppositories in Premature Infants: A Meta-analysis
Livingston MH, Shawyer AC, Rosenbaum PL, et al (McMaster Univ, Hamilton, Ontario, Canada; et al)
Pediatrics 135:1093-1106, 2015

Background and Objective.—Premature infants are often given glycerin enemas or suppositories to facilitate meconium evacuation and transition to enteral feeding. The purpose of this study was to assess the available evidence for this treatment strategy.

Methods.—We conducted a systematic search of Medline, Embase, Central, and trial registries for randomized controlled trials of premature infants treated with glycerin enemas or suppositories. Data were extracted in duplicate and meta-analyzed using a random effects model.

Results.—We identified 185 premature infants treated prophylactically with glycerin enemas in one trial ($n = 81$) and suppositories in two other trials ($n = 104$). All infants were less than 32 weeks gestation and had no congenital malformations. Treatment was associated with earlier initiation of stooling in one trial (2 vs 4 days, $P = .02$) and a trend towards earlier meconium evacuation in another (6.5 vs 9 days, $P = .11$). Meta-analysis demonstrated no effect on transition to enteral feeding (0.7 days faster, $P = .43$) or mortality ($P = 0.50$). There were no reports of rectal bleeding or perforation but there was a trend towards increased risk of necrotizing enterocolitis with glycerin enemas or suppositories (risk ratio = 2.72, $P = .13$). These three trials are underpowered and affected by one or more major methodological issues. As a result, the quality of evidence is low to very low. Three other trials are underway.

Conclusions.—The evidence for the use glycerin enemas or suppositories in premature infants in inconclusive. Meta-analyzed data suggest that treatment may be associated with increased risk of necrotizing enterocolitis. Careful monitoring of ongoing trials is required.

▶ One could argue that conducting a meta-analysis with too few data is not helpful. In the above meta-analysis, not only were there too few data, but also the available data were flawed. And as the authors state, the quality of the evidence is low to very low. For this reason, the conclusion that treatment with glycerine enemas or suppositories may be associated with an increased risk of necrotizing enterocolitis seems gratuitous. Nevertheless, it is surprising that 50 years after the introduction of newborn intensive care, there is still not sufficient evidence to support or refute the use of glycerine enemas or suppositories to facilitate stool passage or improve feeding tolerance in very low birth weight infants. In the discussion section, the authors indicate that there are 2 ongoing clinical trials registered at clinicaltrials.gov concerning the use of glycerine suppositories (NCT 02149407; NCT 01799629). The study population in both studies is very low birth weight infants and the primary outcome is the time to full enteral nutrition. Enrollment in each study is targeted at 220 to 230 infants. In the interim it is probable that clinicians will continue to routinely use glycerine enemas and suppositories.

L. A. Papile, MD

Guidelines for Feeding Very Low Birth Weight Infants
Dutta S, Singh B, Chessell L, et al (McMaster Univ Children's Hosp, Hamilton, Ontario, Canada)
Nutrients 7:423-442, 2015

Despite the fact that feeding a very low birth weight (VLBW) neonate is a fundamental and inevitable part of its management, this is a field which is beset with controversies. Optimal nutrition improves growth and neurological outcomes, and reduces the incidence of sepsis and possibly even retinopathy of prematurity. There is a great deal of heterogeneity of practice among neonatologists and pediatricians regarding feeding VLBW infants. A working group on feeding guidelines for VLBW infants was constituted in McMaster University, Canada. The group listed a number of important questions that had to be answered with respect to feeding VLBW infants, systematically reviewed the literature, critically appraised the level of evidence, and generated a comprehensive set of guidelines. These guidelines form the basis of this state-of-the-art review. The review touches upon trophic feeding, nutritional feeding, fortification, feeding in special circumstances, assessment of feed tolerance, and management of gastric residuals, gastro-esophageal reflux, and glycerin enemas.

▶ There are few areas in neonatal intensive care that involve as much debate based on minimal evidence as how to optimally feed very low birth weight infants. Some of the most common debates involve how quickly we should aim to reach full enteral feeding, frequency of feeds, time to start, how much should be fed, and route of feeding. There are questions as to whether babies should be enterally fed at all if they are on vasoactive medications such as dopamine or they are receiving indomethacin for interventricular hemorrhage prophylaxis, or if they have suffered an episode of hypotension. When and how to fortify human milk, whether thickeners should be used for gastroesophageal reflux, and how to manage gastric residuals are common conundrums.

This article provides feeding guidelines developed by a Canadian working group comprising neonatologists and pediatricians, who systematically reviewed the literature, appraised the level of evidence, and developed a set of guidelines.

I found this to be a valuable review that should be read by anyone caring for preterm infants in a neonatal intensive care unit. It can be valuable in developing individual guidelines based on current best evidence. Not only does it provide evidence, suggestions are actually provided as how to proceed with feedings based on this evidence.

J. Neu, MD

Balancing the risks and benefits of parenteral nutrition for preterm infants: can we define the optimal composition?
Embleton ND, Morgan C, King C (Newcastle Hosps NHS Foundation Trust, UK; Liverpool Women's Hosp, UK; Imperial College Healthcare NHS Trust, London, UK; et al)
Arch Dis Child Fetal Neonatal Ed 100:F72-F75, 2015

Nutrient intakes in preterm infants are frequently inadequate and are associated with worse neurodevelopmental outcome. Preterm infants take time to establish enteral intakes, and parenteral nutrition (PN) is now an integral component of care. Despite this, the evidence base for PN intakes is extremely limited. There remains uncertainty over safe initial and maximum amounts of macronutrients, and the optimal amino acid and lipid composition. Studies have tended to focus on short-term growth measures and there are few studies with long-term follow-up. There may be a tradeoff between improving cognitive outcomes while minimising metabolic harm that means determining the optimal regimen will require long-term follow-up. Given the importance of appropriate nutrition for long-term metabolic and cognitive health, and the associated healthcare costs, optimising the composition of PN deserves to be seen as a research priority in neonatal medicine.

▶ This article provides a critical review of the current status of intravenous nutrition for very low birth weight infants. It underlines the fact that 1 size does not fit all and as an example mentions that what we provide for a preterm infant born at 25 weeks' gestation should be different from that provided to a 32-week gestation preterm who is recovering from necrotizing enterocolitis.

The past few decades of neonatal intensive care have witnessed major changes in survival of very low birth weight infants. Although it is intuitively clear that optimization of early nutrition should improve the long-term physical as well as neurodevelopmental outcome of these survivors, there remains considerable debate about how optimization can best be accomplished. Whereas early enteral nutrition is becoming more common, many extremely low birth weight infants cannot reach full enteral feedings for nearly 2 weeks after birth largely based on gastrointestinal immaturities and adaptations that need to occur to accept a milk diet usually reserved for more mature infants. During this time, parenteral nutrition is needed.

The early days of parenteral nutrition in the neonatal intensive care unit (NICU) usually involved very slow advancement of amino acids and lipids. Studies over the past 2 decades have shown that it appears to be relatively safe to begin with an amino acid infusion rate that will provide quantities that account for accretion (the in utero rate) and losses. The need to provide this in increments has been largely discredited. Likewise, despite common practice of slowly increasing intravenous lipids over several days, this practice also is based on limited substantive data, and thus the infusion of amino acids and lipids likely should be started at approximately 3 to 4 g/kg/d and 3 g/kg/d for most extremely low birth weight infants.

However, as stated in this article, we are far from having optimal amino acid and lipid solutions based on solid evidence. The available solutions were not based on the needs of very low birth weight infants, and the compositions are not optimal. Studies that have been done have had limitations in their outcome criteria and have generally not provided long-term outcome evidence. In the short term, our means of monitoring adequacy and safety remain limited. For example, many NICUs still attempt to monitor triglycerides routinely in preterm infants receiving intravenous lipids without having a strong base of evidence as to what constitutes hypertriglyceridemia in these infants.

This review nicely outlines some of our challenges in optimizing parenteral nutrition to very low birth weight infants and suggests several important areas of uncertainty and ways forward in terms of clinical trials and/or observational studies.

J. Neu, MD

Cow's Milk Contamination of Human Milk Purchased via the Internet
Keim SA, Kulkarni MM, McNamara K, et al (The Research Inst at Nationwide Children's Hosp, Columbus, OH; The Ohio State Univ, Columbus; et al)
Pediatrics 135:e1157-e1162, 2015

Background.—The US Food and Drug Administration recommends against feeding infants human abstract milk from unscreened donors, but sharing milk via the Internet is growing in popularity. Recipient infants risk the possibility of consuming contaminated or adulterated milk. Our objective was to test milk advertised for sale online as human milk to verify its human origin and to rule out contamination with cow's milk.

Methods.—We anonymously purchased 102 samples advertised as human milk online. DNA was extracted from 200 μL of each sample. The presence of human or bovine mitochondrial DNA was assessed with a species-specific real-time polymerase chain reaction assay targeting the nicotinamide adenine dinucleotide (NADH) dehydrogenase subunit 5 gene. Four laboratory-created mixtures representing various dilutions of human milk with fluid cow's milk or reconstituted infant formula were compared with the Internet samples to semiquantitate the extent of contamination with cow's milk.

Results.—All Internet samples amplified human DNA. After 2 rounds of testing, 11 samples also contained bovine DNA. Ten of these samples had a level of bovine DNA consistent with human milk mixed with at least 10% fluid cow's milk.

Conclusions.—Ten Internet samples had bovine DNA concentrations high enough to rule out minor contamination, suggesting a cow's milk product was added. Cow's milk can be problematic for infants with allergy or intolerance. Because buyers cannot verify the composition of milk they purchase, all should be aware that it might be adulterated with cow's milk. Pediatricians should be aware of the online market for human milk and the potential risks.

▶ The American Academy of Pediatrics section on Breastfeeding Medicine recommends the use of donor human milk for premature infants whose mothers are not able to provide a sufficient quantity of their own milk.[1] In hospital settings, donor human milk is purchased from the Human Milk Banking Association of North America (HMBANA), and in most instances informed consent is obtained. HMBANA is a nonprofit organization with strict quality control. All women donating milk to an HMBANA bank are screened for drug use, human immunodeficiency virus, hepatitis B and C, and syphilis. In addition, all milk donated to HMBANA is pasteurized to eliminate potential pathogens.[2] In this ingenious study, Keim et al anonymously purchased human milk from Internet sites and then utilized real-time polymerase chain reaction to determine if the milk purchased via Internet advertising was contaminated with cow's milk protein. Upon analysis of 102 samples advertised as human milk, the authors found that 10% of the samples were contaminated with cow's milk. Furthermore, the amount of bovine DNA was of quantity sufficient to represent a 10% dilution of the human milk with cow's milk. In a previous study, the same group of investigators found high bacterial counts in human milk purchased via the Internet.[3] This study raises serious concerns that go beyond the ingestion of cow's milk protein. If donor human milk is needed, it is imperative that clinicians warn families of the risks of donor milk obtained from sources other than a HMBANA bank, such as the Internet.

L. A. Papile, MD

References

1. Section on Breastfeeding. Breastfeeding and the use of human milk. *Pediatrics.* 2012;129:e827-e841.
2. Human Milk Banking Association of North America. https://www.hmbana.org. Accessed August 24, 2015.
3. Keim SA, Hogan JS, McNamara KA, et al. Microbial contamination of human milk purchased via the internet. *Pediatrics.* 2013;132:e1227-e1235, www.pediatrics.org/cgi/content/full/132/5/e1227.

Cow's Milk Contamination of Human Milk Purchased via the Internet
Keim SA, Kulkarni MM, McNamara K, et al (Nationwide Children's Hosp, Columbus, OH; The Ohio State Univ, Columbus; et al)
Pediatrics 135:e1157-e1162, 2015

Background.—The US Food and Drug Administration recommends against feeding infants human milk from unscreened donors, but sharing milk via the Internet is growing in popularity. Recipient infants risk the possibility of consuming contaminated or adulterated milk. Our objective was to test milk advertised for sale online as human milk to verify its human origin and to rule out contamination with cow's milk.

Methods.—We anonymously purchased 102 samples advertised as human milk online. DNA was extracted from 200 μL of each sample. The presence of human or bovine mitochondrial DNA was assessed with a species-specific real-time polymerase chain reaction assay targeting the nicotinamide adenine dinucleotide (NADH) dehydrogenase subunit 5 gene. Four laboratory-created mixtures representing various dilutions of human milk with fluid cow's milk or reconstituted infant formula were compared with the Internet samples to semiquantitate the extent of contamination with cow's milk.

Results.—All Internet samples amplified human DNA. After 2 rounds of testing, 11 samples also contained bovine DNA. Ten of these samples had a level of bovine DNA consistent with human milk mixed with at least 10% fluid cow's milk.

Conclusions.—Ten Internet samples had bovine DNA concentrations high enough to rule out minor contamination, suggesting a cow's milk product was added. Cow's milk can be problematic for infants with allergy or intolerance. Because buyers cannot verify the composition of milk they purchase, all should be aware that it might be adulterated with cow's milk. Pediatricians should be aware of the online market for human milk and the potential risks.

▶ The use of donor human milk is increasing in the United States and Canada. Donor human milk is most commonly provided to high-risk infants whose mothers are not able to provide sufficient quantity of their own milk. The American Academy of Pediatrics Section on Breastfeeding Medicine recommends the use of donor human milk for premature infants.[1] In hospital settings, informed consent is typically obtained for administration of donor human milk purchased from the Human Milk Banking Association of North America (HMBANA).

HMBANA is a nonprofit organization with strict quality control. Donor milk purchased from a HMBANA bank is pasteurized and cultured for bacteria. All women donating milk to a HMBANA bank are screened for drug use, infectious disease (HIV, hepatitis B or C, and syphilis). In addition, all milk donated to HMBANA is pasteurized to eliminate infectious pathogens.[2] Indeed, the same group of investigators previously found high bacterial counts in human milk purchased via the Internet.[3]

In this ingenious study, Keim et al anonymously purchased human milk from Internet sites and then utilized real-time polymerase chain reaction to determine whether the milk purchased via Internet advertising was contaminated with cow's milk protein. Upon analysis of 102 samples advertised as human milk, the authors found that 10% of the samples were contaminated with cow's milk. Furthermore, the amount of bovine DNA was of quantity sufficient to represent a 10% dilution of the human milk with cow's milk.

Although some infants with milk-protein allergy could be adversely affected by consumption of cow's milk, this study raises serious concerns that go beyond ingestion of cow's milk protein. In situations in which donor milk is provided, the source must be from a milk bank with appropriate accreditation, and clinicians must warn families of the risks of milk obtained from alternate sources such as the Internet.

B. Poindexter, MD, MS

References

1. AAP Section on Breastfeeding. Breastfeeding and the use of human milk. *Pediatrics*. 2012;129:e827-e841.
2. Human Milk Banking Association of North America Website. https://www.hmbana.org. Accessed August 14, 2015.
3. Keim SA, Hogan JS, McNamara KA, et al. Microbial contamination of human milk purchased via the Internet. Pediatrics. 2013;132:e1227-e1235, www.pediatrics.org/cgi/content/full/132/5/e1227.

Network analysis suggests a potentially 'evil' alliance of opportunistic pathogens inhibited by a cooperative network in human milk bacterial communities

(Sam) Ma Z, Guan Q, Ye C, et al (Kunming Inst of Zoology, China; et al)
Sci Rep 5:8275, 2015

The critical importance of human milk to infants and even human civilization has been well established. Yet our understanding of the milk microbiome has been limited to cataloguing OTUs and computation of community diversity. To the best of our knowledge, there has been no report on the bacterial interactions within the milk microbiome. To bridge this gap, we reconstructed a milk bacterial community network based on Hunt et al. Our analysis revealed that the milk microbiome network consists of two disconnected sub-networks. One sub-network is a fully connected *complete graph* consisting of seven genera as nodes and all of its pair-wise interactions among the bacteria are facilitative or cooperative. In contrast, the interactions in the other sub-network of eight nodes are mixed but dominantly cooperative. Somewhat surprisingly, the only 'non-cooperative' nodes in the second sub-network are mutually cooperative *Staphylococcus* and *Corynebacterium* that include some opportunistic pathogens. This potentially 'evil' alliance between *Staphylococcus* and *Corynebacterium* could be inhibited by the remaining nodes that cooperate with one another in the second sub-network. We postulate that the 'confrontation' between the 'evil' alliance and 'benign' alliance and the shifting balance between them may be responsible for dysbiosis of the milk microbiome that permits mastitis.

▶ As with studies in amniotic fluid, placenta, and meconium, breast milk has been found to be a nonsterile habitat.[1-3] The microbes found in these niches are likely to play significant roles in health and disease of not only the fetus and newborn but also the subsequent child and adult. Studies of human milk microbes show that over time in each individual mother's milk, the microbes change slightly but differ considerably when compared with other mothers' milk microbes. The relevance of this finding remains to be determined but is suggestive of a personalized milk microbiome that is transferred from individual mothers to their infants.

New bioinformatics technologies are being applied to the large quantities of data derived from microbial sequencing, and this article describes novel approaches to evaluate the microbiome data from the study by Hunt et al[3] to evaluate interactions between bacteria using "network analysis." This method employs newly developed mathematics theories and network analysis software to evaluate how well the networks of microbes are connected. In this study, it was found that 2 distinct networks of bacteria were found that were not closely related to one another. The first of these contained 8 genera and the second contained 7. The first of these also contained 2 genera usually thought of as being pathogens, namely *Staphylococcus* and *Corynebacterium*. The network analysis showed that every other bacterium in the milk opposes these 2 microbes in a noncooperative relationship. The authors speculate that these community members team up against these 2 microbial genera to suppress the "evil alliance" these may have with one another and thus prevent disease.

This network analysis approach is still novel, and we are in the early phases of learning to employ this tool. It is a fascinating example of the world of evaluating systems rather than individual perturbations. With these paradigm shifts, we will need to adjust the way we think about testing individual hypotheses and think about interactions of microbes, proteins, metabolites, and so on.

J. Neu, MD

References

1. Funkhouser LJ, Bordenstein SR. Mom knows best: the universality of maternal microbial transmission. *PLoS Biol.* 2013;11:e1001631.
2. Jeurink PV, van Bergenhenegouwen J, Jimenez E, et al. Human milk: a source of more life than we imagine. *Benef Microbes*. 2013;4:17-30.
3. Hunt KM, Foster JA, Forney LJ, et al. Characterization of the diversity and temporal stability of bacterial communities in human milk. *PLoS One*. 2011;6: e21313.

Utility of Gastrointestinal Fluoroscopic Studies in Detecting Stricture After Neonatal Necrotizing Enterocolitis
Wiland EL, South AP, Kraus SJ, et al (Cincinnati Children's Hosp Med Ctr, OH)
J Pediatr Gastroenterol Nutr 59:789-794, 2014

Objectives.—We report our institution's 5-year experience with upper gastrointestinal study with small bowel follow-through (UGI-SBFT) and contrast enema (CE) for the diagnosis of a post-necrotizing enterocolitis (NEC) stricture. We hypothesized that sensitivity and specificity of UGISBFT and CE were <85% in diagnosing a post-NEC stricture.

Methods.—A retrospective observational cohort study was performed. Included patients were neonates diagnosed as having Bell's modified stage 2 or 3 NEC who had undergone UGI-SBFT and/or CE to evaluate for a stricture. Exploratory laparotomy was used to definitively determine the stricture presence, which was confirmed by pathology. An infant was categorized as having no stricture if no surgical intervention occurred or if no stricture was reported on pathology following surgical resection.

Results.—A total of 56 patients met inclusion criteria, with 51 UGI-SBFT and 85 CE performed. A total of 25 patients were diagnosed as having a stricture. For small bowel (SB) strictures, CE compared with UGI-SBFT has a higher sensitivity (0.667 vs 0.00) and a similar specificity (0.857 vs 0.833). For SB and/or colonic strictures, CE has a sensitivity of 0.667 and a specificity of 0.951. Strictures were more likely to be found on imaging in symptomatic infants compared with those in asymptomatic infants (28% vs 8%, $P = 0.002$).

Conclusions.—CE should be the initial study in the diagnostic workup for a post-NEC stricture because this test has a higher likelihood of detecting a stricture if it is present. As a result of low sensitivity of UGI-SBFT and/or CE in the diagnosis of a post-NEC stricture, a negative study should not rule out the diagnosis of a stricture in persistently symptomatic patients.

▶ A common complication of necrotizing enterocolitis (NEC) in the neonate is intestinal stricture. This complication occurs fairly commonly after NEC (up to 30% of cases) and can present with severe feeding intolerance, sepsis, and abdominal distension. Definitive treatment is with resection of the stenotic area. Before surgery, contrast studies are commonly done to determine whether a stricture is present. These include an upper gastrointestinal (GI) with small bowel follow-through study and/or a contrast enema. There is often confusion as to which of these procedures should be performed, and an upper GI study is commonly done first. This study shows that greatest specificity and sensitivity can be obtained with the use of the contrast enema because the majority of these strictures occur in the colon (80%) or distal small bowel (that can be reached with a contrast enema). The authors provide several caveats, which include that stricture formation is a dynamic process and a contrast study may need to be repeated to provide a more definitive diagnosis. This is a practical retrospective study that guides us to use the contrast enema first if there is a suspicion of stricture; however, if symptoms continue or worsen, one should consider repeat of the contrast enema and also doing an upper GI-small bowel follow-through study to find those lesions that are continuing to evolve or that are in a more proximal site.

J. Neu, MD

Fecal Short-Chain Fatty Acids of Very-Low-Birth-Weight Preterm Infants Fed Expressed Breast Milk or Formula
Pourcyrous M, Nolan VG, Goodwin A, et al (Univ of Memphis, TN)
J Pediatr Gastroenterol Nutr 59:725-731, 2014

Objectives.—In preterm infants, the metabolic responses of gastrointestinal (GI) bacteria to different diets are poorly understood despite the possible effects on GI health. Therefore, we tested the hypothesis that diet influences bacterial metabolism by measuring short-chain fatty acids (SCFAs) in stool samples from very-low-birth-weight (VLBW) preterm infants without GI disorder as surrogate biomarkers of bacterial metabolism.

Methods.—Ion chromatography was used to measure fecal SCFAs (acetate, formate, propionate, butyrate, and isobutyrate), lactate, and chloride in fresh stool samples collected from 32 preterm infants (without major congenital anomalies, GI disorders, or a recent history of antibiotic administration and on full feed of either expressed maternal breast milk [EBM; n = 13] or a formula for preterm infants [Similac Special Care Formula; preterm formula, PTF; n = 19]).

Results.—The mean birth weight was 972 g, the mean gestational age was 27 weeks, and the mean postnatal age at first stool sample was 36 days. When adjusted for gestational age, the stools of EBM infants had higher concentrations (micromoles per gram of stool) of total SCFA (128 vs 68; $P = 0.002$), acetate (41 vs 13; $P = 0.005$), propionate (15.1 vs 4.4; $P = 0.003$), and chloride (21,814 vs 10,652; $P = 0.02$). Interactions between postnatal age and diet were detected for lactate ($P = 0.05$), propionate ($P = 0.03$), and butyrate ($P = 0.03$).

Conclusions.—Diets fed to VLBW preterm infants influence fecal SCFA profiles, and hence the metabolism of the GI bacteria, and potentially the health of preterm infants. The responses of bacterial metabolism to diet are influenced with postnatal age and gestational age at birth.

▶ There are numerous products of microbial metabolism in the gastrointestinal tract. Among these are the highly bioactive 2, 3, and 4 carbon short chain fatty acids (SCFAs) acetate, propionate, and butyrate. These exert numerous effects in the gastrointestinal tract, including proliferation, differentiation, tightening inters epithelial junctions, exerting effects on the immune system, and, in the case of butyrate, being the major fuel for the colonic epithelium.

The microbial ecology of human milk-fed infants is known to differ from that of formula-fed infants, and thus the authors quantified SCFA in fortified expressed breast milk (EBM) versus preterm formula (PTF). Infants who had reached full enteral feedings were included, thus most preterm infants were evaluated later than those born less preterm. Total fecal SCFA was almost twice as high in the EBM infants throughout the evaluation period. However, when the individual SCFAs were evaluated, propionate started slightly higher in the EBM infants and the increment increased over time. Butyrate concentration started much higher in EBM-fed infants but converged to similar concentrations as in the PTF-fed infants at about 60 postnatal days, then appeared to actually become lower. The differences in total SCFA make a lot of sense when one considers that the EBM contains endogenous microbes that may seed the intestine and result in metabolism to SCFA, whereas PTF does not contain these microbes. The question is raised here about donor milk, which is pasteurized and does not contain microbes. Will it have a similar metabolic profile as the PTF?

The differences in propionate and butyrate concentrations over time are difficult to explain, but it is possible that over time a different microbial ecology exerts differential effects on individual SCFA production, with butyrate producing bacterial decreasing over time in comparison to those involved in propionate production.

Although the authors mention necrotizing enterocolitis as a possible result of the differences in these metabolic products from EBM versus PTF, this is certainly possible, but proof of this hypothesis will require more extensive experimentation.

J. Neu, MD

Long-Chain Polyunsaturated Fatty Acids and Cognition in VLBW Infants at 8 years: an RCT

Almaas AN, Tamnes CK, Nakstad B, et al (Univ of Oslo, Norway; et al)
Pediatrics 135:972-980, 2015

Objective.—To test the hypothesis that supplementation with the long chain polyunsaturated fatty acids docosahexaenoic acid (DHA) and arachidonic acid (AA) to very low birth weight (VLBW) infants would improve long-term cognitive functions and influence neuroanatomical volumes and cerebral cortex measured by MRI.

Methods.—The current study is a follow-up of a randomized, double-blinded, placebo-controlled study of supplementation with high-dose DHA (0.86%) and AA (0.91%) to 129 VLBW infants fed human milk. Ninety-eight children participated at 8 years follow-up and completed a broad battery of cognitive tests. Eighty-one children had cerebral MRI scans of acceptable quality.

Results.—There were no significant differences between the intervention group and the control group on any of the cognitive measures. Equally, MRI data on segmental brain volumes and cerebral cortex volume, area, and thickness suggested no overall group effect.

Conclusions.—This study is the first long-term follow-up of a randomized controlled trial with supplementation of DHA and AA to human milk fed VLBW infants investigating both cognitive functions and brain macrostructure measured by MRI. No cognitive or neuroanatomical effects of the supplementation were detected at 8 years of age.

▶ Long-chain polyunsaturated fatty acids (PUFA), specifically docosahexaenoic acid (DHA) and arachidonic acid (AA), are essential for the development of the central nervous system. Because major accumulation of DHA and AA in the brain occurs during the last trimester and the first postnatal months, infants who are born preterm are deprived of this accumulation prenatally. Although human milk and preterm formulas contain DHA and AA, the amounts are much less than those in the intrauterine supply.

The above study is a follow-up to the original small clinical trial in which very low birth weight infants who were fed human milk were randomly assigned to receive either high doses of DHA and AA or placebo. Two previous reports noted a positive effect on cognition and attention when the cohort was 6 months and 20 months corrected age, respectively.[1,2] The above study includes developmental outcome data on 76% of eligible participants and MRI of the brain information on 63%. The neuropsychological evaluation at 8 years of age included an extensive battery of tests, including measures of general intellectual ability, short and working memory, learning and memory, and motor skills. MRI analyses included the measurement of neuro-anatomic volumes.

The long-term outcome of another large multicenter, randomized trial of PUFA supplementation showed no benefit of supplementing the diets of preterm infants with high-dose DHA.[3] At 7 years of age, neuropsychological test data did not differ between the DHA supplemented and placebo cohort. In contrast to the above study, the latter trial included both human milk-fed and formula-fed infants and larger and more mature preterm infants. The similar findings in the 2 trials that high-dose PUFA supplementation does not confer an advantage regarding brain development and function in childhood suggest supplementation with PUFA is not needed.

L. A. Papile, MD

References

1. Henriksen C, Haugholt K, Lingren M, et al. Improved cognitive outcome among preterm infants attributable to early supplementation of human milk with docosahexaenoic and arachnidonic acid. *Pediatrics.* 2008;121:1137.
2. Westerberg AC, Schei R, Henriksen C, et al. Attention among very low birth weight infants following early supplementation with docosahexaenoic and arachnidonic acid. *Axta Paediatr.* 2011;100:47.
3. Collins CT, Gibson RA, Anderson PJ, et al. Neurodevelopmental outcomes at 7 years' corrected age in pretrm infants who were fed high-dose docosahexaenoic acid to term equivalent: a follow-up of a randomized controlled trial. *BMJ Open.* 2015;5:e007314.

Hirschsprung disease in the premature newborn: A population based study and 40-year single center experience
Downey EC, Hughes E, Putnam AR, et al (Univ of Utah, Salt Lake City)
J Pediatr Surg 50:123-125, 2015

Background/Purpose.—Understanding of Hirschsprung disease (HD) in premature newborns (PHD) is anecdotal. We have sought in this study to identify the demographic and clinical features of PHD.

Methods.—All patients with HD 1970—2011 treated at our tertiary care children's hospital were identified. Patients with biopsy confirmed HD and EGA <37 weeks were selected for further review. Prenatal and birth data, demographics, clinical signs, radiologic and pathologic data, and operative interventions were examined. The occurrence of PHD was observed using data from the Utah Department of Health database 1997—2011.

Results.—404 patients with HD from 1970 to 2011 were treated. Twenty-seven (6.7%) had PHD. Mean birth weight in PHD was 2196 grams and mean gestational age 34 (range 29—36) weeks. Seven patients had Down syndrome. Nonchromosomal anomalies occurred in 25%. Median time from birth to biopsy diagnosis was 42 days (range 2–316 days). The most common presenting signs were abdominal distension and bilious emesis. The HD incidence in Utah for all births was 1/4322 (0.023%) and for premature infants 1/3885 (0.027%).

Conclusions.—PHD are similar to term infants with HD. Diagnosis of HD is often delayed in premature newborns, and associated anomalies are more common.

▶ Most single-institution case series have taken their rightful place next to the dinosaurs in the museum. I included this series on Hirschsprung disease (HD) because it reinforced a few important diagnostic points when considering HD in preterm infants. First, the prevalence is similar to term infants; second, preterm infants are more likely to be recognized later and present with bilious vomiting rather than obstipation, because delayed and irregular passage of stool is so common in preterm infants; and finally, we are reminded of the high association of trisomy 21 with HD in preterm infants. Everyone recognizes that bilious vomiting in newborns is an urgent condition that requires immediate attention. Bilious vomiting, with or without abdominal distention, is an initial sign of intestinal obstruction in newborns, although many infants with bilious vomiting will not turn out to have an obstruction. Duodenal atresia, midgut malrotation and volvulus, jejunoileal atresia, meconium ileus, and necrotizing enterocolitis are the most common causes of neonatal intestinal obstruction. However, HD must be ruled out, especially in preterm infants.

When a neonate vomits bile, gastric decompression to prevent further vomiting and aspiration should be accomplished before any diagnostic or therapeutic maneuvers. For those optimists who had hoped that HD could be recognized prenatally, abnormal sonographic findings of fetal bowel were absent in the vast majority of fetuses who are diagnosed with HD after birth.[1]

What about the outcomes with surgery? The Finnish group reported their outcomes on a population-based series of 146 patients with HD after transanal mucosectomy.[2] The level of disease was rectosigmoid in 83%, long segment in 7%, total colonic in 4%, and extending up to the small bowel in 6%; 29% had an associated syndrome. No patients were lost to follow-up, and overall survival was 98%. At the latest follow-up, 42% had occasional soiling, 12% had frequent soiling, and 46% had no soiling. Constipation occurred in 9%. An associated syndrome was the only predictor for soiling or constipation (odds ratio [OR] 4.3, 95% CI 1.5-12). Forty-four percent developed recurrent postoperative enterocolitis, which was predicted by extended aganglionosis (OR 6.9, 95% CI 2.4-20) and syndromic disease (OR 2.4, 95% CI 1.2-5.0). Hence extended aganglionosis and associated syndromes were significant risk factors for recurrent postoperative enterocolitis. HD remains an interesting diagnostic dilemma.

A. A. Fanaroff, MBBCh, FRCPE

References

1. Jakobson-Setton A, Weissmann-Brenner A, Achiron R, Kuint J, Gindes L. Retrospective analysis of prenatal ultrasound of children with Hirschsprung disease. *Prenat Diagn.* 2015 [Epub ahead of print].
2. Neuvonen MI, Kyrklund K, Lindahl HG, Koivusalo AI, Rintala RJ, Pakarinen MP. A population-based, complete follow-up of 146 consecutive patients after transanal mucosectomy for Hirschsprung disease. *J Pediatr Surg.* 2015 [Epub ahead of print].

Nutritional outcomes in survivors of congenital diaphragmatic hernia (CDH)—Factors associated with growth at one year

Bairdain S, Khan FA, Fisher J, et al (Boston Children's Hosp, MA; et al)
J Pediatr Surg 50:74-77, 2015

Background.—Malnutrition is prevalent among congenital diaphragmatic hernia (CDH) survivors. We aimed to describe the nutritional status and factors that impact growth over the 12-months following discharge from the pediatric intensive care unit (PICU) in this cohort.

Methods.—CDH survivors, who were discharged from the PICU from 2000 to 2010 with follow-up of at least 12 months, were included. Nutritional intake, anthropometric, and clinical variables were recorded. Multivariable linear regression was used to determine factors associated with weight-for-age Z-scores (WAZ) at 12 months.

Results.—Data from 110 infants, 67% male, 50% patch repair, were analyzed. Median (IQR) WAZ for the cohort was -1.4 (-2.4 to -0.3) at PICU discharge and -0.4 (-1.3 to 0.2) at 12-months. The percentage of infants with significant malnutrition (WAZ <-2) decreased from 26% to 8.5% ($p < 0.001$). Patch repair ($p = 0.009$), protein intake <2.3 g/kg/day ($p = 0.014$), and birth weight (BW) <2.5 kg ($p < 0.001$) were associated with lower WAZ at 12-months.

Conclusions.—CDH survivors had a significantly improved nutritional status in the 12-months after PICU discharge. Patch repair, lower BW, and inadequate protein intake were significant predictors of lower WAZ at 12-months. A minimum protein intake in the PICU of 2.3 g/kg/day was essential to ensure optimal growth in this cohort.

▶ This retrospective single institutional study evaluated growth over the first year of life among 110 congenital diaphragmatic hernia (CDH) survivors over a 10-year period. Nutritional intake, anthropometrics, and clinical variables were among the data collected. A multivariable linear regression was used to determine factors associated with weight-for-age *Z* scores (WAZ) at 12 months.

At this institution, infants with CDH were admitted to the pediatric intensive care unit (PICU). A stepwise enteral nutrition advancement algorithm was used based on the literature, and commitment to the plan is evidenced by intensive educational efforts, discussion of nutritional strategies on daily rounds, and regular audits to ensure adherence to stay on course with the agreed-on algorithm.

A dedicated dietician was integrally involved and prescribed macronutrient goals. There was detailed assessment of intake and nutritional status as part of the multidisciplinary CDH follow-up clinic, but there was no nutritional data collection performed in the postdischarge period.

The multivariate predictive model for lower WAZ at 12 months of age included patch repair for the CDH, protein intake < 2.3 g/k/d, and birth weight < 2.5 kg as independent predictors. This multidisciplinary quality improvement initiative at a single institution to standardize nutritional approach to a single subset of infants appeared to be effective in reducing growth failure.

Standardizing nutritional approach has been successful in the neonatal intensive care unit (NICU) as well. Multiple studies have shown fewer days to full feedings, better growth, and even reduction in necrotizing enterocolitis (NEC) as groups of health care providers agreed on an evidence-based approach to nutritional strategies. In the CDH study, as seen in many NICU subsets of infants like very low-birth-weight infants or specifically infants with NEC or bronchopulmonary dysplasia, degree of illness, protein intake, and birth weight and growth restriction at birth all play an important role in determining growth success.

Protein is the sentinel nutrient that defines lean growth and especially its relationship to energy or the protein/energy ratio. In this study, learning more about head circumference and developmental outcomes related to growth would have been interesting to see the relationship between catch-up growth and outcome. Also, a specific postdischarge strategy with additional protein would have perhaps added even more catch-up growth.

Very encouraging was the fact that the study, using greater than -2 WAZ to define "malnutrition," saw a reduction in this diagnosis from 26% at discharge from PICU to 8.5% at 1 year of age. This shows the importance of "catch-up" growth during the first year of life and is programmed by protein during the neonatal course and then extended by nutrient enhancement at the first year of life.

D. H. Adamkin, MD

10 Hematology and Bilirubin

Why do four NICUs using identical RBC transfusion guidelines have different gestational age-adjusted RBC transfusion rates?
Henry E, Christensen RD, Sheffield MJ, et al (The Women and Newborn's Clinical Program, Salt Lake City, UT; et al)
J Perinatol 35:132-136, 2015

Objective.—To compare neonatal red blood cell (RBC) transfusion rates in four large Intermountain Healthcare NICUs, all of which adhere to the same RBC transfusion guidelines.

Study Design.—This retrospective analysis was part of a transfusion-management quality-improvement project. De-identified data included RBC transfusions, clinical and laboratory findings, the anemia-prevention strategies in place in each NICU, and specific costs and outcomes.

Result.—Of 2389 NICU RBC transfusions given during the 4-year period studied, 98.9 ± 2.1% (mean ± s.d.) were compliant with our transfusion guidelines, with no difference in compliance between any of the four NICUs. However, RBC transfusion rates varied widely between the four, with averages ranging from 4.6 transfusions/1000 NICU days to 21.7/1000 NICU days ($P < 0.00001$). Gestational age-adjusted transfusion rates were correspondingly discordant ($P < 0.00001$). The lower-transfusing NICUs had written anemia-preventing guidelines, such as umbilical cord milking at very low birth weight delivery, use of cord blood for admission laboratory studies, and darbepoetin dosing for selected neonates. Rates of Bell stage ≥2 necrotizing enterocolitis and grade ≥3 intraventricular hemorrhage were lowest in the two lower-transfusing NICUs ($P < 0.0002$ and $P < 0.0016$). Average pharmacy costs for darbepoetin were $84/dose, with an average pharmacy cost of $269 per transfusion averted. With a cost of $900/RBC transfusion, the anemia-preventing strategies resulted in an estimated cost savings to Intermountain Healthcare of about $6970 per 1000 NICU days, or about $282 300 annually.

Conclusion.—Using transfusion guidelines has been shown previously to reduce practice variability, lower transfusion rates and diminish transfusion costs. Based on our present findings, we maintain that even when transfusion guidelines are in place and adhered to rigorously, RBC transfusion rates are reduced further if anemia-preventing strategies are also in place.

▶ Christensen and colleagues evaluated several strategies to increase red cell mass and decrease neonatal transfusions with the goal of maintaining/improving outcomes at a decreased cost. They previously showed that transfusion guidelines reduce practice variability, lower transfusion rates, and diminish transfusion costs. The current study by Henry and colleagues evaluated implementing anemia-reducing strategies to further reduce transfusions and costs. They compared 4 similarly sized neonatal intensive care units (NICUs) in Utah that followed the same transfusion guidelines. They identified 5 additional policies implemented in some of the NICUs to decrease red cell loss and increase red cell production: delayed cord clamping or cord milking, drawing initial laboratory specimens from the fetal circulation in the placenta, administering darbepoetin, limiting phlebotomy losses, and administering supplemental iron to very low birth weight infants.

The NICUs with all of the listed policies in place had more than a 4-fold decrease in the number of transfusions administered (4.6 transfusions per 1000 NICU days compared with 21.7 transfusions per 1000 NICU days), and significantly lower incidences of stage ≥2 necrotizing enterocolitis and grade ≥3 intracranial hemorrhage. These improvements were achieved in the face of decreased hospital costs, with an estimated cost savings of approximately $7000 per 1000 NICU days. The data reported in this study were analyzed retrospectively from a large data repository. If confirmed in a generalized NICU population, the cost savings and improved outcomes represent an outstanding advance in neonatal care that could be easily implemented.

R. Ohls, MD

Early Discharge of Infants and Risk of Readmission for Jaundice
Lain SJ, Roberts CL, Bowen JR, et al (Univ of Sydney, Australia; Royal North Shore Hosp, Sydney, Australia)
Pediatrics 135:314-321, 2015

Objectives.—To examine the association between early discharge from hospital after birth and readmission to hospital for jaundice among term infants, and among infants discharged early, to investigate the perinatal risk factors for readmission for jaundice.

Methods.—Birth data for 781 074 term live-born infants born in New South Wales, Australia from 2001 to 2010 were linked to hospital admission data. Logistic regression models were used to investigate the association between postnatal length of stay (LOS), gestational age (GA), and readmission for jaundice in the first 14 days of life. Other significant perinatal risk factors associated with readmission for jaundice were examined for infants discharged in the first 2 days after birth.

Results.—Eight per 1000 term infants were readmitted for jaundice. Infants born at 37 weeks' GA with an LOS at birth of 0 to 2 days were over 9 times (adjusted odds ratio [aOR] 9.43; 95% CI, 8.34–10.67) and at 38 weeks' GA were 4 times (aOR 4.05; 95% CI, 3.62–4.54) more likely to be readmitted for jaundice compared with infants born at 39 weeks' GA with an LOS of 3 to 4 days. Other significant risk factors for readmission for jaundice for infants discharged 0 to 2 days after birth included vaginal birth, born to mothers from an Asian country, born to first-time mothers, or being breastfed at discharge.

Conclusions.—This study can inform guidelines or policy about identifying infants at risk for readmission for jaundice and ensure that appropriate post-discharge follow-up is received.

▶ In otherwise healthy newborn infants, serum bilirubin values typically peak at 3 to 5 postnatal days in term infants and later in preterm infants, regardless of whether they have been discharged to home. As a result, some newborns are discharged before their bilirubin level peaks and may require readmission for phototherapy. In this large, contemporary, population-based analysis from New South Wales, Australia, Lain et al linked birth data to hospital admission data to examine the association of length of stay and gestational age with readmission for jaundice during the first 14 days of age.

In this population, 8 per 1000 infants were readmitted for jaundice and likely received phototherapy. Not surprisingly, odds of readmission increased with decreasing gestational age and shorter length of stay. No data are available on phototherapy use during the birth hospitalization and it is unclear if these infants were included in the analyses. The association of vaginal birth and readmission may reflect shorter hospital stay in those infants, and it is possible that the higher risk for readmission in first-time mothers reflects less established breast feeding at discharge than in multiparous mothers. According to their calculations, 31 infants born at 37 weeks' gestation or 83 born at 38 weeks' gestation would require 3 or more days of birth hospitalization to prevent one readmission for jaundice.

The Australian data are striking in that only 33% of infants had length of stay (LOS) less than 2 days, whereas LOS of 3 to 4 days or more than 4 days were 43% and 23%, respectively. In contrast, in a US multicenter, prospective, observational study of healthy newborns 35 or more weeks' gestation, the median age at discharge was 56 hours.[1] In that report, of 982 infants, 4.2% received phototherapy during their birth hospitalization, and 3.5% were treated after discharge, likely influenced by including lower gestational age infants than in the Australian study.

Unlike the United States, Canada, and other countries, Australia does not have national guidelines regarding predischarge screening of newborns for risk of severe hyperbilirubinemia development. Although home follow-up visits for newborns are supported, the timing and frequency are variable. As the authors state, a systematic approach supported by clinical guidelines would ensure a safe start for all newborns and may reduce readmissions for jaundice.

A. R. Stark, MD

Reference

1. Bhutani VK, Stark AR, Lazzeroni LC, et al. Predischarge screening for severe neonatal hyperbilirubinemia identifies infants who need phototherapy. *J Pediatr.* 2013; 162:477-482.e1.

Early Discharge of Infants and Risk of Readmission for Jaundice

Lain SJ, Roberts CL, Bowen JR, et al (Univ of Sydney, New South Wales, Australia; Royal North Shore Hosp, Sydney, New South Wales, Australia)
Pediatrics 135:314-321, 2015

Objectives.—To examine the association between early discharge from hospital after birth and readmission to hospital for jaundice among term infants, and among infants discharged early, to investigate the perinatal risk factors for readmission for jaundice.

Methods.—Birth data for 781 074 term live-born infants born in New South Wales, Australia from 2001 to 2010 were linked to hospital admission data. Logistic regression models were used to investigate the association between postnatal length of stay (LOS), gestational age (GA), and readmission for jaundice in the first 14 days of life. Other significant perinatal risk factors associated with readmission for jaundice were examined for infants discharged in the first 2 days after birth.

Results.—Eight per 1000 term infants were readmitted for jaundice. Infants born at 37 weeks' GA with an LOS at birth of 0 to 2 days were over 9 times (adjusted odds ratio [aOR] 9.43; 95% CI, 8.34–10.67) and at 38 weeks' GA were 4 times (aOR 4.05; 95% CI, 3.62–4.54) more likely to be readmitted for jaundice compared with infants born at 39 weeks' GA with an LOS of 3 to 4 days. Other significant risk factors for readmission for jaundice for infants discharged 0 to 2 days after birth included vaginal birth, born to mothers from an Asian country, born to first-time mothers, or being breastfed at discharge.

Conclusions.—This study can inform guidelines or policy about identifying infants at risk for readmission for jaundice and ensure that appropriate post-discharge follow-up is received.

▶ Several studies have been published dealing with this question, but the results have been conflicting, even though it is intuitive to expect a lower readmission rate for jaundice in infants who stay longer. One explanation for the differences in outcome in the existing published studies could be that they were all conducted in individual hospitals or, at the most, in hospital systems, whereas the study by Lain et al is the first population-based study of this question. The very large sample of some 781 000 term infants allowed these investigators to analyze the relevant risk factors that might be responsible for the development of jaundice of sufficient severity to merit readmission and the results are not surprising. Although several other investigators have documented the well-known and powerful association between decreasing gestation and an increased risk of hyperbilirubinemia,[1] none have looked at this question in relationship to the length of stay. Nevertheless, given the well-known association between ineffective lactation and jaundice and the fact that early-term infants are much less likely to nurse adequately than their full-term counterparts, it is not surprising to find that it is the early-term infants, discharged in the first 2 days, who are most likely to be readmitted to hospital for jaundice.

M. J. Maisels, MB, BCh, DSc

Reference

1. Maisels MJ, Newman TB. The epidemiology of neonatal hyperbilirubinemia. In: Stevenson DK, Maisels MJ, Watchko JF, eds. *Care of the Jaundiced Neonate.* New York, NY: McGraw Hill; 2012:97-113.

Discrepancies Between Transcutaneous and Serum Bilirubin Measurements
Taylor JA, for the Better Outcomes through Research for Newborns Network (Univ of Washington, Seattle; et al)
Pediatrics 135:224-231, 2015

Objective.—To characterize discrepancies between transcutaneous bilirubin (TcB) measurements and total serum bilirubin (TSB) levels among newborns receiving care at multiple nursery sites across the United States.

Methods.—Medical records were reviewed to obtain data on all TcB measurements collected during two 2-week periods on neonates admitted to participating newborn nurseries. Data on TSB levels obtained within 2 hours of a TcB measurement were also abstracted. TcB − TSB differences and correlations between the values were determined. Data on demographic information for individual newborns and TcB screening practices for each nursery were also collected. Multivariate regression analysis was used to identify characteristics independently associated with the TcB − TSB difference.

Results.—Data on 8319 TcB measurements were collected at 27 nursery sites; 925 TSB levels were matched to a TcB value. The mean TcB − TSB difference was 0.84 ± 1.78 mg/dL, and the correlation between paired measurements was 0.78. In the multivariate analysis, TcB − TSB differences were 0.67 mg/dL higher in African-American newborns than in neonates of other races ($P < .001$). The TcB − TSB difference also varied significantly based on brand of TcB meter used and hour of age of the infant. For 2.2% of paired measurements, the TcB measurement underestimated the TSB level by ≥3 mg/dL.

Conclusions.—During routine clinical care, TcB measurement provided a reasonable estimate of TSB levels in healthy newborns.

Discrepancies between TcB and TSB levels were increased in African-American newborns and varied based on brand of meter used.

▶ Transcutaneous bilirubin (TcB) measurements have been used throughout the world for some 30 years, and a recent monograph[1] discusses, in detail, the history, physics, and biology of this assay, as well as the data documenting our experience with this technique. Although the published data consistently confirm that we can rely on the TcB as a screening measurement, most of these data come from research studies in a single or a few hospitals, where measurements are performed by research staff and careful attention is given to detail and quality control. Taylor et al ask whether the data generated in these studies is applicable to the "real world" of clinical practice, where measurements are typically made by any one of a number of overworked and harried nursing staff and where careful attention to detail and quality control is much less likely to occur.

To answer this question, they gathered retrospective data from 38 newborn nurseries located in academic medical centers or community hospitals. These nurseries are part of the 82 nursery Better Outcomes through Research for Newborns network, located in 35 states. In these nurseries, almost all newborns were routinely screened with a TcB level before discharge, and some 925 total serum bilirubin (TSB) levels were linked to the TcB measurements. They found that 2.2% of TcB measurements underestimated the TSB by ≥3.0 mg/dL. Because a falsely low (false-negative) TcB measurement could result in failure to treat an infant who meets the criteria for phototherapy, we need to know whether this difference between TcB and TSB measurements in 2% of newborns is clinically important.

The first question to be asked is whether the apparent error lies in the TcB measurement. In almost all of the published data, the TSB measurement has been considered the gold standard, but surveys by the American College of Pathologists have shown that TSBs measured by several established laboratory methods were 2 to 5 mg/dL higher than the reference method.[2] So what appear to be falsely low TcB levels could, in some cases, be due to erroneously high TSB measurements.

The second question is: if the TSB is actually > 3 mg/dL above the TcB, is this likely to cause a serious problem? The primary purpose of phototherapy in infants ≥35 weeks' gestation is to prevent the need for an exchange transfusion. We have no evidence that phototherapy in this population has changed any infant's developmental outcome. Currently recommended phototherapy levels in well infants are ~4.5 to 7 mg/dL below exchange transfusion levels.[3] Although not extinct, kernicterus in the Western world is rare and generally seen only at TSB levels > 35 mg/dL.[4-6] Because the currently recommended levels for phototherapy in infants ≥35 weeks are at least 10 to 20 mg/dL below these thresholds, it seems there is ample margin for error.

If the primary concern is that TcB levels might underestimate the TSB, it is a simple matter to set TcB cut points below the TSB level that might warrant investigation or treatment. In a study we performed in 5 office-based pediatric practices,[7] and in which 70 of 118 (59%) of TSBs were ≥15 mg/dL, none of 33 infants who had a TcB < 14 mg/dL had a TSB of ≥17 mg/dL (negative predictive value = 1; 95% confidence interval 0.87–1.0). So if we measure the TSB whenever the TcB is ≥13 or 14 mg/dL, the chance of missing the need for phototherapy in a 4-day-old infant is very low.

Transcutaneous bilirubinometers measure the bilirubin in the extravascular tissue and not in the blood, so a TcB measurement is not a substitute for the TSB. Nevertheless, the TcB can tell us (1) when to worry about an infant and (2) when to get a TSB. We have used TcB measurements in our nurseries and outpatient clinics for more than 2 decades, and pediatricians in 5 of our affiliated practices have been using these measurements for the past 6 years. We measure the TSB whenever the TcB exceeds the 95th percentile on our TCB nomogram,[8] and we have yet to encounter a significant problem with TcBs.

As we noted in a recent commentary,[9] "as long as common sense, clinical judgment, and appropriate follow-up are employed, the likelihood of a bad outcome resulting from an erroneous TcB measurement seems small, whereas the benefits to infants, patients, and care providers of an instantaneous, noninvasive estimate of the TSB level, are abundant."

M. J. Maisels, MB, BCh, DSc

References

1. De Luca D, Engle W, Jackson G. *Transcutaneous Bilirubinometry: Hepatology Research and Clinical Developments.* New York: Nova Biomedical; 2013.
2. Lo SF, Doumas BT. The status of bilirubin measurements in U.S. laboratories: why is accuracy elusive? *Semin Perinatol.* 2011;35:141-147.
3. Maisels MJ, Baltz RD, Bhutani V, et al. Management of hyperbilirubinemia in the newborn infant 35 or more weeks of gestation. *Pediatrics.* 2004;114:297-316.
4. Vandborg P, Hansen B, Griesen G, Mathiasen R, Kasper F, Ebbesen F. Follow up of extreme neonatal hyperbilirubinaemia in 5 to 10 year old children: a Danish population based study. *Dev Med Child Neurol.* 2015;57:378-384.
5. Ebbesen F, Bjerre JV, Vandborg PK. Relation between serum bilirubin levels > 450 μmol/L and bilirubin encephalopathy; a Danish population-based study. *Acta Paediatr.* 2012;101:384-389.
6. Kuzniewicz MW, Wickremasinghe AC, Wu YW, et al. Incidence, etiology, and outcomes of hazardous hyperbillirubinemia in newborns. *Pediatrics.* 2014;134:504-509.
7. Maisels MJ, Engle W, Wainer S, Jackson GL, McManus S, Artinian F. Transcutaneous bilirubin levels in an outpatient and office population. *J Perinatol.* 2011;31:621-624.
8. Maisels MJ, Deridder JM, Kring EA, Balasubramaniam M. Routine transcutaneous bilirubin measurements combined with clinical risk factors improve the prediction of subsequent hyperbilirubinemia. *J Perinatol.* 2009;29:612-617.
9. Maisels MJ. Transcutaneous bilirubin measurement: does it work in the real world? *Pediatrics.* 2015;135:364-366.

Peanut, milk, and wheat intake during pregnancy is associated with reduced allergy and asthma in children
Bunyavanich S, Rifas-Shiman SL, Platts-Mills TA, et al (Icahn School of Medicine at Mount Sinai, NY; Harvard Pilgrim Health Care Inst, Boston, MA; Univ of Virginia Health System, Charlottesville; et al)
J Allergy Clin Immunol 133:1373-1382, 2013

Background.—Maternal diet during pregnancy may affect childhood allergy and asthma.

Objective.—We sought to examine the associations between maternal intake of common childhood food allergens during early pregnancy and childhood allergy and asthma.

Methods.—We studied 1277 mother-child pairs from a US prebirth cohort unselected for any disease. Using food frequency questionnaires administered during the first and second trimesters, we assessed maternal intake of common childhood food allergens during pregnancy. In mid-childhood (mean age, 7.9 years), we assessed food allergy, asthma, allergic rhinitis, and atopic dermatitis by questionnaire and serum-specific IgE levels. We examined the associations between maternal diet during pregnancy and childhood allergy and asthma. We also examined the cross-sectional associations between specific food allergies, asthma, and atopic conditions in mid-childhood.

Results.—Food allergy was common (5.6%) in mid-childhood, as was sensitization to at least 1 food allergen (28.0%). Higher maternal peanut intake (each additional z score) during the first trimester was associated with 47% reduced odds of peanut allergic reaction (odds ratio [OR], 0.53; 95% CI, 0.30-0.94). Higher milk intake during the first trimester was associated with reduced asthma (OR, 0.83; 95% CI, 0.69-0.99) and allergic rhinitis (OR, 0.85; 95% CI, 0.74-0.97). Higher maternal wheat intake during the second trimester was associated with reduced atopic dermatitis (OR, 0.64; 95% CI, 0.46-0.90). Peanut, wheat, and soy allergy were each cross-sectionally associated with increased childhood asthma, atopic dermatitis, and allergic rhinitis (ORs, 3.6 to 8.1).

Conclusion.—Higher maternal intake of peanut, milk, and wheat during early pregnancy was associated with reduced odds of mid-childhood allergy and asthma.

▶ Many clinicians believe delayed introduction to the mother during pregnancy and lactation of potentially allergenic foods such as milk, eggs, peanuts, and wheat prevents atopic diseases. Systematic reviews do not support these restrictions, nor do guidelines from the American Academy of Pediatrics. Recent studies in infants who had peanuts introduced within the first year after birth actually suggest decreased subsequent allergy to peanuts. Nevertheless, these are small studies, and several larger studies are underway that will provide additional guidance in terms of food introduction during infancy.

This article addresses the question of whether maternal allergen intake during the first or second trimesters of pregnancy result in increased or decreased allergies after the child is born and reaches midchildhood. Using a Food Frequency Questionnaire modified for pregnancy, dietary intake was evaluated during different stages of early pregnancy. This differed from previous studies that evaluated diets during the later stages of pregnancy. Using strict criteria for food allergy diagnosis, the authors found that higher maternal peanut intake during the first trimester was associated with a 47% reduced odds of allergic reactions to peanuts. Similarly, higher milk intake was associated with reduced asthma and allergic rhinitis. During the second trimester, higher maternal wheat intake was associated with reduced atopic dermatitis. This makes sense mechanistically because these antigens can readily be delivered to the fetus through the maternal circulation, and the fetus has dendritic cells and other functioning cell types that could support mechanisms that lead to subsequent tolerance.

This study supports current guidelines that state that restriction of any of these foods is not necessary during pregnancy. However, there are still limitations because of the retrospective nature of this study, and additional, better controlled prospective studies as well as studies that make mechanistic sense are needed before we make recommendations for increasing intake of such allergens during early pregnancy.

J. Neu, MD

Thrombocytopenia in late preterm and term neonates after perinatal asphyxia
Christensen RD, Baer VL, Yaish HM (Univ of Utah School of Medicine, Salt Lake City)
Transfusion 55:187-196, 2015

Background.—A recent NHLBI conference concluded that platelet (PLT) transfusions of neonates must become more evidence based. One neonatal disorder for which transfusions are given is a poorly defined entity, the "thrombocytopenia of perinatal asphyxia." To expand the evidence base for this entity, we performed a multicentered, retrospective analysis of neonates with perinatal asphyxia.

Study Design and Methods.—We analyzed records of term and late preterm neonates with perinatal asphyxia defined by a cord blood pH of not more than 6.99 and/or base deficit of at least 16 mmol/L. From these we identified neonates with at least two PLT counts of fewer than $150 \times 10^9/L$ in the first week of life and described the severity, nadir, and duration of the thrombocytopenia.

Results.—Thrombocytopenia occurred in 31% (117/375) of neonates with asphyxia versus 5% of matched nonasphyxiated controls admitted to a neonatal intensive care unit ($p < 0.0001$). Twenty-one of the 117 asphyxiated neonates were excluded from the remaining analysis due to disseminated intravascular coagulation or extracorporeal membrane oxygenation. Nadir PLT counts of the remaining 96 were on Day 3 ($75 \times 10^9/L$; 90% confidence interval, 35.7×10^9-$128.6 \times 10^9/L$) and normalized by Days 19 to 21. PLT counts after asphyxia roughly correlated inversely with elevated nucleated red blood cell count (NRBC) counts at birth. Thirty of the 96 received at least one PLT transfusion, all given prophylactically, none for bleeding.

Conclusions.—We maintain that the thrombocytopenia of perinatal asphyxia is an authentic entity. Its association with elevated NRBC counts suggests that hypoxia is involved in the pathogenesis. Because PLT counts are only moderately low, the condition is transient, and bleeding problems seem rare, we speculate that PLT transfusions should not be needed for most neonates with this condition.

▶ Whenever I encounter a decreasing platelet count in a newborn who suffered perinatal asphyxia, my number one concern is disseminated intravascular coagulopathy (DIC), followed by the possibility of occult organ injury where platelet consumption is underway. This report convinced me that my differential diagnosis should be expanded.

In an effort to provide a better evidence base for transfusion practice in thrombocytopenic infants following perinatal asphyxia, the authors build a compelling argument that thrombocytopenia of perinatal asphyxia (TPA) is an authentic entity that is not associated with platelet consumption but rather is caused by reduced platelet production in the bone marrow. This diagnosis was characterized by a declining platelet count over the first week of life, reaching a nadir on day 3, in the moderate range of thrombocytopenia: $75 \times 10^9/L$; confidence interval, 35.7×10^9-$128.6 \times 10^9/L$, and gradually normalizing by 3 weeks. Interestingly, low platelet counts after asphyxia roughly correlated inversely with elevated nucleated red cell counts at birth, which begs the question of whether hypoxia may be a causal link between these 2 bone marrow aberrations.[1]

Thrombocytopenia occurred in 31% (117 of 375) of neonates with asphyxia versus 5% of matched nonasphyxiated controls. Only some of these infants (N = 21) were eliminated because of confounding platelet consumption from DIC or extracorporeal membrane oxygenation.

Of the remaining 96 infants meeting criteria for TPA, 30 received platelet transfusions, all given prophylactically in the absence of bleeding. These transfusions incremented the platelet counts very well in treated infants, contrary to what is seen in consumptive coagulopathy or neonatal alloimmune thrombocytopenia. The authors suggest that the moderate thrombocytopenia seen in TPA posed no bleeding risk. Furthermore, none of the 11 deaths among those with TPA involved active bleeding or hemorrhagic complications.

The last group studied was infants treated with therapeutic hypothermia (91 of 374) for neonatal asphyxia. In a previous study of 10 neonates with hypoxic-ischemic encephalopathy who were treated with hypothermia, Christensen et al[2] reported no appreciable decrease in platelet numbers but a significant prolongation in bleeding time during cooling, which completely reversed once the infants were rewarmed. In this study, those who received therapeutic hypothermia showed decline in platelet counts over the first 3 to 4 days of life in the same proportion to noncooled asphyxiated infants who subsequently had thrombocytopenia.

Platelet transfusion strategies for term and near-term neonates currently lack a strong evidence base.[3] This retrospective study describes a common, fairly benign, and self-resolving course of thrombocytopenia in most affected infants who meet criteria for perinatal asphyxia. Unlike those with DIC, platelet transfusions are unlikely to be helpful.

E. K. Stork, MD

References

1. Christensen RD, Henry E, Andres RL, Bennett ST. Reference ranges for blood concentrations of nucleated red blood cells in neonates. *Neonatology.* 2011;99: 289-294.
2. Christensen RD, Sheffield MJ, Lambert DK, Baer VL. Effect of therapeutic hypothermia in neonates with hypoxic-ischemic encephalopathy on platelet function. *Neonatology.* 2012;101:91-94.
3. Christensen RD. Platelet transfusion in the neonatal intensive care unit: benefits, risks, alternatives. *Neonatology.* 2011;100:311-318.

Thrombocytopenia in late preterm and term neonates after perinatal asphyxia

Christensen RD, Baer VL, Yaish HM (Univ of Utah School of Medicine, Salt Lake City)
Transfusion 55:187-196, 2015

Background.—A recent NHLBI conference concluded that platelet (PLT) transfusions of neonates must become more evidence based. One neonatal disorder for which transfusions are given is a poorly defined entity, the "thrombocytopenia of perinatal asphyxia." To expand the evidence base for this entity, we performed a multicentered, retrospective analysis of neonates with perinatal asphyxia.

Study Design and Methods.—We analyzed records of term and late preterm neonates with perinatal asphyxia defined by a cord blood pH of not more than 6.99 and/or base deficit of at least 16 mmol/L. From these we identified neonates with at least two PLT counts of fewer than 150×10^9/L in the first week of life and described the severity, nadir, and duration of the thrombocytopenia.

Results.—Thrombocytopenia occurred in 31% (117/375) of neonates with asphyxia versus 5% of matched nonasphyxiated controls admitted to a neonatal intensive care unit ($p < 0.0001$). Twenty-one of the 117 asphyxiated neonates were excluded from the remaining analysis due to disseminated intravascular coagulation or extracorporeal membrane oxygenation. Nadir PLT counts of the remaining 96 were on Day 3 (75×10^9/L; 90% confidence interval, 35.7×10^9 - 128.6×10^9/L) and normalized by Days 19 to 21. PLT counts after asphyxia roughly correlated inversely with elevated nucleated red blood cell count (NRBC) counts at birth. Thirty of the 96 received at least one PLT transfusion, all given prophylactically, none for bleeding.

Conclusions.—We maintain that the thrombocytopenia of perinatal asphyxia is an authentic entity. Its association with elevated NRBC counts suggests that hypoxia is involved in the pathogenesis. Because PLT counts are only moderately low, the condition is transient, and bleeding problems seem rare, we speculate that PLT transfusions should not be needed for most neonates with this condition.

▶ In this retrospective, multicenter observational study, Christensen and colleagues investigated the natural history of platelet counts in infants who had significant metabolic acidosis in cord blood, presumably from perinatal asphyxia. Nearly one-third of these infants (30%) developed thrombocytopenia compared with 5% of matched controls without acidoses. Platelet counts showed a steady decline over the first 3 days of life, followed by a slow return to normal levels by days 16 to 18. The authors suggest that thrombocytopenia following asphyxia is a transient, self-limited phenomenon generally not accompanied by coagulopathy and should infrequently require transfusion therapy. Platelet counts did not appear to be any lower in infants treated with neuroprotective hypothermia compared with those who were not.

Thrombocytopenia was also associated with elevations in the nucleated red blood cell (NRBC) count, a marker of intrauterine hypoxia. This suggests that the thrombocytopenia in this population could result from erythropoietic overproduction/platelet underproduction, as well as platelet consumption as part of the hypoxic cascade, or both. Nevertheless, the value of this study is to get us to think before we transfuse.

S. M. Donn, MD

11 Renal, Metabolism, and Endocrine Disorders

Clinically stable very low birthweight infants are at risk for recurrent tissue glucose fluctuations even after fully established enteral nutrition
Mola-Schenzle E, Staffler A, Klemme M, et al (Ludwig Maximilian Univ Munich-Grosshadern, Germany; Regional Hosp Bolzano, Italy)
Arch Dis Child Fetal Neonatal Ed 100:F126-F131, 2015

Objective.—In previous cases, we have observed occasional hypoglycaemic episodes in preterm infants after initial intensive care. In this prospective study, we determined the frequency and severity of abnormal tissue glucose (TG) in clinically stable preterm infants on full enteral nutrition.

Methods.—Preterm infants born at <1000 g (n = 23; G1) and birth weight 1000−1500 g (n = 18; G2) were studied at a postmenstrual age of 32 ± 2 weeks (G1) and 33 ± 2 weeks (G2). Infants were fed two or three hourly, according to a standard bolus-nutrition protocol, and continuous subcutaneous glucose measurements were performed for 72 h. Normal glucose values were assumed at ≥2.5 mmol/L (45 mg/dL) and ≤8.3 mmol/L (150 mg/dL). Frequency, severity and duration of glucose values beyond normal values were determined.

Results.—We observed asymptomatic low TG values in 39% of infants in G1 and in 44% in G2. High TG values were detected in 83% in G1 and 61% in G2. Infants in G1 experienced prolonged and more severe low TG episodes, and also more frequent and severe high TG episodes. In G1 and G2, 87% and 67% of the infants, respectively, showed glucose fluctuations characterised by rapid glucose increase followed by a rapid glucose drop after feeds. In more mature infants, glucose fluctuations were less pronounced and less dependent on enteral feeds.

Conclusions.—Clinically stable well-developing preterm infants beyond their initial period of intensive care show interstitial glucose instabilities exceeding values as low as 2.5 mmol/L and as high as 8.3 mmol/L. This novel observation may play an important role for the susceptibility of these high-risk infants for the development of the metabolic syndrome.

Trial Registration Number.—German trial registration number DRKS00004590.

▶ It has been well established that preterm infants are at risk for the metabolic syndrome (hypertension, diabetes, obesity, and coronary artery disease) later in life.[1] Attention has been directed to their early nutrition, and the major thrusts are to avoid early malnutrition, provide adequate protein from as early as day 1, nourish with human milk, and avoid too rapid weight gain in the first months of life to avoid sowing the seeds for the metabolic syndrome.[2] Before the publication abstracted here, little to no attention had been paid to fluctuations in blood sugar. Sure, physicians recognized that preterm infants and especially growth-restricted preterm infants were at risk for hypoglycemia, but they were monitored and steps were taken to prevent or treat hypoglycemia. On the other hand, hyperglycemia was recognized in sick preterm infants, particularly after being treated with postnatal steroids, excess glucose administration, babies with fungal sepsis, and the rare infant with transient neonatal diabetes. By applying the newer technology that enables continuous monitoring of tissue blood sugar, Mola-Schenzle and colleagues have demonstrated for the first time that metabolic instabilities may persist beyond the first month of life in clinically stable infants on full enteral nutrition. By using Continuous Glucose Monitoring System, they were able to assess the duration of glucose values beyond the normal range. Almost one-quarter of the low-glucose episodes lasted between 30 and 60 minutes, whereas the more frequent high-glucose episodes lasted usually between 10 and 30 minutes, and in 17%, > 60 minutes. Because high glucose values in the first week of life are associated with increased mortality and white matter reduction, it is disturbing to document these values beyond the first week of life.

As noted by the authors, there is no precedent for interpreting these data. There is a large body of literature attesting to the risks of hypoglycemia for loss of IQ points if not full-blown neurodevelopmental impairment. But what happens if it occurs in clinically stable, growing, asymptomatic infants? Time alone will tell. This is a small sample, but there is no doubt that this report will stimulate further investigations accompanied by more complex metabolic measurements and imaging studies. Follow-up of the current subjects is mandatory.

A. A. Fanaroff, MBBCh, FRCPE

References

1. Parkinson JR, Hyde MJ, Gale C, et al. Preterm birth and the metabolic syndrome in adult life: a systematic review and meta-analysis. *Pediatrics.* 2013;131: e1240-e1263.
2. Singhal A, Cole TJ, Fewtrell M, Deanfield J, Lucas A. Is slower early growth beneficial for long-term cardiovascular health? *Circulation.* 2004;109:1108-1113.

Preterm Birth Is Associated with Higher Uric Acid Levels in Adolescents
Washburn LK, Nixon PA, Russell GB, et al (Wake Forest Univ, Winston-Salem, NC)
J Pediatr 167:76-80, 2015

Objective.—To compare serum uric acid levels in adolescents born prematurely and adolescents born at term and to assess the correlation between serum uric acid and blood pressure (BP) in those born prematurely.

Study Design.—In this observational cohort study, 124 adolescents born prematurely and 44 adolescents born at term were studied at 14 years of age. Multivariate analyses were used to describe the relationship of premature birth to serum uric acid while adjusting for confounding variables. Pearson correlation was used to describe the relationship between uric acid and systolic BP among those born prematurely.

Results.—Adjusting for race, sex, maternal hypertension, and fetal growth, we found that preterm adolescents had greater serum uric acid levels than adolescents born at term (adjusted mean difference 0.46, 95% CI 0.10-0.81 mg/dL; 27.4, 6-48.2 μmol/L; $P=.012$). Among those born prematurely, uric acid was positively correlated with systolic BP (Pearson correlation coefficient: 0.29, 0.12-0.44; $P=.0013$).

Conclusions.—Serum uric acid levels are greater in adolescents born prematurely than in those born at term, and this difference could contribute to greater BP among individuals born prematurely.

▶ Many studies have found that preterm infants are at higher risk of essential hypertension than their term-born counterparts. In this study, Washburn et al analyzed serum uric acid concentrations at 14 years of age in 124 former preterm infants and 44 full-term controls. In their case—control study, they found that the children born preterm had higher blood pressure and higher serum uric acid levels (adjusted mean difference was 0.46 mg/dL [0.10-0.81], 27.4 mmol/L [6-48.2]; $P=.012$). The authors' hypothesis was that renal alterations during early development in preterm infants lead to higher uric acid, which in turn leads to hypertension. It is difficult in this cross-sectional study to determine whether the hypertension results from higher uric acid or whether uric acid is simply a marker for impaired renal function, and thus uric acid excretion is impaired. Nonetheless, this important study again highlights the importance of closer monitoring of blood pressure among former preterm infants during childhood than is typically done during the course of pediatric care. These authors call for further work to determine the etiology of hypertension (including elevated uric acid) in preterm infants for the purpose of developing targeted therapies.

H. H. Burris, MD, MPH

Neonatal Citrullinemia: Novel, Reversible Neuroimaging Findings Correlated With Ammonia Level Changes

Ruder J, Legacy J, Russo G, et al (Univ of Central Florida College of Medicine, Orlando; PA and the Pediatric Epilepsy Ctr of Central Florida)
Pediatr Neurol 51:553-556, 2014

Background.—Citrullinemia type I is an autosomal recessive disorder of the urea cycle in which a patient lacks the cytosolic enzyme, argininosuccinic acid synthetase. This enzyme deficiency results in elevated levels of ammonia, glutamine, and citrulline. The accumulation of ammonia and glutamine causes neurodegenerative changes that are detectible on magnetic resonance imaging. This is the first case report of citrullinemia with repeat magnetic resonance images and electroencephalographs in the acute phase of hyperammonemia.

Case.—This 3800 g white boy was born at 40 weeks 4 days gestation to a 25-year-old mother. He was delivered at home to a certified midwife with no reported complications. He was doing well until day of life 4, when the mother reported he would no longer latch to feed. He was observed to have markedly elevated ammonia levels and ultimately diagnosed with citrullinemia type I. The initial magnetic resonance image was markedly abnormal. After aggressive medical management, his repeat magnetic resonance image revealed marked improvement in the acute setting.

Conclusion.—Early and aggressive management of hyperammonemia can result in improved magnetic resonance imaging findings in the acute setting. It is too early to know if this will translate to an improved clinical outcome. Clinical suspicion must remain high for urea cycle disorders in neonates with magnetic resonance image changes similar to those resulting from hypoxic-ischemic injury.

▶ This article describes a term newborn who developed clinical findings compatible with hyperammonemia secondary to the urea cycle defect, citrullinemia type 1. The baby was treated with supportive therapy; sodium benzoate, phenylacetate, and arginine; and hemodialysis to control the hyperammonemia. The authors were fortunate to obtain magnetic resonance imaging (MRI) brain scans on days of life 6 and 17, which demonstrated the presumed effects of hyperammonemia and elevated glutamate and its improvement with aggressive treatment. The authors carefully cautioned not to extrapolate long-term outcome from the structural changes demonstrated on neuroimaging.

I took 2 messages from this case report. First, this potentially lethal genetic disorder indeed produces restricted diffusion during the acute phases of hyperammonemia, which improves with treatment and time. Second, it reinforces the concept that the earlier the treatment, the better, which is not a new concept.[1-3] In the case reported, the infant presented on the fourth postnatal day with nonspecific findings of poor feeding, hypothermia, and, appropriately, concern for sepsis. It was not until day 6, and after the initial MRI, that metabolic disease was considered and ammonia concentration was measured.

The key to successful treatment of urea cycle disorders is the prompt diagnosis and treatment of the hyperammonemia. To diagnose metabolic disease, the clinician has to think about metabolic disease in the differential diagnoses of infants presenting on the third or fourth postnatal day, usually with lethargy, poor feeding, vomiting, and seizures. Unfortunately, the relative rarity of these disorders often results from omission in the differential diagnosis, as happened in this case.

S. M. Donn, MD

References

1. Donn SM, Swartz RD, Thoene JG. Comparison of exchange transfusion, peritoneal dialysis, and hemodialysis for the treatment of hyperammonemia in an anuric newborn infant. *J Pediatr.* 1979;95:67-70.
2. Donn SM, Banagale RC. Neonatal hyperammonemia. *Pediatr Rev.* 1984;5:203-208.
3. Donn SM, Thoene JG. Prospective prevention of neonatal hyperammonaemia in argininosuccinic aciduria by arginine therapy. *J Inherit Metab Dis.* 1985;8:18-20.

12 Miscellaneous

Comparison of four near-infrared spectroscopy devices shows that they are only suitable for monitoring cerebral oxygenation trends in preterm infants
Schneider A, Minnich B, Hofstätter E, et al (Paracelsus Med Univ, Salzburg, Austria; Univ of Salzburg, Austria)
Acta Paediatr Int J Paediatr 103:934-938, 2014

Aim.—Measuring cerebral oxygenation using near-infrared spectroscopy (NIRS) has taken on an increasingly important role in the field of neonatology. Several companies have already developed commercial devices, and more publications are reporting absolute boundary values or percentiles for neonates. We compared four commercially used devices to discover whether they provided consistent results in the same patients.

Methods.—We recruited nine preterm infants and tested them for 2 h, using sensors from two different devices. The measurements were carried out six times on each child, so that all four devices were compared with each other. A total of 54 measurements were conducted. The following devices were compared: the NIRO 200 (Hamamatsu Photonics K.K), the INVOS 5100c (Somanetics), the Fore-Sight (CAS Med.) and the SenSmart X-100 (NONIN).

Results.—The cerebral tissue oxygenation data yielded by the individual devices differed significantly from each other, ranging from a minimum difference of 2.93% to a maximum difference of 12.66%.

Conclusion.—The commercially available NIRS devices showed highly significant differences in local cerebral tissue oxygenation levels, to the extent that the industry cannot agree on uniform and reproducible standards. Therefore, NIRS should only be used for trend measurements in preterm infants.

▶ Clinical application of near-infrared spectroscopy (NIRS) to monitor cerebral oxygenation in preterm infants continues to expand in the intensive care setting. Differences between commercially available NIRS devices no doubt account for measurable variability in absolute cerebral oxygenation values as the authors demonstrate. For example, 1 manufacturer uses a laser-based light source with generation of 4 narrow wavelengths, another manufacturer uses a single LED-based emitter with 2 wider wavelengths, and a third device uses a dual LED emitter with 4 wavelengths. Differences also exist in the frequency of measurements per minute, spatial resolution technique, and algorithm to calculate regional saturation values based on weighting of oxygenated to deoxygenated hemoglobin.

However, it would be premature to discard NIRS technology. A growing body of literature has demonstrated the utility of trend measurements in preterm infants for recognition of a hemodynamically significant patent ductus arteriosus, disrupted cerebral autoregulation, and risk for cerebral hypoxemia. One could arguably establish "normal" absolute cerebral oxygenation values and expected values for specific conditions by focusing efforts on a designated type of NIRS device and learning how to use this selected device well. Further development of this technology will better standardize the optimal type of commercially available NIRS device in the future, but current device differences should not prevent NIRS monitoring from becoming a useful adjunct to improve care for preterm infants at high risk for impaired brain oxygenation.

V. Y. L. Chock, MD

Comparison of four near-infrared spectroscopy devices shows that they are only suitable for monitoring cerebral oxygenation trends in preterm infants

Schneider A, Minnich B, Hofstätter E, et al (Paracelsus Med Univ, Salzburg, Austria; Univ of Salzburg, Austria)
Acta Paediatr 103:934-938, 2014

Aim.—Measuring cerebral oxygenation using near-infrared spectroscopy (NIRS) has taken on an increasingly important role in the field of neonatology. Several companies have already developed commercial devices, and more publications are reporting absolute boundary values or percentiles for neonates. We compared four commercially used devices to discover whether they provided consistent results in the same patients.

Methods.—We recruited nine preterm infants and tested them for 2 h, using sensors from two different devices. The measurements were carried out six times on each child, so that all four devices were compared with each other. A total of 54 measurements were conducted. The following devices were compared: the NIRO 200 (Hamamatsu Photonics K.K), the INVOS 5100c (Somanetics), the Fore-Sight (CAS Med.) and the SenSmart X-100 (NONIN).

Results.—The cerebral tissue oxygenation data yielded by the individual devices differed significantly from each other, ranging from a minimum difference of 2.93% to a maximum difference of 12.66%.

Conclusion.—The commercially available NIRS devices showed highly significant differences in local cerebral tissue oxygenation levels, to the extent that the industry cannot agree on uniform and reproducible standards. Therefore, NIRS should only be used for trend measurements in preterm infants.

▶ There is a great deal of enthusiasm for introducing near-infrared spectroscopy (NIRS) measurement to neonatal intensive care, especially for the measurement of cerebral tissue oxygenation. Measuring local tissue oxygenation using NIRS uses the same basic technology as measuring peripheral arterial oxygen saturation by pulse oximetry. To compare data obtained with various oximetry instruments, technical standards and the option to check or gauge the devices were developed. As illustrated by the clinical observational study described here, the commercial NIRS devices that are currently available provide cerebral tissue oxygenation measurements at different levels, with some of the differences big enough to have a probable effect on clinical management. Thus, it would appear that the devices do not measure the same thing and do not give the same answers in the same infants. Until there are valid reference systems and perhaps more standardized algorithms for the whole NIRS technology, it cannot be considered a reliable tool to be used in the clinical management of very preterm infants. As the authors note, at this juncture, it should only be used for trend measurements.

L. A. Papile, MD

Refractive Outcomes Following Bevacizumab Monotherapy Compared With Conventional Laser Treatment: A Randomized Clinical Trial
Geloneck MM, Chuang AZ, Clark WL, et al (The Univ of Texas Health Science Ctr—Houston Med School; Palmetto Health Baptist Med Ctr, Columbia, SC; et al)
JAMA Ophthalmol 132:1327-1333, 2014

Importance.—Children born prematurely who develop retinopathy of prematurity (ROP) often develop myopia, and those who require laser treatment may develop very high myopia, which has considerable clinical consequences.

Objective.—To report refractive outcomes in preterm infants who developed ROP in zone I or zone II posterior as stage 3+ ROP or aggressive posterior ROP (APROP).

Design, Setting, and Participants.—All infants received intravitreal bevacizumab or laser therapy in a prospective, stratified, randomized, controlled, masked, multicenter clinical trial, Bevacizumab Eliminates the Angiogenic Threat for ROP (BEAT-ROP). Children who received intravitreal bevacizumab or laser in the BEAT-ROP clinical trial, with treatment randomized by infant, underwent cycloplegic retinoscopic refraction at a mean age of 2½ years. Fifteen centers with both pediatric and vitreoretinal ophthalmologists participating in level 3 neonatal intensive care units in academic centers with institutional review board approval were included in the trial. Of the originally enrolled 150 infants (300 eyes) in the BEAT-ROP clinical trial, 13 infants (26 eyes) died (6 received intravitreal bevacizumab; 7 received laser) and 19 eyes had intraocular surgery (6 infants bilaterally). Thus, 45 eyes (19 infants bilaterally) were excluded, leaving 131 infants (255 eyes, including 21 eyes that received a successful second treatment for recurrence).

Interventions.—Follow-up of the BEAT-ROP cohort.

Main Outcomes and Measures.—Spherical equivalent refractive outcomes and their distribution by ROP zone and treatment.

Results.—Refractions were available for 109 of 131 eligible infants (83.2%) and 211 of 255 eyes (82.7%). Mean (SD) spherical equivalent refractions were as follows: zone I, −1.51 (3.42) diopters (D) in 52 eyes that received intravitreal bevacizumab and −8.44 (7.57) D in 35 eyes that received laser treatment ($P < .001$); and zone II posterior, −0.58 (2.53) D in 58 eyes that received intravitreal bevacizumab and −5.83 (5.87) D in 66 eyes that received laser treatment ($P < .001$). Very high myopia (≥ -8.00 D) occurred in zone I in 2 of 52 (3.8%) eyes that received intravitreal bevacizumab and in 18 of 35 (51.4%) eyes that received laser treatment ($P < .001$). Very high myopia occurred in zone II posterior in 1 of 58 (1.7%) eyes that received intravitreal bevacizumab and in 24 of 66 (36.4%) eyes that received laser treatment ($P < .001$).

Conclusions and Relevance.—More very high myopia was found in eyes that received laser treatment than in eyes that received intravitreal bevacizumab. This difference is possibly related to anterior segment development that is present with intravitreal bevacizumab but minimal or absent following laser treatment.

Trial Registration.—clinicaltrials.gov Identifier: NCT00622726.

▶ Over the past several years the intravitreal instillation of bevacizumab, an antivascular endothelial growth factor, has gained acceptance as the preferred treatment for severe retinopathy of prematurity (ROP). Its popularity relates in part to the ease of use and relatively low cost compared with laser ablation. However, the consequences of bevacizumab therapy, particularly in comparison to those associated with laser ablation, have not been described.

This study is a follow-up to the BEAT-ROP multicenter clinical trial in which 150 extremely low birth weight infants with ROP in Zone I or Zone II posterior with stage 3+ ROP or aggressive posterior ROP in both eyes were randomized to receive treatment in both eyes of either intravitreal bevacizumab or near confluent laser therapy.[1] At a mean age of 2.5 years, the reported frequency of myopia for laser-treated eyes was 1.6-fold (Zone II posterior) to 1.7-fold (Zone I) higher than in the bevacizumab-treated group. In addition, the distribution of the severity of myopia for both Zone I and Zone II ROP was skewed toward emmetropia for the bevacizumab treatment, whereas laser ablation demonstrated a bimodal distribution with peaks at very high myopia and low myopia. Of note, there was no significant difference in the severity of myopia between Zone I and Zone II ROP within each treatment arm. It should be noted that because the refractions were performed by unmasked ophthalmologists, many of whom participated in the original trial, there may be an inherent bias in the data. Although the results are encouraging, additional information is needed.

L. A. Papile, MD

Reference

1. Mintz-Hittner HA, Kennedy KA, Chuang AZ, BEAT-ROP Cooperative Group. Efficacy of intravitreal bevacizumab for stage 3+ retinopathy of prematurity. *N Engl J Med.* 2011;364:603-615.

Between-Hospital Variation in Treatment and Outcomes in Extremely Preterm Infants

Rysavy MA, for the Eunice Kennedy Shriver National Institute of Child Health and Human Development Neonatal Research Network (Univ of Iowa; et al)
N Engl J Med 372:1801-1811, 2015

Background.—Between-hospital variation in outcomes among extremely preterm infants is largely unexplained and may reflect differences in hospital practices regarding the initiation of active lifesaving treatment as compared with comfort care after birth.

Methods.—We studied infants born between April 2006 and March 2011 at 24 hospitals included in the Eunice Kennedy Shriver National Institute of Child Health and Human Development Neonatal Research Network. Data were collected for 4987 infants born before 27 weeks of gestation without congenital anomalies. Active treatment was defined as any potentially lifesaving intervention administered after birth. Survival and neurodevelopmental impairment at 18 to 22 months of corrected age were assessed in 4704 children (94.3%).

Results.—Overall rates of active treatment ranged from 22.1% (interquartile range [IQR], 7.7 to 100) among infants born at 22 weeks of gestation to 99.8% (IQR, 100 to 100) among those born at 26 weeks of gestation. Overall rates of survival and survival without severe impairment ranged from 5.1% (IQR, 0 to 10.6) and 3.4% (IQR, 0 to 6.9), respectively, among children born at 22 weeks of gestation to 81.4% (IQR, 78.2 to 84.0) and 75.6% (IQR, 69.5 to 80.0), respectively, among those born at 26 weeks of gestation. Hospital rates of active treatment accounted for 78% and 75% of the between-hospital variation in survival and survival without severe impairment, respectively, among children born at 22 or 23 weeks of gestation, and accounted for 22% and 16%, respectively, among those born at 24 weeks of gestation, but the rates did not account for any of the variation in outcomes among those born at 25 or 26 weeks of gestation.

Conclusions.—Differences in hospital practices regarding the initiation of active treatment in infants born at 22, 23, or 24 weeks of gestation explain some of the between-hospital variation in survival and survival without impairment among such patients. (Funded by the National Institutes of Health.)

▶ Understanding differences in hospital-specific practices regarding the initiation of either active treatment or comfort care at the time of birth for the extremely low gestational age infant and how this influences survival and morbidity has been a gap in the literature. This recent study, conducted by the Eunice Kennedy Shriver National Institute of Child Health and Human Development Neonatal Research Network, evaluated and reported the between-hospital variation in initiation of active treatment of extremely preterm infants at birth and the associations with survival and other outcomes including survival without impairment among these infants. Active treatment was defined as interventions including surfactant therapy and other standard measures for resuscitation and respiratory support.

Overall, the study found that there were significant differences in the initiation of active treatment at the time of birth among extremely low gestational age infants. These differences were most notable in the lowest gestational ages and less so in the higher gestational ages, where nearly all infants received active treatment at the time of birth (ie, 24, 25, and 26 weeks).

Gestational Age Active Treatment Administered	(95% Confidence Interval)
22 weeks 22.1%	18.1−26.8
23 weeks 71.8%	68.5−74.9
24 weeks 97.1%	96.0−98.0
25 weeks 99.6%	99.1−99.8
26 weeks 99.8%	99.4−100.0

The data on initiation of active treatment were significantly higher in both 22- and 23-week infants who were born on day 5 or day 6 of the specific gestational week compared with infants who were born at the beginning of the same week. The authors suggest that this might be explained by both the family and the clinical team tending to "round up" toward the end of the week when making decisions about whether to initiate active treatment. This finding is curious in light of the fact that outside the setting of in vitro fertilization, best estimates of gestational age are not 100% precise, with a margin of error of at least 5 days.[1]

The decision to intervene with active treatment in the extremely low gestational age infant is complex and influenced by many nuanced factors. The study reported by Rysavy and colleagues is novel because it provides new information about clinical outcomes for the extremely low gestational age infant based on whether active treatment was initiated at the time of birth. This information is most notable in the lower gestational age groups, where the outcomes were most different based on the difference between infants who received active treatment and all infants. For example, the survival, survival without severe impairment, and survival without moderate or severe impairment, in all infants at 22 weeks of gestation were on average 5.1 (95% confidence interval: 3.2−7.9), 3.4 (1.9−5.9), and 2.0 (0.9−4.1), respectively. This was in contrast to 23.1 (14.9−34.0), 15.4 (8.8−25.4), and 9.0 (4.3−17.9) in infants who received active treatment. Notable differences in the same outcomes were also observed in infants born at 23 weeks but not in the infants born at 24, 25, and 26 weeks of gestation, because the majority of infants who are born at these gestational ages received active treatment.

When we account for the type of treatment provided at the time of birth and early in the neonatal period, the clinical outcomes, which are still influenced negatively by gestational age, are better in infants who received active treatment. We still have a great deal to learn about caring for the extremely low gestational age infant at the time of birth and how to council families who are in our care under these difficult circumstances. These study findings may inform our collective decision making about initiation of active treatment at the time of birth for some infants.

K. E. Gregory

Reference

1. Kramer MS, McLean FH, Boyd ME, Usher RH. The validity of gestational age estimation by menstrual dating in term, preterm, and postterm gestations. JAMA. 1988;260:3306-3308.

Pigmentary Lines of the Newborn: A Case Report and Review of the Literature
Fosse N, Itin P (Univ of Basel, Switzerland; Univ Hospital Basel, Switzerland)
Dermatology 228:198-201, 2014

Various diseases of pigmentation in the newborn are known, such as congenital or acquired linear hyperpigmentation. Pigmentary lines of the newborn are counted among the transient benign cutaneous lesions in the newborn and appear to be rather rare. This paper reports on a newborn with pigmentary lines in the creases of the abdomen. The 5-month-old boy is the first case observed so far in the University Hospital of Basel in Switzerland. He was born at term and healthy, without any congenital abnormalities. The horizontally arranged linear hyperpigmentation appeared shortly after birth and faded spontaneously after 5 months. Pigmentary lines of the newborn are rare and the non-hormonal cause may be flexion in utero or other mechanically induced stimulation. So far, only eight similar cases have been reported, which are listed in a table.

▶ There are numerous conditions related to skin pigmentation that can be seen in the neonatal period. Common entities include linea nigra, transient pustular melanosis, a dark scrotum or vulva, darkly pigmented nipples, and Mongolian spots. Some of these are hormonal in origin but generally benign. Other pigmented lesions such as the so-called giant hairy nevus or congenital melanocytic nevus may not only cause serious disfiguration but also place the infant at higher risk for malignant degeneration into melanoma. In such cases, the nevi are removed electively.

This article describes a newborn with horizontal pigmentary lines in the creases of the abdomen. The lines were horizontally arranged and faded spontaneously after 5 months. The authors discuss hyper- and hypopigmentation disorders and their etiology. Pigmentary lines are not associated with any other anomalies and are not thought to be due to hormonal stimulation. They are seldom seen in white infants, and because they are found on the flexural lines, they may relate to irritation experienced in utero.

Although there are only a few case reports on this entity, it may be much more common; it is important for the clinician to remember that these are benign and reassurance may be all that is needed.

J. Neu, MD

Origins of the breast milk-derived cells; an endeavor to find the cell sources
Sani M, Hosseini SM, Salmannejad M, et al (Shiraz Univ of Med Sciences, Iran)
Cell Biol Int 39:611-618, 2015

Fresh human breast milk consists of a heterogeneous population of cells that may offer a non-invasive source of cells for therapeutic proposes. The aims of this study were to characterize the breast milk-derived cells cultured in vitro. To do this, the cells from human breast milk were cultured and the expression of the CD markers along with the embryonic stem cell markers, endothelial and luminal mammary epithelial cell markers was evaluated by flow cytometry and immunofluorescence. The presence of fetal microchimerism among the isolated cells was also determined by the presence of SRY gene. They were also differentiated into adipocytes and osteoblasts. The results showed that a remarkable number of cells expressed the mesenchymal stem cell (MSC) markers such as CD90, CD44, CD271, and CD146. A subpopulation of the human breast milk-derived cells (HBMDC) also expressed the embryonic stem cell markers, such as TRA 60−1, Oct4, Nanog and Sox2 but not SSEA1 or 4. The frequencies of the cells which expressed the endothelial, hematopoietic cell markers were negligible. SRY gene was not detected in the breast milk isolated cells. A subpopulation of the cells also expressed cytokeratin 18, the marker of luminal mammary epithelial cells. These cells showed the capability to differentiate into adipocytes and osteoblasts. In conclusion, these finding highlighted the presence of cells with various sources in the breast milk. Different stem cells including MSCs or embryonic stem cell-like cell along with the exfoliated cells from luminal epithelial cells were found among the isolated cells. The breast milk-derived stem cells might be considered as a non-invasive source of the stem cells for therapeutic purpose.

▶ We appear to be on the precipice of a new generation of research into human milk. In the previous generation of research, various macro- and micronutrient properties were evaluated. These properties have been used by industry as a gold standard for developing commercial preparations with similarities to human milk. Additionally, the presence of immunologic molecules, cells, lipases, nucleotides, certain long chain lipids, free amino acids, and other biochemical agents were found in appreciable quantities and have been subjects of considerable investigation.

In the current generation of human milk research, the microbiome,[1] metabolome,[2] and epigenome[3] of human milk have stimulated interest. In addition, microRNAs that may be responsible for controlling transcription of various proteins in human milk are being discovered.[4] This article involves another of these new-generation areas of human milk research, that is, stem cells.

Although it has been known for several years that cells suggestive of having stem cell properties were present in human milk, this area has only recently generated major excitement. One group found that stem cells in human milk have embryonic stem cell-like properties and have the capability to differentiate into neuron-like cells as well as several other cell types.[5] The current study evaluates these cells in further detail, also supporting their embryonic stem cell-like properties, without being embryonic stem cells. They also determine whether these cells may be chimeras with, looking for the *SRY* gene that would be found in mothers who have male offspring. This was not found, thus likely negating this hypothesis. The cells found in this study had the capability to differentiate into osteoblasts and adipocytes, but no mention is made about differentiation into neural cells, as in the aforementioned article.

Although this is a new area where considerable work is needed, the potential of having a ready source of embryonic-like pluripotential stem cells with the capability to differentiate into cell types for use in regenerative medicine is exciting. Whether these cells also play a role in the newborn enhancing development is an area of tremendous interest.

J. Neu, MD

References

1. Hunt KM, Foster JA, Forney LJ, et al. Characterization of the diversity and temporal stability of bacterial communities in human milk. *PLoS One*. 2011;6: e21313.
2. Fanos V, Van den Anker J, Noto A, Mussap M, Atzori L. Metabolomics in neonatology: fact or fiction? *Semin Fetal Neonatal Med*. 2013;18:3-12.
3. Verduci E, Banderali G, Barberi S, et al. Epigenetic effects of human breast milk. *Nutrients*. 2014;6:1711-1724.
4. Yu ZB, Guo XR. A new component of breast milk: microRNA. *Zhongguo Dang Dai Er Ke Za Zhi*. 2012;14:719-723 [in Chinese].
5. Twigger A-J, Hodgetts S, Filgueira L, Hartmann PE, Hassiotou F. From breast milk to brains: the potential of stem cells in human milk. *J Hum Lact*. 2013;29: 136-139.

Diagnostic Yield of Sonography in Infants With Suspected Hip Dysplasia: Diagnostic Thinking Efficiency and Therapeutic Efficiency
Ashby E, Roposch A (UCL Inst of Child Health, London, UK)
Am J Roentgenol 204:177-181, 2015

Objective.—The purpose of this study is to determine the impact of sonographic information on surgeons' diagnostic thinking and decision making in the management of infants with a possible diagnosis of developmental dysplasia of the hip (DDH).

Subjects and Methods.—Five experienced orthopedic surgeons examined 66 hips of infants who were referred for a possible diagnosis of DDH and reported for each hip a confidence level about the diagnosis of DDH using a visual analog scale (VAS) before and after hip sonography was obtained. In addition, they reported a management plan. We determined the efficiency in diagnostic thinking by calculating the mean gain in diagnostic confidence as the percentage change in VAS scores and the impact of sonography on the management plan (therapeutic efficiency).

Results.—Sonography led to a change in diagnosis in 52% (34/66) of hips. The management plan changed in 32% (21/66) of hips. The mean gain in reported diagnostic confidence was 19.4% (95% CI, 17.3−21.5%), but it was 46.0% (95% CI, 30.5−60.8%) in cases where the management changed as a result of sonography (difference, 37.7%; $p < 0.0001$). The greatest yield of sonography was found in hips showing limited abduction. Sonography obviated further follow-up in 23% (15/66) of cases.

Conclusion.—Sonography refined the diagnostic thinking of clinicians and led to a change in diagnosis in 52% of cases. Management plans changed in 32% of cases.

▶ An integral part of the newborn physical is the hip check, looking for physical evidence of developmental dysplasia of the hip (DDH). Because the child's hip will not develop normally if it remains unstable and anatomically abnormal by walking age, the careful physical examination is complemented by an ultrasound evaluation that is done either routinely in some centers or selectively in others. In a center with universal ultrasound screening Kolb et al[1] evaluated 5356 hips in the first 2 weeks of life and found sonographic signs of DDH in 0.24% of the newborns in keeping with expected finding of 1-2 in 1000 births. The ideal time for ultrasound screening appears to be 6 to 8 weeks, which is when routine ultrasound is recommended. MRI is increasingly used because it is a noninvasive imaging modality that offers excellent anatomic detail, enabling the differentiation of ossified and unossified components of the hip.[2]

What is the impact of ultrasound on clinical decision making? This excellent article by Ashby and Roposch shows that it is significant. Members of an expert panel changed their diagnosis and as a result their management plan in more than half of the patients after the addition of ultrasonography data. Ultrasonography was helpful in reassuring almost a quarter of the subjects who needed no further follow-up and was most helpful for patients referred for limitations with abduction. This study emphasizes how clinicians use technology to make better clinical decisions. This is beneficial for the patients, cost-effective, and good for the clinicians.

A. A. Fanaroff, MBBCh, FRCPE

References

1. Kolb A, Schweiger N, Mailath-Pokorny M, et al. Low incidence of early developmental dysplasia of the hip in universal ultrasonographic screening of newborns: analysis and evaluation of risk factors. *Int Orthop.* 2015 [Epub ahead of print].
2. Starr V, Ha BY. Imaging update on developmental dysplasia of the hip with the role of MRI. *AJR Am J Roentgenol.* 2014;203:1324-1335.

A comparison of the direct cost of care in an open-bay and single-family room NICU

Stevens DC, Thompson PA, Helseth CC, et al (Sanford Children's Hosp, Sioux Falls, SD; Sanford School of Medicine of the Univ of South Dakota, Vermillion; et al)
J Perinatol 34:830-835, 2014

Objective.—This research examined the proposition that the direct costs of care were no different in an open-bay (OPBY) as compared with a single-family room (SFR) neonatal intensive care (NICU) environment.

Study Design.—This was a sequential cohort study.

Result.—General linear models were implemented using clinical and cost data for all neonates admitted to the two cohorts studied. Costs were adjusted to year 2007 U.S. dollars. Models were constructed for the unadjusted regression and subsequently by adding demographic variables, treatment variables, length of respiratory support and length of stay. With the exception of the last, none were found to achieve significance. The full model had $R^2 = 0.799$ with $P = 0.0095$ and predicted direct costs of care less in the SFR NICU.

Conclusion.—For the time, location and administrative practices in place, this study demonstrates that care can be provided in the SFR NICU at no additional cost as compared with OPBY NICU.

▶ In this article, the authors use a complex economic modeling methodology to compare the direct costs of care between their older open-bay room structure with the newer single-room care. They conclude that the costs are comparable and should not discourage institutions contemplating this switch from doing so. Although I found this to be a worthwhile undertaking, I wonder whether these conclusions are generally exportable. In our own institution, we were not able to replicate what these investigators did in using the same number of nurses to care for the same number of patients. Depending on space and configuration, it might be possible for smaller units. Removing multiples (twins, triplets, etc) from the analysis may also be a methodological flaw, particularly for centers in which multifetal gestation is common and where there is an active assisted reproduction program.

It is also critical that other cost issues be considered in addition to the direct costs. Parents seem to genuinely like single-room care. They are reluctant to accept back transport to other facilities that cannot offer single-room care and thus present lost opportunity costs for more critically ill babies when census is high. Stress levels among care providers seem to be higher at times in the single-room format. Alarm fatigue, increased physical requirements to care for patients who might be separated by a distance a lot greater than under the open-bay format, and additional stress from other evolving practices (such as electronic medical records) may affect nurse retention, and the cost of training new nurses must then be factored into the analysis.

Single-room care is a popular fad of the new millennium. We are, as a nation, spending huge sums to convert open-bay rooms or build new facilities with single-room care. Will it last, or will the pendulum lose its momentum and swing back to the more efficient open-bay model? Time will tell.

S. M. Donn, MD

Evacuation of a Neonatal Intensive Care Unit in a Disaster: Lessons From Hurricane Sandy

Espiritu M, Patil U, Cruz H, et al (Univ School of Medicine, NY)
Pediatrics 134:e1662-e1669, 2014

NICU patients are among those potentially most vulnerable to the effects of natural or man-made disaster on a medical center. The published data on evacuations of NICU patients in the setting of disaster are sparse. In October of 2012, New York University Langone Medical Center was evacuated during Hurricane Sandy in the setting of a power outage secondary to a coastal surge. In this setting, 21 neonates were safely evacuated from the medical center's NICU to receiving hospitals within New York City in a span of 4.5 hours. Using data recorded during the evacuation and from staff debriefings, we describe the challenges faced and lessons learned during both the power outage and vertical evacuation. From our experience, we identify several elements that are important to the functioning of an NICU in a disaster or to an evacuation that may be incorporated into future NICU-focused disaster planning. These include a clear command structure, backups (personnel, communication, medical information, and equipment), establishing situational awareness, regional coordination, and flexibility as well as special attention to families and to the availability of neonatal transport resources.

▶ It has been 10 years since Hurricane Katrina (2005), and US hospitals have made significant improvements in disaster preparedness. Espiritu et al describe their experience at New York University Langone Medical Center during another devastating hurricane (Sandy) 7 years after Katrina. Again, heroic and resourceful medical providers prevented morbidity and mortality to the neonatal patients in their charge. We should be reminded that hospital evacuations are not a rare occurrence. The US Federal Emergency Management Agency (FEMA) states that approximately 1 hospital per week has to be evacuated for some natural or manmade disaster. The Joint Commission (JCAHO) now has national emergency management standards (E.C. 4.10—4.20) and requires hospitals to demonstrate proper plans and response mechanisms to potential disasters with twice-yearly testing of the emergency operation plan. Six areas are emphasized: communications, supplies, security, staff (responsibilities and command structure), and utilities for self-sufficiency and maintaining clinical care, especially for vulnerable populations. However, we as neonatologists recognize that our patients represent a unique population that challenges even the most well-conceived disaster plan.

Specialized disaster plans for neonatal intensive care units (NICUs) should include separate "shelter-in-place" and evacuation plans. A shelter-in-place plan must have complete provisions of self-sufficiency for 96 hours. When transferring patients to functioning units, we should be able to transfer providers and equipment as well to lessen a potentially dangerous surge of patients in the receiving hospitals. This may require an emergency declaration that allows any licensed provider to practice in any hospital in the state to circumvent the cumbersome credentialing process. Integration of hospitals in a state or region may help identify where the best place will be for patients at various levels of illness acuity. Such a plan, as suggested by Cohen et al, the Triage Resource Allocation in Neonatology (T.R.A.I.N), identifies acuity levels of patients and available resources from every participating NICU in the region on a daily basis.

Several states (eg, California, Illinois) have put together exceptional NICU evacuation guidelines and state disaster plans. No area of the country is immune from some type of disaster, and we could all learn from the experiences described in this and other articles recounting disaster experiences to help lessen the impact on our patients when the next disaster occurs.

J. P. Goldsmith, MD

13 Pharmacology

Antenatal magnesium sulfate and spontaneous intestinal perforation in infants less than 25 weeks gestation
Rattray BN, Kraus DM, Drinker LR, et al (Duke Univ Med Ctr. Durham, NC)
J Perinatol 34:819-822, 2014

Objective.—Evaluate spontaneous intestinal perforation (SIP)/death among extremely low birthweight (ELBW) infants before, during and after initiation of an antenatal magnesium for neuroprotection protocol (MgPro).

Study Design.—We tested associations between SIP/death and magnesium exposure, gestational age (GA) and interactions with GA and magnesium exposure in a cohort of inborn ELBW infants before, during and after MgPro.

Result.—One hundred and fifty-five ELBW infants were included, 81 before, 23 during and 51 after MgPro. ELBW infants (78.3%) were exposed to Mg during MgPro compared with 50.6% and 60.8% before and after, respectively. Incidence of SIP on protocol was 30.4% vs 12.9% off protocol ($P = 0.03$). GA was strongly associated with SIP ($P < 0.01$). Antenatal Mg dose was also associated with SIP/death regardless of epoch (odds ratio 9.3 (1.04–104.6)), but increased SIP/death was limited to those <25 weeks gestation.

Conclusion.—Higher Mg dose was associated with higher SIP and death risk among infants with the lowest birthweights. Validation of this observation in larger populations is warranted.

▶ It may be true that no good deed goes unpunished. In this report, the authors raise the question of whether neurodevelopmental benefits of antepartum treatment of women with threatened preterm delivery with magnesium comes at the cost of an increased risk of spontaneous intestinal perforation (SIP). Following up on an incidental observation that rates of SIP seemed to be high during an interval in which a trial of magnesium for neuroprotection was in progress at their center, these authors identified statistically significant associations between SIP and estimated gestational age < 25 weeks and large cumulative doses of magnesium. These conclusions depend heavily on the outcomes of the 23 infants born during the trial period, however. In that group, all 7 infants who developed SIP (and no others) died, compared with only 6 of 17 infants with SIP before and after the trial period ($P = .004$). Statistical significance of the reported association was achieved only with pooling of data from the periods before and after the trial and only for SIP and death as separate outcomes.

The complete concordance of death and SIP during the trial biases this analysis because separation of the outcomes lowers their rates outside, but not during, the trial period. Those reservations notwithstanding, associations of the combined outcome with estimated gestational age < 25 weeks and cumulative magnesium dose were also evident in logistic regression modeling, which demonstrated the strongest associations with large magnesium doses in infants < 25 weeks' gestation (as an interaction term), as well as with postnatal exposure to hydrocortisone, but the details of that regression analysis are not provided. Interaction analysis demonstrated no effects of magnesium exposure in infants ≥25 weeks' gestation. This provocative analysis should be considered to be hypothesis generating, not hypothesis testing or confirmatory. Although vigilance for SIP in the most immature infants (those < 25 weeks' gestational age)—and especially those exposed to postnatal hydrocortisone as well as large doses of antepartum magnesium—appears to be an appropriate response to these data, independent confirmation of this putative association is required before it is applied to limit antenatal magnesium exposure in this high-risk population.

W. E. Benitz, MD

Diuretic Exposure in Premature Infants from 1997 to 2011
Laughon MM, Chantala K, Aliaga S, et al (Univ of North Carolina at Chapel Hill; et al)
Am J Perinatol 32:49-56, 2015

Objective.—Diuretics are often prescribed off-label to premature infants, particularly to prevent or treat bronchopulmonary dysplasia. We examined their use and safety in this group.

Study Design.—Retrospective cohort study of infants < 32 weeks gestation and < 1,500 g birth weight exposed to diuretics in 333 neonatal intensive care units from 1997 to 2011. We examined use of acetazolamide, amiloride, bumetanide, chlorothiazide, diazoxide, ethacrynic acid, furosemide, hydrochlorothiazide, mannitol, metolazone, or spironolactone combination. Respiratory support and fraction of inspired oxygen on the first day of each course of diuretic use were identified.

Results.—About 37% (39,357/107,542) infants were exposed to at least one diuretic; furosemide was the most commonly used (93% with ≥ 1 recorded dose), followed by spironolactone, chlorothiazide, hydrochlorothiazide, bumetanide, and acetazolamide. About 74% patients were exposed to one diuretic at a time, 19% to two diuretics simultaneously, and 6% to three diuretics simultaneously. The most common combination was furosemide/spironolactone, followed by furosemide/chlorothiazide and chlorothiazide/spironolactone. Many infants were not receiving mechanical ventilation on the first day of each new course of furosemide (47%), spironolactone (69%), chlorothiazide (61%), and hydrochlorothiazide (68%). Any adverse event occurred on 42 per 1,000 infant-days for any diuretic and 35 per 1,000 infant-days for furosemide. Any serious adverse event occurred in 3.8 for any diuretic and 3.2 per 1,000 infant-days for furosemide. The most common laboratory abnormality associated with diuretic exposure was thrombocytopenia.

Conclusion.—Despite no Food and Drug Administration (FDA) indication and little safety data, over one-third of premature infants in our population were exposed to a diuretic, many with minimal respiratory support.

▶ Among the most commonly used drugs in neonatal intensive care are antibiotics, but not far behind are diuretics. As shown in this retrospective cohort study of 107 642 infants less than 32 weeks' gestational age and weighing less than 1500 grams discharged from 1 of 333 neonatal intensive care units, 37% were exposed to at least 1 diuretic, with furosemide the most commonly used. Despite this widespread use, there is no Food and Drug Administration indication for use of these drugs and few safety data.

Several salient features are seen in this study. Infants with the greatest exposure were the most immature: 66% of the infants weighing less than 1000 grams were exposed to diuretics. The use has increased by about 10% from 1997 to 2005 but remained stable until 2011. Many of these infants received the diuretic for more than a month. Several adverse events were associated with the use of diuretics, the most common of which was thrombocytopenia. However, it appears that some adverse events that may be more severe, such as severe osteopenia with bone fractures, were not evaluated, or at least not mentioned, but these are known adverse effects associated with calcium loss secondary to diuretic usage.

As stated in the article, the most common reason for use of diuretic was for bronchopulmonary dysplasia. Although physiologic data support that diuretics remove excess fluid and allow for improved gas exchange, guidance for when and how we should be using diuretics is largely lacking. When the variation of use between centers may range between 4% and 86% as seen in a previous smaller study,[1] there is something wrong: there is obviously no standard of care. There is no evidence that shows that their use results in decreased ventilator days or decreased length of stay. On the other hand, adverse events related to their use are common, and the result is vicious cycles of diuretic use, electrolyte abnormalities, response to these electrolyte abnormalities (eg, adding NaCl to the intravenous solution), and then greater use of diuretics. It is often unclear what response is expected when diuretics are used, and often there is no response but the diuretics are continued.

This is certainly an area of neonatal intensive care that requires more attention with clinical trials and quality improvement projects that help guide the clinician as to most judicious use of these agents.

J. Neu, MD

Reference

1. Slaughter JL, Stenger MR, Reagan PB. Variation in the use of diuretic therapy for infants with bronchopulmonary dysplasia. *Pediatrics.* 2013;131:716-723.

Azithromycin in Early Infancy and Pyloric Stenosis

Eberly MD, Eide MB, Thompson JL, et al (Uniformed Services Univ of the Health Sciences, Bethesda, MD)
Pediatrics 135:483-488, 2015

Background and Objective.—Use of oral erythromycin in infants is associated with infantile hypertrophic pyloric stenosis (IHPS). The risk with azithromycin remains unknown. We evaluated the association between exposure to oral azithromycin and erythromycin and subsequent development of IHPS.

Methods.—A retrospective cohort study of children born between 2001 and 2012 was performed utilizing the military health system database. Infants prescribed either oral erythromycin or azithromycin as outpatients in the first 90 days of life were evaluated for development of IHPS. Specific diagnostic and procedural codes were used to identify cases of IHPS.

Results.—A total of 2466 of 1 074 236 children in the study period developed IHPS. Azithromycin exposure in the first 14 days of life demonstrated an increased risk of IHPS (adjusted odds ratio [aOR], 8.26; 95% confidence interval [CI], 2.62–26.0); exposure between 15 and 42 days had an aOR of 2.98 (95% CI, 1.24–7.20). An association between erythromycin and IHPS was also confirmed. Exposure to erythromycin in the first 14 days of life had an aOR of 13.3 (95% CI, 6.80–25.9), and 15 to 42 days of life, aOR 4.10 (95% CI, 1.69–9.91). There was no association with either macrolide between 43 and 90 days of life.

Conclusions.—Ingestion of oral azithromycin and erythromycin places young infants at increased risk of developing IHPS. This association is strongest if the exposure occurred in the first 2 weeks of life, but persists although to a lesser degree in children between 2 and 6 weeks of age.

▶ In medicine there are many instances of double-edged swords. On the one hand, a therapy may be beneficial, but on the other, the price of the benefit is an adverse side effect. Macrolide antibiotics are an example of a double-edged sword in the perinatal period. They are effective antibiotics in pregnancy, but if administered to the baby in the first 2 weeks of life, they significantly increase the chance that the infant will require surgery for infantile hypertrophic pyloric stenosis (IHPS). Add to the complex equation the fact that they effectively increase gut motility because preterm babies have diminished to absent motility. Azithromycin has superseded erythromycin for many prescribers, and thus Eberly and colleagues conducted this study to see whether administration in the first weeks of life increased the risk of pyloric stenosis. Not surprisingly, it did. The following discussion confirms this finding on examination of large databases.

Lund et al[1] used a nationwide Danish register from 1996 to 2011 to assess the association between use of macrolide antibiotics in mothers and infants from pregnancy onset until 120 days after birth and IHPS. The impressive database included 999 378 liveborn singletons, more than 30 000 mothers who had macrolide prescriptions during pregnancy, 21 557 mothers after birth, and 6591 prescriptions for babies. These were linked to the need for surgery for IHPS: 880

infants developed IHPS, 0.9 cases per 1000 births. There was almost a 30-fold increase in IHPS in infants exposed to macrolides in the first 2 weeks of life and a greater than a 3-fold incidence of IHPS in infants who used macrolides between days 14 through 120. Maternal use in the first 2 weeks also increased the risk 3-fold. The logical conclusion is that macrolide antibiotics were strongly associated with IHPS and should be prescribed "only if treatment benefits outweigh the risk."

Using an Israeli database, Bahat Dinur et al[2] looked at the risk of birth defects among 1033 women exposed to macrolide antibiotics in the first trimester. There was no association between macrolides and either major malformations (odds ratio 1.08; 95% confidence interval 0.84-1.38) or specific malformations, after accounting for maternal age, parity ethnicity, prepregnancy diabetes, and year of exposure. They also concluded that "exposure in the third trimester is not likely to increase neonatal risks for pyloric stenosis or intussusception in a clinically meaningful manner." Källén et al[3] using the Swedish database, concluded that erythromycin use during the first trimester was associated with an increase in cardiac malformations.

A. A. Fanaroff, MBBCh, FRCPE

References

1. Lund M, Pasternak B, Davidsen RB, et al. Use of macrolides in mother and child and risk of infantile hypertrophic pyloric stenosis: nationwide cohort study. *BMJ.* 2014;348:g1908.
2. Bahat Dinur A, Koren G, Matok I, Wiznitzer A. Fetal safety of macrolides. *Antimicrob Agents Chemother.* 2013;57:3307-3311.
3. Källén BA, Otterblad Olausson P, Danielsson BR. Is erythromycin therapy teratogenic in humans? *Reprod Toxicol.* 2005;20:209-214.

A Randomized, Controlled Trial of Oral Propranolol in Infantile Hemangioma
Léauté-Labrèze C, Hoeger P, Mazereeuw-Hautier J, et al (Centre Hospitalier Universitaire (CHU), Bordeaux, France; Kinderkrankenhaus Wilhelmstift, Hamburg, Germany; Hôpital des Enfants, Toulouse, France; et al)
N Engl J Med 372:735-746, 2015

Background.—Oral propranolol has been used to treat complicated infantile hemangiomas, although data from randomized, controlled trials to inform its use are limited.

Methods.—We performed a multicenter, randomized, double-blind, adaptive, phase 2—3 trial assessing the efficacy and safety of a pediatric-specific oral propranolol solution in infants 1 to 5 months of age with proliferating infantile hemangioma requiring systemic therapy. Infants were randomly assigned to receive placebo or one of four propranolol regimens (1 or 3 mg of propranolol base per kilogram of body weight per day for 3 or 6 months). A preplanned interim analysis was conducted to identify the regimen to study for the final efficacy analysis. The primary end point was success (complete or nearly complete resolution of the target hemangioma) or failure of trial treatment at week 24, as assessed by independent, centralized, blinded evaluations of standardized photographs.

Results.—Of 460 infants who underwent randomization, 456 received treatment. On the basis of an interim analysis of the first 188 patients who completed 24 weeks of trial treatment, the regimen of 3 mg of propranolol per kilogram per day for 6 months was selected for the final efficacy analysis. The frequency of successful treatment was higher with this regimen than with placebo (60% vs. 4%, $P < 0.001$). A total of 88% of patients who received the selected propranolol regimen showed improvement by week 5, versus 5% of patients who received placebo. A total of 10% of patients in whom treatment with propranolol was successful required systemic retreatment during follow-up. Known adverse events associated with propranolol (hypoglycemia, hypotension, bradycardia, and bronchospasm) occurred infrequently, with no significant difference in frequency between the placebo group and the groups receiving propranolol.

Conclusions.—This trial showed that propranolol was effective at a dose of 3 mg per kilogram per day for 6 months in the treatment of infantile hemangioma. (Funded by Pierre Fabre Dermatologie; ClinicalTrials.gov number, NCT01056341.)

▶ Infantile hemangiomas are common, occurring in up to 10% of infants. The course of most lesions is uncomplicated, although approximately 12% of lesions require specialist referral. Systemic glucocorticoids represent standard therapy for complicated infantile hemangioma with interferon alfa and vincristine reserved for refractory cases. These treatments result in variable efficacy and frequent adverse effects. Recently, several authors have reported the successful resolution of infantile hemangioma with propranolol therapy. Given the favorable adverse effect profile of this nonselective β-adrenergic receptor-blocking agent, it has become standard therapy despite limited examination in small randomized trials. In this article, Leaute-Labreze and colleagues randomized 460 infants at 1 to 5 months of age with proliferating infantile hemangioma requiring systemic therapy to propranolol or placebo to assess the efficacy and safety of this therapy. An adaptive trial design allowed for selection of the optimal regimen (3 mg per kilogram per day over 1 mg per kilogram per day) and duration of therapy (6 months over 3 months) after interim analysis. A regimen of 3 mg per kilogram per day resulted in a higher rate of successful resolution compared with placebo at 24 weeks (60% vs 4%, $P < .001$). No difference in serious adverse events was observed between the propranolol and placebo groups. Important mild to moderate adverse effects more frequently observed in patients randomized to propranolol included bronchospasm, bradycardia, hypotension, and hypoglycemia. The results of this trial confirm the utility of propranolol as first-line therapy for complicated infantile hemangioma. Although the adverse effect profile of propranolol is not benign, the lack of serious adverse events is reassuring and represents a substantial advantage over previous standards of care.

C. McPherson

Phthalates and critically ill neonates: device-related exposures and non-endocrine toxic risks
Mallow EB, Fox MA (Risk Sciences and Public Policy Inst, Baltimore, MD)
J Perinatol 34:892-897, 2014

Objective.—To assess the types and magnitudes of non-endocrine toxic risks to neonates associated with medical device-related exposures to di(2-ethylhexyl)phthalate (DEHP).

Study Design.—Dose-response thresholds for DEHP toxicities were determined from published data, as were the magnitudes of DEHP exposures resulting from neonatal contact with polyvinyl chloride (PVC) devices. Standard methods of risk assessment were used to determine safe levels of DEHP exposure in neonates, and hazard quotients were calculated for devices individually and in aggregate.

Result.—Daily intake of DEHP for critically ill preterm infants can reach 16 mg/kg per day, which is on the order of 4000 and 160,000 times higher than desired to avoid reproductive and hepatic toxicities, respectively. The non-endocrine toxicities of DEHP are similar to complications experienced by preterm neonates.

Conclusion.—DEHP exposures in neonatal intensive care are much higher than estimated safe limits, and might contribute to common early and chronic complications of prematurity. Concerns about phthalates should be expanded beyond endocrine disruption.

▶ In this article, Mallow and Fox described the types and severities of nonendocrine toxic risks in newborns exposed to di(2-ethylhexyl)phthalate (DEHP) derived from exposure to medical devices with polyvinyl chloride. Chemical risk assessments were derived from published data. They described the role of DEHP and its metabolites in oxidative stress, airspace reduction, cholestasis, hippocampal neuronal loss, and disordered retinal development. Sources of DEHP include blood products, intravenous tubing, endotracheal tubes, feeding tubes, and other devices. Estimates of typical exposures were made and correlated with illness severity and length of exposure. They concluded that DEHP exposures can exceed the estimated safe levels by 3 to 5 orders of magnitude.

Although neonatologists have gotten better at controlling known risks, especially through measuring serum concentrations and monitoring toxicities, this article serves as a reminder that there are also unknown risks that can contribute to illness severity and create additional complications. This is not new, but without surveys such as this, it is easily overlooked. Sedman et al described aluminum toxicity from parenteral nutrition solutions,[1] and Shehab et al similarly described exposure to the excipients benzyl alcohol and propylene glycol, common vehicles used in pharmaceuticals delivered to critically ill newborns.[2] We would be wise to heed these messages.

S. M. Donn, MD

References

1. Sedman AB, Klein GL, Merritt RJ, et al. Evidence of aluminum loading in infants receiving intravenous therapy. *N Engl J Med*. 1985;312:1337-1343.
2. Shehab N, Lewis CL, Streetman DD, Donn SM. Exposure to the pharmaceutical excipients benzyl alcohol and propylene glycol among critically ill neonates. *Pediatr Crit Care Med*. 2009;10:256-259.

Reduction in Developmental Coordination Disorder with Neonatal Caffeine Therapy

Doyle LW, on behalf of the Caffeine for Apnea of Prematurity Trial investigators (Univ of Melbourne, Victoria, Australia; et al)
J Pediatr 165:356-359.e2, 2014

Objective.—To determine the effect of neonatal caffeine treatment on rates of developmental coordination disorder (DCD).

Study Design.—Children in the Caffeine for Apnea of Prematurity trial were assessed for motor performance (Movement Assessment Battery for Children [MABC]), clinical signs of cerebral palsy, and Full-Scale IQ at 5 years of age by staff who were unaware of the children's treatment group. DCD was defined as MABC <5th percentile in children with a Full-Scale IQ >69 who did not have a diagnosis of cerebral palsy.

Results.—There were 1433 children with known MABC corrected-age percentile as well as known Full-Scale IQ at 5 years and cerebral palsy status, of whom 735 had been randomly assigned to caffeine and 698 to placebo therapy. The rate of DCD was lower in those treated with caffeine (11.3%) than in the placebo group (15.2%) (OR adjusted for center and baseline covariates, 0.71, 95% CI, 0.52-0.97; $P = .032$).

Conclusions.—Neonatal caffeine therapy for apnea of prematurity reduces the rate of DCD at 5 years of age. As more children have DCD than have cerebral palsy, this is an important additional benefit from neonatal caffeine treatment.

▶ Nearly a decade ago, the Caffeine for Apnea of Prematurity (CAP) trial demonstrated that caffeine therapy initiated within the first 10 days of life lowers the rates of cerebral palsy and cognitive delay at 18 to 21 months of age in infants born preterm. Despite these early benefits, caffeine therapy had no significant impact on the incidence of major motor or cognitive impairment at a corrected age of 5 years. This loss of effect may be attributable to the lower incidence of major impairment at 5 years compared with 18 months. However, developmental coordination disorder without cerebral palsy occurs more frequently in children born very preterm and has important implications for behavior, social skills, and self-esteem. In this follow-up study of CAP trial patients, the authors investigate motor performance with the Movement Assessment Battery for Children in 1433 children at 5 years' corrected age. The rate of developmental coordination disorder was lower in patients treated with caffeine as preterm infants compared with those randomized to placebo (11.3% vs 15.2%, $P = .032$). This trial highlights an important ongoing benefit of neonatal caffeine therapy, despite the loss of significance with respect to major impairments. Of great interest, the authors have already embarked on developmental follow-up of the entire CAP cohort and magnetic resonance imaging of a subgroup of patients at 11 years of age. Developmental outcomes will provide further insight on the long-term impact of caffeine therapy. MRI analysis has the potential to elucidate the neuroanatomic underpinnings of the benefits observed at 5 years of age and potentially beyond. Follow-up of the CAP trial cohort continues to yield invaluable data and establishes a benchmark for all future randomized trials conducted in the field of neonatology.

C. McPherson

Morphine Versus Clonidine for Neonatal Abstinence Syndrome
Bada HS, Sithisarn T, Gibson J, et al (Univ of Kentucky, Lexington; Kentucky Children's Hosp, Lexington; et al)
Pediatrics 135:e383-e391, 2015

Objective.—The study goal was to determine whether clonidine treatment of neonatal abstinence syndrome (NAS) would result in a better neurobehavioral performance compared with morphine.

Methods.—This pilot study prospectively enrolled infants ≥35 weeks' gestational age admitted for treatment of NAS. After informed consent was obtained, infants were randomized to receive morphine (0.4 mg/kg per day) or clonidine (5 µg/kg per day) divided into 8 doses. A 25% dose escalation every 24 hours was possible per protocol (maximum of 1 mg/kg per day for morphine and 12 µg/kg per day for clonidine). After control of symptoms, the dose was tapered by 10% every other day. Clinical staff monitored infants by using Finnegan scoring. Masked research staff administered the NICU Network Neurobehavioral Scale (NNNS) at 1 week and at 2 to 4 weeks after initiation of treatment and the Bayley Scales III, and Preschool Language Scale IV, at 1-year adjusted age. Analyses included descriptive statistics, repeated measures analysis of variance, and Wilcoxon tests.

Results.—Infants treated with morphine ($n = 15$) versus clonidine ($n = 16$) did not differ in birth weight or age at treatment. Treatment duration was significantly longer for morphine (median 39 days) than for clonidine (median 28 days; $P = .02$). NNNS summary scores improved significantly with clonidine but not with morphine. On subsequent assessment, those receiving clonidine had lower height of arousal and excitability ($P < .05$). One-year motor, cognitive, and language scores did not differ between groups.

Conclusions.—Clonidine may be a favorable alternative to morphine as a single-drug therapy for NAS. A multicenter randomized trial is warranted.

▶ Opioid use represents a growing epidemic in the United States, leading to a dramatic increase in the prevalence of neonatal abstinence syndrome (NAS). Standard treatment regimens generally use opioids, despite concerns regarding the long-term outcomes of neonates after prolonged in utero and ex utero opioid exposure. Clonidine represents a promising alternative therapy, lessening the manifestations of withdrawal through inhibition of the release of noradrenaline in the locus coeruleus. Several recent trials have evaluated clonidine as an adjunct to opioid therapy; Bada and colleagues performed the first randomized trial comparing clonidine to morphine as monotherapy for NAS. In this trial, infants admitted for treatment of NAS were randomized to morphine (0.4 mg/kg/day divided every 3 hours) or clonidine (5 mcg/kg/day divided every 3 hours). Daily escalations were permitted by 25% to a maximum of 1 mg/kg/day of morphine or 12 mcg/kg/day of clonidine. After symptom control, the dose was tapered by 10% every other day. Demographic characteristics did not differ between the clonidine group (n = 16) and the morphine group (n = 15). Treatment duration was significantly shorter for clonidine-treated infants (median 28 days vs 39 days, $P = .02$). Clonidine-treated infants had lower height of arousal and excitability on the NICU Network Neurobehavioral Scale (NNNS) at discharge or during clinic follow-up ($P < .05$). NNNS profiles have previously been associated with behavioral and cognitive outcomes in later childhood, highlighting the promise of these pilot results. Further investigation is necessary, including larger randomized controlled trials, potentially with a higher initial dose of clonidine and more rapid weaning schedule. This pilot trial lays the foundation for future investigations seeking to improve the outcome of infants exposed to opioids in utero.

C. McPherson

14 Postnatal Growth and Development/ Follow-up

Between-Hospital Variation in Treatment and Outcomes in Extremely Preterm Infants
Rysavy MA, for the Eunice Kennedy Shriver National Institute of Child Health and Human Development Neonatal Research Network (Univ of Iowa; et al)
N Engl J Med 372:1801-1811, 2015

Background.—Between-hospital variation in outcomes among extremely preterm infants is largely unexplained and may reflect differences in hospital practices regarding the initiation of active lifesaving treatment as compared with comfort care after birth.

Methods.—We studied infants born between April 2006 and March 2011 at 24 hospitals included in the Eunice Kennedy Shriver National Institute of Child Health and Human Development Neonatal Research Network. Data were collected for 4987 infants born before 27 weeks of gestation without congenital anomalies. Active treatment was defined as any potentially lifesaving intervention administered after birth. Survival and neurodevelopmental impairment at 18 to 22 months of corrected age were assessed in 4704 children (94.3%).

Results.—Overall rates of active treatment ranged from 22.1% (interquartile range [IQR], 7.7 to 100) among infants born at 22 weeks of gestation to 99.8% (IQR, 100 to 100) among those born at 26 weeks of gestation. Overall rates of survival and survival without severe impairment ranged from 5.1% (IQR, 0 to 10.6) and 3.4% (IQR, 0 to 6.9), respectively, among children born at 22 weeks of gestation to 81.4% (IQR, 78.2 to 84.0) and 75.6% (IQR, 69.5 to 80.0), respectively, among those born at 26 weeks of gestation. Hospital rates of active treatment accounted for 78% and 75% of the between-hospital variation in survival and survival without severe impairment, respectively, among children born at 22 or 23 weeks of gestation, and accounted for 22% and 16%, respectively, among those born at 24 weeks of gestation, but the rates did not account for any of the variation in outcomes among those born at 25 or 26 weeks of gestation.

Conclusions.—Differences in hospital practices regarding the initiation of active treatment in infants born at 22, 23, or 24 weeks of gestation explain some of the between-hospital variation in survival and survival without impairment among such patients. (Funded by the National Institutes of Health.)

▶ The question of the right approach to resuscitation of infants at the margin of viability has long troubled both health care providers and families. Where outcomes are uncertain, approaches will surely differ. Rysavy and colleagues report on survival and neurodevelopment at 2 years in a cohort of almost 5000 infants born between 220 and 266 weeks of gestation in 24 National Institute of Child Health and Human Development Neonatal Research Network hospitals. They found that variability in hospital approach to active resuscitation of infants at 22 to 23 weeks of gestation accounted for about 75% of the variation in survival in these infants. By 24 weeks of gestation, variation in hospital approach accounted for only 20% of the variability, and at higher gestations it was not a factor. It seems logical that until the threshold of viability is actually crossed, active support of more infants should result in survival of more infants. Even so, survival rates for infants actively supported averaged only 23% at 22 weeks of gestation, and 33% at 23 weeks of gestation, with only 9% and 16% of infants born at those gestation times surviving without moderate or severe neurodevelopmental impairment when tested at age 2.

One might ask: does this increase in survival result in survival of more infants with significant neurodevelopmental impairment or without? The answer is both—keeping in mind the limited predictive ability of neurodevelopmental testing at age 2. The result of providing active support to more infants is that more infants survive in each category. For the entire cohort, of every 100 infants born at 22 weeks of gestation, an average of 5 survived, of whom, 3 had moderate or severe impairment and 2 did not. For every 100 of those infants receiving active support at delivery, an average of 23 survived, of whom, 35% had severe impairment, 26% had moderate impairment, and 39% had neither. So, active support would result in an average of 18 additional survivors, about evenly split between those categories. At 23 weeks of gestation, an average of 24 of 100 survived in the overall sample: 25% with severe impairment, 29% with moderate impairment, and 46% with neither. For every 100 infants provided active support, about 9 more survived, with the same proportions of neurodevelopmental outcomes.

A second question might then be: do the hospitals with the highest survival rates at 22 and 23 weeks have improved neurodevelopmental outcomes in the survivors? In other words, does an optimistic outlook translate to higher percentage of "intact" survival? The adjusted risk rates shown in Fig 2 in the original article suggest that is not the case; the percentage of infants surviving with moderate-to-severe neurodevelopmental impairment increases in step with the survival rate.

So how might these data be of use in counseling parents? First, as Neil Marlow says in his accompanying editorial, these data highlight the importance of providing parents with more specific and relevant data regarding outcomes of infants born at the margin of viability—not just the overall percentage of survival but the survival rate and outcomes of infants for whom active resuscitation was provided.[1] Second, we know that gestational age is far from the only variable affecting outcomes, and we should remember the limitations of counseling based only on gestational age. And third, we should remember that in adulthood, these children and their parents rate their quality of life and outcomes more favorably than those who care for them in the neonatal intensive care unit might expect.[2]

So is the glass half full or half empty? Do we resuscitate all, as several hospitals in this network did? Or none at certain gestations as others chose? No categorical approach would seem to make sense when outcomes are so uncertain and when the chance of survival without moderate or severe impairment hovers around 10% to 20% at 22 to 23 weeks of gestation. With this level of uncertainty, parents deserve our best information and support in their choices for their family, both before birth and thereafter.

K. Watterberg

References

1. Marlow N. The elephant in the delivery room. *N Engl J Med.* 2015;372: 1856-1857.
2. Saigal S, Stoskopf B, Boyle M, et al. Comparison of current health, functional limitations, and health care use of young adults who were born with extremely low birth weight and normal birth weight. *Pediatrics.* 2007;119:e562-e573.

Bayley-III Cognitive and Language Scales in Preterm Children
Spencer-Smith MM, Spittle AJ, Lee KJ, et al (Monash Univ, Melbourne, Australia; Murdoch Childrens Research Inst, Melbourne, Australia; et al)
Pediatrics 135:e1258-e1265, 2015

Background.—This study aimed to assess the sensitivity and specificity of the *Bayley Scales of Infant and Toddler Development, Third Edition* (Bayley-III), Cognitive and Language scales at 24 months for predicting cognitive impairments in preterm children at 4 years.

Methods.—Children born <30 weeks' gestation completed the Bayley-III at 24 months and the *Differential Ability Scale, Second Edition* (DAS-II), at 4 years to assess cognitive functioning. Test norms and local term-born reference data were used to classify delay on the Bayley-III Cognitive and Language scales. Impairment on the DAS-II Global Conceptual Ability, Verbal, and Nonverbal Reasoning indices was classified relative to test norms. Scores < −1 SD relative to the mean were classified as mild/moderate delay or impairment, and scores < −2 SDs were classified as moderate delay or impairment.

Results.—A total of 105 children completed the Bayley-III and DAS-II. The sensitivity of mild/moderate cognitive delay on the Bayley-III for predicting impairment on DAS-II indices ranged from 29.4% to

38.5% and specificity ranged from 92.3% to 95.5%. The sensitivity of mild/moderate language delay on the Bayley-III for predicting impairment on DAS-II indices ranged from 40% to 46.7% and specificity ranged from 81.1% to 85.7%. The use of local reference data at 24 months to classify delay increased sensitivity but reduced specificity. Receiver operating curve analysis identified optimum cut-point scores for the Bayley-III that were more consistent with using local reference data than Bayley-III normative data.

Conclusions.—In our cohort of very preterm children, delay on the Bayley-III Cognitive and Language scales was not strongly predictive of future impairments. More children destined for later cognitive impairment were identified by using cut-points based on local reference data than Bayley-III norms.

▶ The Bayley Scales of Infant and Toddler Development (BSID) was designed to assess developmental delay. The first and second version of the BSID provided only 2 broad developmental indices: the Mental Developmental Index, which assessed early cognitive and language development, and the Psychomotor Developmental Index, which evaluated early fine and gross motor development. These broad measures lacked the ability to differentiate specific delays in either cognitive and language development or in fine and gross motor development. The most recent edition, BSID-III, has been restructured to include scores for cognitive, language, and fine and gross motor domains. It was hoped that the changes would improve its capacity to identify specific developmental problems in high-risk infants.

Although the BSID was not intended to predict future cognitive function, it is often used across research and clinical settings in this manner. However, as has been shown by others[1,2] and reemphasized in the report featured here, the BSID scores do not strongly predict later neurodevelopmental impairment. The positive and negative predictive values (95% confidence interval [CI]) of the BSID-III Cognitive scale for later mild/moderate cognitive delay were 50% (18.7%-81.3%) and 87.1% (78.5%-93.2%), and those of the Language scale were 36.8% (16.3%-61.6%) and 90% (81.2%-95.6%), respectively. When a local reference group of term-born infants rather than test norms was used to define developmental delay, positive and negative predictive values (95% CI) for mild/moderate delay were 37.1% (21.5%-51.1%) and 94.1% (85.6%-98.4%) for the Cognitive scale, and 27.8% (14.2%-45.2%) and 92.1% (82.4%-97.4%) for the Language scale. Thus, even when a local reference group is used and despite a refinement of the BSID, some at-risk children are not being classified as delayed and accordingly might not receive the level of monitoring or early intervention that is needed.

L. A. Papile, MD

References

1. Spittle AJ, Spencer-Smith MM, Eeles AL, et al. Does the Bayley-III motor scale at 2 years predict motor outcome at 4 year in very preterm children? *Dev Med Child Neurol.* 2013;55:448-452.

2. Woods PL, Rieger I, Wocadio C, Gordon A. Predicting the outcome of a specific language impairment at 5 years of age through early developmental assessment in preterm infants. *Early Hum Dev.* 2014;90:613-619.

International standards for newborn weight, length, and head circumference by gestational age and sex: the Newborn Cross-Sectional Study of the INTERGROWTH-21st Project

Villar J, for the International Fetal and Newborn Growth Consortium for the 21st Century (INTERGROWTH-21St) (Univ of Oxford, UK; et al)
Lancet 384:857-868, 2014

Background.—In 2006, WHO published international growth standards for children younger than 5 years, which are now accepted worldwide. In the INTERGROWTH-21St Project, our aim was to complement them by developing international standards for fetuses, newborn infants, and the postnatal growth period of preterm infants.

Methods.—INTERGROWTH-21st is a population-based project that assessed fetal growth and newborn size in eight geographically defined urban populations. These groups were selected because most of the health and nutrition needs of mothers were met, adequate antenatal care was provided, and there were no major environmental constraints on growth. As part of the Newborn Cross-Sectional Study (NCSS), a component of INTERGROWTH-21st Project, we measured weight, length, and head circumference in all newborn infants, in addition to collecting data prospectively for pregnancy and the perinatal period. To construct the newborn standards, we selected all pregnancies in women meeting (in addition to the underlying population characteristics) strict individual eligibility criteria for a population at low risk of impaired fetal growth (labelled the NCSS prescriptive subpopulation). Women had a reliable ultrasound estimate of gestational age using crown—rump length before 14 weeks of gestation or biparietal diameter if antenatal care started between 14 weeks and 24 weeks or less of gestation. Newborn anthropometric measures were obtained within 12 h of birth by identically trained anthropometric teams using the same equipment at all sites. Fractional polynomials assuming a skewed t distribution were used to estimate the fitted centiles.

Findings.—We identified 20 486 (35%) eligible women from the 59 137 pregnant women enrolled in NCSS between May 14, 2009, and Aug 2, 2013. We calculated sex-specific observed and smoothed centiles for weight, length, and head circumference for gestational age at birth. The observed and smoothed centiles were almost identical. We present the 3rd, 10th, 50th, 90th, and 97th centile curves according to gestational age and sex.

Interpretation.—We have developed, for routine clinical practice, international anthropometric standards to assess newborn size that are intended to complement the WHO Child Growth Standards and allow comparisons across multiethnic populations.

▶ The World Health Organization (WHO) growth curves, published in 2006, are the international standard for monitoring growth of children up to 5 years of age. The WHO curves, however, begin at birth and are only appropriate for infants at term corrected gestation. Funded by the Bill and Melinda Gates Foundation, the International Fetal and Newborn Growth Consortium for the 21st Century (INTERGROWTH-21st) Project is an ambitious, multinational population-based study with the goal of developing international standards for fetuses, newborn infants, and postnatal growth of infants born prematurely.

The Newborn Cross-Sectional Study, a substudy of the INTERGROWTH-21st Project, was designed to develop an international standard for classification of small-for-gestational-age (SGA) as these infants are at greater risk of morbidity and mortality. Anthropometric measurements were obtained in more than 20 000 infants from 8 countries within 12 hours of birth by trained examiners using identical equipment and measurement procedures. The study population was unique in that strict inclusion criteria were applied to ensure inclusion of pregnancies and newborn infants of women at low risk of fetal growth impairment. The overall rate of preterm birth in the cohort was 5.5%, and neonatal mortality was quite low. Remarkably, 88% of the cohort was exclusively breastfed at time of hospital discharge.

Smoothed centile curves for weight, length, and head circumference according to gestational age (lower limit 33 weeks) and gender are provided. The lower limit of 33 weeks' gestation is a limitation but not surprising given the strict attention given to selecting a healthy population for inclusion.

The investigators also plan to construct curves based on serial ultrasound examinations of the healthy women who delivered at term to compare estimated fetal weight with actual measurements obtained from premature infants. Given the inherent limitations of birth weight-based growth curves for preterm infants, this approach will be a much-needed tool once validated.

This study also demonstrates the feasibility of obtaining newborn length measurements. From a global perspective, obtaining accurate length measurements at birth is a crucial to efforts to diagnose and reduce growth stunting during the first 1000 days of life.

The INTERGROWTH-21st Project not only provides growth curves that should become the new standard for identifying SGA infants at birth but also offers methods to obtain anthropometric measurements that can be used globally to improve growth outcomes.

B. Poindexter, MD, MS

Nature and origins of mathematics difficulties in very preterm children: a different etiology than developmental dyscalculia
Simms V, Gilmore C, Cragg L, et al (Univ of Leicester, UK; Loughborough Univ, UK; Univ of Nottingham, UK; et al)
Pediatr Res 77:389-395, 2015

Background.—Children born very preterm (<32 wk) are at high risk for mathematics learning difficulties that are out of proportion to other academic and cognitive deficits. However, the etiology of mathematics difficulties in very preterm children is unknown. We sought to identify the nature and origins of preterm children's mathematics difficulties.

Methods.—One hundred and fifteen very preterm children aged 8—10 y were assessed in school with a control group of 77 term-born classmates. Achievement in mathematics, working memory, visuospatial processing, inhibition, and processing speed were assessed using standardized tests. Numerical representations and specific mathematics skills were assessed using experimental tests.

Results.—Very preterm children had significantly poorer mathematics achievement, working memory, and visuospatial skills than term-born controls. Although preterm children had poorer performance in specific mathematics skills, there was no evidence of imprecise numerical representations. Difficulties in mathematics were associated with deficits in visuospatial processing and working memory.

Conclusion.—Mathematics difficulties in very preterm children are associated with deficits in working memory and visuospatial processing not numerical representations. Thus, very preterm children's mathematics difficulties are different in nature from those of children with developmental dyscalculia. Interventions targeting general cognitive problems, rather than numerical representations, may improve very preterm children's mathematics achievement.

▶ Math problems are the only kind for which double negatives can turn out positive, so don't count these kids out yet!

Serious difficulties in mathematical skills are common among children who were born preterm, even in the absence of general cognitive delay. Although the etiology of these math problems is unknown, many have speculated that dyscalculia, a learning disorder characterized by poor approximate number system acuity and abnormal numerical representation, may be responsible. In children with dyscalculia, there is a dysfunction in the representation and manipulation of quantity information, resulting in problems with magnitude comparison tasks. This study is an important contribution to our understanding of the specific nature and origin of the mathematical difficulties in very preterm children, suggesting that these problems originate from deficits in visuospatial processing and working memory rather than from imprecise numerical representation. A similar observation was reported by a recent large prospective German study of 922 children ranging from 23 to 41 weeks' gestation. In the

German cohort, the risk of math impairment increased with decreasing gestational age but was not associated with dyscalculia.[1]

Deficits in basic numerical representation associated with dyscalculia have been linked to structural and functional abnormalities in the bilateral intraparietal sulci. In contrast, brain development after preterm birth reflects a combination of developmental and destructive influences on many areas of the brain, typically associated with other neurocognitive deficits. This study suggests that interventions targeting both working memory and visuospatial abilities alongside math-specific skills may be beneficial for preterm children. Recent advances in neuroimaging have demonstrated task-specific links between school age math proficiency and functional MRI signal within distinct regions of the parietal lobes.[2] Further research correlating MRI structure with specific mathematical function may "add up to" targeted interventions that "count" to end the mysterious mathematical misunderstanding among preterm survivors. In the meantime, we may heed this advice from Albert Einstein: "Don't worry about your difficulties in understanding math; I assure you that mine are greater."

D. Costello-Wilson, MD

References

1. Jaekel J, Wolke D. Preterm birth and dyscalculia. *J Pediatr.* 2014;164:1327-1332.
2. Klein E, Moeller K, Kiechl-Kohlendorfer U, et al. Processing of intentional and automatic number magnitudes in children born prematurely: evidence from fMRI. *Dev Neuropsychol.* 2014;39:342-364.

Referral of Very Low Birth Weight Infants to High-Risk Follow-Up at Neonatal Intensive Care Unit Discharge Varies Widely across California

Hintz SR, Gould JB, Bennett MV, et al (Stanford Univ School of Medicine, CA; et al)
J Pediatr 166:289-295, 2015

Objectives.—To determine rates and factors associated with referral to the California Children's Services high-risk infant follow-up (HRIF) program among very low birth weight (BW) infants in the California Perinatal Quality of Care Collaborative.

Study Design.—Using multivariable logistic regression, we examined independent associations of demographic and clinical variables, neonatal intensive care unit (NICU) volume and level, and California region with HRIF referral.

Results.—In 2010-2011, 8071 very low BW infants were discharged home; 6424 (80%) were referred to HRIF. Higher odds for HRIF referral were associated with lower BW (OR 1.9, 95% CI 1.5-2.4; ≤750 g vs 1251-1499 g), higher NICU volume (OR 1.6, 1.2-2.1; highest vs lowest quartile), and California Children's Services Regional level (OR 3.1, 2.3-4.3, vs intermediate); and lower odds with small for gestational age (OR

0.79, 0.68-0.92), and maternal race African American (OR 0.58, 0.47-0.71) and Hispanic (OR 0.65, 0.55-0.76) vs white. There was wide variability in referral among regions (8%-98%) and NICUs (<5%-100%), which remained after risk adjustment.

Conclusions.—There are considerable disparities in HRIF referral, some of which may indicate regional and individual NICU resource challenges and barriers. Understanding demographic and clinical factors associated with failure to refer present opportunities for targeted quality improvement initiatives.

▶ The California Perinatal Quality of Care Collaborative (CPQCC) is a population-based dataset of perinatal variables and short-term outcomes for greater than 95% of infants discharged from newborn intensive care units (NICUs) in the State of California. In 2009, the CPQCC partnered with the California Children's Services (CCS) to create the CPQCC-CCS High-Risk Infant Follow-up Quality of Care Initiative (CPQCC-CCS HRIF). The above report, which is the initial report of the initiative, summarizes data related to the demographic and medical characteristics of very low birth weight infants who were and were not referred for HRIF at the time of discharge from the hospital. It is noteworthy that overall, 80% of eligible infants were referred for HRIF at hospital discharge. It is not surprising that a greater proportion of the smallest and sickest babies, those cared for in large centers, and a lower proportion of black and Hispanic infants were enrolled in HRIF. The cost of maintaining a multidisciplinary follow-up team that includes dieticians, occupational and physical therapists, and social workers, in addition to medical personnel team, is quite high, and although CCS subsidizes some HRIF services, most probably the cost far exceeds any reimbursement. Thus, infants who most likely have additional sources of revenue, such as the smallest and sickest infants and those whose families have private insurance, may be referred preferentially for HRIF. The authors have launched a statewide survey to gain a more granular understanding of the factors influencing referral to HRIF programs, including HRIF coordination and communication with NICUs and personnel and funding sources. The results will be most helpful in pinpointing barriers to HRIF, not only in California, but also throughout the United States.

L. A. Papile, MD

Cardiorespiratory events in extremely low birth weight infants: neurodevelopmental outcome at 1 and 2 years
Greene MM, Patra K, Khan S, et al (Rush Univ Med Ctr, Chicago, IL)
J Perinatol 34:562-565, 2014

Objective.—To examine the association between cardiorespiratory events (CRE) and neurodevelopmental (ND) outcome at 8 and 20 months corrected age (CA) in a contemporary extremely low birth weight (ELBW) cohort.

Study Design.—Retrospective chart review of 98 ELBW infants born in 2009 to 2010 who completed ND assessments at 8 and 20 months CA. Neonatal, sociodemographic, CRE and ND data were collected. ND outcome measures included neurologic examination and results from the Bayley Scales of Infant and Toddler Development-III. Multiple regression analyses adjusted for the impact of neonatal risk factors on ND outcome.

Result.—After adjusting for neonatal and social variables, greater frequency of CRE was related to worse language scores at 8 months, while CRE of greater severity were related to worse language at 20 months CA.

Conclusion.—CRE in ELBW infants have impact on language development in the first two years of life.

▶ The "cardiorespiratory events" (CRE) that characterize apnea and bradycardia of prematurity are pervasive in every intensive care nursery, but responses of care providers to those events are highly diverse. For some neonatologists, apnea/bradycardia events are part of the background noise of the unit and are accepted with equanimity. For others, they are a threat to neurological integrity, and many interventions are brought to bear to suppress them. These differences in approach reflect a range in beliefs about the significance of CRE, from sanguinity that no harms accrue from them, to great anxiety about long-term adverse effects, including spastic diplegia from periventricular leukomalacia, as well as more subtle developmental outcomes such as those discussed in this article. As always in instances of widely divergent views, there is little evidence to guide best practice. This report attempts to bring some clarity to that conversation, providing evidence of statistical associations between number and severity of CRE and language development at age 8 and 20 months, respectively. Although the abstract suggests that "CRE in ELBW [extremely low birth weight] infants have impact on language development," the conclusion in the text makes the more circumspect observation that "this investigation revealed an association between greater frequency of CRE and lower developmental scores." This distinction is important because these results, although worrisome, cannot address the causal role that CRE might have in compromised language development in early childhood. Even a confirmatory randomized controlled trial demonstrating improvement in cognitive or language performance in subjects for whom measures to reduce CRE were applied would not fully resolve this uncertainty because it remains possible that both are independent effects of the intervention. Nonetheless, the hypothesis of a causal relationship is quite plausible. For example, reduction in apnea events could account for improvement in early neurodevelopmental outcomes associated with caffeine use in very low birth weight preterm infants. Although we may never be able to resolve this mechanistic question, the observations reported in this article provide a potential target for interventions to optimize developmental outcomes, and they should not be too glibly dismissed. If treatments that reduce CRE result in better outcomes, it may not matter exactly what the mechanisms are that allow that result to be achieved.

W. E. Benitz, MD

Developmental outcomes at 3 years of age following major non-cardiac and cardiac surgery in term infants: A population-based study

Walker K, Loughran-Fowlds A, Halliday R, et al (Univ of Sydney, New South Wales, Australia; et al)
J Paediatr Child Health, 2015 [Epub ahead of print]

Objective.—The objective of this study was to determine whether there remain developmental differences between term infants at 3 years of age following major non-cardiac surgery (NCS) and cardiac surgery (CS) compared with healthy control infants in New South Wales (NSW), Australia.

Study Design.—Between 2006 and 2008, term infants who required NCS or CS within the first ninety days of life were enrolled in a prospective population-based study. Their developmental outcome was then compared with a cohort of healthy term infants. Infants initially assessed at 1 year of age were then re-assessed at 3 years of age using the Bayley scales of infant and toddler development (version-III).

Results.—Of the 539 term infants assessed at 1 year of age, 417 returned for the 3-year assessment, with 378 complete assessments. The mean scores for the infants who underwent CS ($P < 0.001$) were significantly lower in all subscales of the assessment compared with the controls, while the mean scores for the infants who underwent NCS were significantly lower in three of the subscales ($P < 0.05$). The infants who underwent CS scored significantly lower in four of the subscales ($P < 0.05$), compared with the infants who underwent NCS.

Conclusion.—The second phase of this unique population-based study provides further data on the outcomes of infants who underwent major NCS and CS. Major surgery in infants continues to be associated with developmental delay at 3 years of age compared with control infants; however the majority of the delay is mild. The risk remains higher in CS group with the pattern and severity of delay similar to that observed in the first study.

▶ Decades ago, Anand and colleagues[1] showed that the addition of deep anesthesia to analgesia during intraoperative management of infants undergoing cardiac surgery was associated with reduced physiological markers of stress, lower perioperative mortality, and improved postoperative outcomes. More recently, the recognition of potential adverse effects of anesthesia on the developing brain has raised concern regarding outcomes following neonatal surgery. In this follow-up component of a previously reported study on 1-year outcomes of an Australian cohort of infants with or without exposure to major surgery,[2] Walker and colleagues explored neurodevelopmental outcomes at age 3 among infants who underwent cardiac or noncardiac surgery. The investigators found that compared with control infants, infants exposed to either major cardiac or noncardiac surgery were at increased risk of neurodevelopmental deficits with scores on 5 of 5 Bayley subscales significantly lower than those of control infants. Children who underwent cardiac surgery were at greatest risk, scoring significantly lower on 4 of 5 Bayley subscales than infants undergoing noncardiac surgery. Associated exposures and mechanisms producing this vulnerability have yet to be fully identified. Anesthesia might be a contributor[3]; however, the antecedents of the neurologic effects of surgery are likely to be multifactorial, and the excess disability among infants exposed to cardiac surgery, compared with those undergoing major noncardiac surgery, might in part relate to greater severity of illness, underlying cardiac anomalies and associated preoperative hypoxemia, or altered brain perfusion before or during cardiac surgery. Biological underpinnings aside, neonatal and pediatric caregivers must be sensitive to these vulnerabilities, avoid unnecessary neonatal surgery, and be vigilant in assessing the neurodevelopment of infants who have undergone surgery. The authors propose applying newer tools, such as the General Movements Assessment, to identify neurological signs as early as 3 months of age.

L. J. Van Marter, MD, MPH

References

1. Anand K, Hickey P. Halothane-morphine compared with high-dose sufentanil for anesthesia and postoperative analgesia in neonatal cardiac surgery. *N Engl J Med.* 1992;326:1-9.
2. Walker K, Badawi N, Halliday R, et al. Early developmental outcomes following major noncardiac and cardiac surgery in term infants: a population-based study. *J Pediatr.* 2012;161:748-752.
3. Sinner B, Becke K, Engelhard K. General anaestheics and the developing brain: an overview. *Anaesthesia.* 2014;69:1009-1022.

In Utero and Childhood Polybrominated Diphenyl Ether Exposures and Body Mass at Age 7 Years: The CHAMACOS Study

Erkin-Cakmak A, Harley KG, Chevrier J, et al (Univ of California, Berkeley; et al)
Environ Health Perspect 123:636-642, 2015

Background.—Polybrominated diphenyl ethers (PBDEs) are lipophilic flame retardants that bioaccumulate in humans. Child serum PBDE concentrations in California are among the highest worldwide. PBDEs may be associated with obesity by disrupting endocrine systems.

Objective.—In this study, we examined whether pre- and postnatal exposure to the components of pentaBDE mixture was associated with childhood obesity in a population of Latino children participating in a longitudinal birth cohort study in the Salinas Valley, California.

Methods.—We measured PBDEs in serum collected from 224 mothers during pregnancy and their children at 7 years of age, and examined associations with body mass index (BMI) at age 7 years.

Results.—Maternal PBDE serum levels during pregnancy were associated with higher BMI z-scores in boys (BMI z-score $\beta_{adjusted} = 0.26$; 95% CI: -0.19, 0.72) but lower scores in girls (BMI z-score $\beta_{adjusted} = -0.41$; 95% CI: -0.87, -0.05) at 7 years of age ($p_{interaction} = 0.04$). In addition, child's serum BDE-153 concentration ($\log_{10}$), but not other pentaBDE congeners, demonstrated inverse associations with BMI at age 7 years (BMI z-score $\beta_{adjusted} = -1.15$; 95% CI: $-1.53, -0.77$), but there was no interaction by sex.

Conclusions.—We estimated sex-specific associations with maternal PBDE levels during pregnancy and BMI at 7 years of age, finding positive associations in boys and negative associations in girls. Children's serum BDE-153 concentrations were inversely associated with BMI at 7 years with no difference by sex. Future studies should examine the longitudinal trends in obesity with PBDE exposure and changes in hormonal environment as children transition through puberty, as well as evaluate the potential for reverse causality.

▶ The CHAMACOS Study is a longitudinal birth cohort based in the Salinas Valley, California, made up of Latino children whose parents are primarily farm workers. The study team has historically evaluated associations of pesticides and other toxins and child health. In the current analysis, maternal polybrominated diphenyl ether (PBDE) exposure was measured in mothers during pregnancy and in offspring at 7 years of age. Among the 224 mother–child pairs, maternal PBDE serum levels were associated with higher age 7 body mass index (BMI) z-scores in boys (0.26, 95% confidence interval [CI] −0.19 to 72) but lower in girls (−0.41, 95% CI −0.87 to −0.05). Child levels of a subtype of PDBEs (BDE-156) were associated with lower BMI at age 7 in both girls and boys. Sex-specific effects of maternal exposures in pregnancy and offspring outcomes are not uncommon and may be due to differences hormonal response to endocrine disrupting chemicals. Such studies raise the question as to whether some of the sex-specific risks of respiratory distress syndrome or neurodevelopmental impairments observed in preterm infants might also be due to differences in endocrine disrupting chemicals' effects following exposure in-utero and in the neonatal intensive care units.

H. H. Burris, MD, MPH

Neurodevelopmental outcomes of preterm singletons, twins and higher-order gestations: a population-based cohort study
Gnanendran L, for the NICUS Network (Canberra Hosp, Garran, Australia; et al)
Arch Dis Child Fetal Neonatal Ed 100:F106-F114, 2015

Objective.—To study the neurodevelopmental outcomes of multiple (twins, triplets, quads) compared with singleton extremely preterm infants <29 weeks gestation.

Design.—Population-based retrospective cohort study.

Setting.—A network of 10 neonatal intensive care units in a geographically defined area of New South Wales and the Australian Capital territory.

Patients.—1473 infants <29 weeks gestation born between 1 January 1998 and 31 December 2004.

Intervention.—At 2–3 years of corrected age, a neurodevelopmental assessment was conducted using either the Griffiths Mental Developmental Scales or the Bayley Scales of Infant Development II.

Main Outcome Measure.—Moderate–severe functional disability was defined as developmental delay (Griffiths Mental Developmental Scales General Quotient or Bayley Scales of Infant Development-II Mental Development Index >2 SDs below the mean), moderate cerebral palsy (unable to walk without aids), sensorineural or conductive deafness (requiring amplification) or bilateral blindness (visual acuity <6/60 in the better eye).

Results.—Of the 1081 singletons and 392 multiples followed-up, singletons demonstrated higher rates of systemic infections, steroid treatment for chronic lung disease and birth weight <10th percentile. Moderate–severe functional disability did not differ significantly between singletons and multiples (15.8% vs 17.6%, OR 1.14; 95% CI 0.84 to 1.54; $p = 0.464$). Further subgroup analysis of twins, higher-order gestations, 1st-born multiples, 2nd or higher-born multiples, same and unlike gender multiples, did not demonstrate statistically higher rates of functional disability compared with singletons.

Conclusions.—Premature infants from multiple gestation pregnancies appear to have comparable neurodevelopmental outcomes to singletons.

▶ The advent of artificial reproductive technology has led to an increased rate of multiple gestations. In 1980, 1 in every 53 babies born in the United States was a twin, compared with 1 in every 30 babies in 2011, a 76% jump in the twin birth rate. The neurodevelopmental outcomes of multiple gestations, particularly those born preterm, compared with singletons, is a controversial issue. In the above retrospective analysis of prospectively collected data, the investigators compared the 2- to 3-year corrected age developmental outcomes of twins and triplets who were less than 29 weeks' gestational age at birth with those of a comparable gestational age cohort of singletons and concluded that preterm infants from multiple gestation pregnancies do not appear to have an increased risk for poor neurodevelopmental outcomes.

From the data presented, it is obvious that the singletons and multiples were not comparable. The multiples were older (mean, 26.7 ± 1.3 vs 26.5 ± 1.4) and heavier (mean, 974.72 ± 24.4 vs 940 ± 225.0) at birth compared with singletons, and the rate of small for gestational age was almost 2-fold higher in the singletons (11.8% vs 6.1%). The higher rates of pregnancy-induced hypertension in the mothers of singletons (20.7% vs 9.4%) may explain some of these differences. At birth, singletons were significantly more likely to have a 5-minute Apgar score less than 7 (21.4% vs 13.6%), and as newborns they had significantly higher rates of systemic infections (42% vs 36%) and steroid treatment for chronic lung disease (29.3% vs 23.2%). The increase in individual infant risks for poor neurodevelopmental outcomes in singletons most likely biased the data in favor of the multiples group and may have led to the authors' optimistic conclusion regarding the outcomes of preterm multiples.

L. A. Papile, MD

An Update on the Impact of Postnatal Systemic Corticosteroids on Mortality and Cerebral Palsy in Preterm Infants: Effect Modification by Risk of Bronchopulmonary Dysplasia

Doyle LW, Halliday HL, Ehrenkranz RA, et al (Univ of Melbourne, Parkville, Australia; Queen's Univ, Belfast, NI; Yale Univ School of Medicine, New Haven, CT)
J Pediatr 165:1258-1260, 2014

Infants at higher risk of bronchopulmonary dysplasia had increased rates of survival free of cerebral palsy after postnatal corticosteroid treatment in a previous metaregression of data from 14 randomized controlled trials. The relationship persists and is stronger in an updated analysis with data from 20 randomized controlled trials.

▶ In 2005, Lex Doyle and his colleagues took a major step forward in evaluating benefits and risks of a therapeutic intervention in neonatology when they performed a meta-regression of the effects of dexamethasone on the outcome of "death or cerebral palsy (CP)" in preterm infants enrolled in studies of dexamethasone to prevent or treat bronchopulmonary dysplasia (BPD).[1] Rather than considering all studies to be the same, they evaluated the effect of dexamethasone on death or CP in relationship to the risk of BPD in the placebo group. They concluded that dexamethasone was associated with an increased risk for death or CP in populations with a BPD rate of less than about 50% in the placebo group but a decrease in the risk of death or CP in populations with a baseline BPD risk greater than 50%. This evaluation highlighted the need to weigh both benefit and risk when a disease is itself a risk factor for the adverse outcome of interest.

Now, 10 years later, these authors have updated their meta-regression with 6 new studies (3 dexamethasone, 3 hydrocortisone) and have come to the same conclusion: a net benefit in the outcome of death or CP for postnatal steroid treatment in studies with an incidence of BPD greater than 46% in the placebo group (95% confidence interval, 33%-60%) and a net harm less than that point. Of note, however, is that with the exception of a difference of one patient in one study, all the new studies were either neutral or favored corticosteroid treatment, regardless of the placebo group risk for BPD, which ranged from 32% to 83%. The new studies also all used a lower glucocorticoid dose than most of the previously reported studies. In fact, with the exception of that one patient, all of the studies reporting a higher incidence of death or CP in the treated group used a starting dexamethasone dose of 0.5 mg/kg/d.

So perhaps less really is more? This new meta-regression may provide encouragement for investigators to re-examine the use of glucocorticoids for BPD with new studies that use lower drug doses and to restrain their enthusiasm until at least the 2-year neurodevelopmental outcomes are known.

K. Watterberg

Reference

1. Doyle LW, Halliday HL, Ehrenkranz RA, Davis PG, Sinclair JC. Impact of postnatal systemic corticosteroids on mortality and cerebral palsy in preterm infants: effect modification by risk for chronic lung disease. *Pediatrics*. 2005;115: 655-661.

Effects of Hypothermia for Perinatal Asphyxia on Childhood Outcomes
Azzopardi D, for the TOBY Study Group (King's College London, UK; et al)
N Engl J Med 371:140-149, 2014

Background.—In the Total Body Hypothermia for Neonatal Encephalopathy Trial (TOBY), newborns with asphyxial encephalopathy who received hypothermic therapy had improved neurologic outcomes at 18 months of age, but it is uncertain whether such therapy results in longer-term neurocognitive benefits.

Methods.—We randomly assigned 325 newborns with asphyxial encephalopathy who were born at a gestational age of 36 weeks or more to receive standard care alone (control) or standard care with hypothermia to a rectal temperature of 33 to 34°C for 72 hours within 6 hours after birth. We evaluated the neurocognitive function of these children at 6 to 7 years of age. The primary outcome of this analysis was the frequency of survival with an IQ score of 85 or higher.

Results.—A total of 75 of 145 children (52%) in the hypothermia group versus 52 of 132 (39%) in the control group survived with an IQ score of 85 or more (relative risk, 1.31; $P = 0.04$). The proportions of children who died were similar in the hypothermia group and the control group (29% and 30%, respectively). More children in the hypothermia group than in the control group survived without neurologic abnormalities (65 of 145 [45%] vs. 37 of 132 [28%]; relative risk, 1.60; 95% confidence interval, 1.15 to 2.22). Among survivors, children in the hypothermia group, as compared with those in the control group, had significant reductions in the risk of cerebral palsy (21% vs. 36%, $P = 0.03$) and the risk of moderate or severe disability (22% vs. 37%, $P = 0.03$); they also had significantly better motor-function scores. There was no significant between-group difference in parental assessments of children's health status and in results on 10 of 11 psychometric tests.

Conclusions.—Moderate hypothermia after perinatal asphyxia resulted in improved neurocognitive outcomes in middle childhood.

▶ This is the third large randomized clinical trial of induced hypothermia for neonatal encephalopathy to report on the long-term outcomes of enrolled trial infants. In the Eunice Kennedy Shriver National Institute of Child Health and Human Development (NICHD) trial surviving children in the hypothermia group had a lower rate of death than those in the control group.[1] However, there were no significant differences in the rate of disability or cognitive outcomes. The CoolCap trial showed that outcome in childhood was similar to that noted at 18 months of age, although the study did not include a structured neuropsychological evaluation but rather relied on questionnaire data from parents.[2]

Unlike the previous 2 reports, this study noted that induced hypothermia was associated with a significant improvement in neurocognitive outcomes and a lower frequency of moderate-to-severe disability. The results, although encouraging, need to be taken in perspective. Of the 229 eligible children, 184 (80%) participated in the follow-up evaluation. Full-scale IQ testing was available for 140 children and 179 were assessed for disability, 62% and 78%, respectively, of the eligible cohort. It has been shown that the results of studies in which the follow-up rate is low may underestimate the frequency of a poor outcome. Thus, the results of NICHD trial follow-up study in which more than 90% of the cohort underwent extensive formal evaluation may reflect a true estimate of neuropsychological outcome of children who were treated with induced hypothermia as newborns.

L. A. Papile, MD

References

1. Shankaran S, Pappas A, McDonald SA, et al. Childhood outcomes after hypothermia for neonatal encephalopathy. *N Engl J Med.* 2012;366:2085-2092.
2. Guillet R, Edwards AD, Thoresen M, et al. Seven-to eight-year follow-up of the CoolCap trial of head cooling for neonatal encephalopathy. *Pediatri Res.* 2012; 71:205-209.

Association of Low Birth Weight and Preterm Birth With the Incidence of Knee and Hip Arthroplasty for Osteoarthritis
Hussain SM, Wang Y, Wluka AE, et al (Monash Univ and Alfred Hosp, Melbourne, Victoria, Australia; et al)
Arthritis Care Res (Hoboken) 67:502-508, 2015

Objective.—Low birth weight (LBW) and preterm birth have been associated with adverse adult outcomes, including hypertension, insulin resistance, cardiovascular disease, and reduced bone mass. It is unknown whether LBW and preterm birth affect the risk of osteoarthritis (OA). This study aims to examine whether LBW and preterm birth were associated with the incidence of knee and hip arthroplasty for OA.

Methods.—A total of 3,604 participants of the Australian Diabetes, Obesity and Lifestyle Study who reported their birth weight and history of preterm birth and were age >40 years at the commencement of arthroplasty data collection comprised the study sample. The incidence of knee and hip replacement for OA during 2002–2011 was determined by linking cohort records to the Australian Orthopaedic Association National Joint Replacement Registry.

Results.—One hundred and sixteen participants underwent knee arthroplasty and 75 underwent hip arthroplasty for OA. LBW (yes versus no; hazard ratio [HR] 2.04, 95% confidence interval [95% CI] 1.11–3.75, $P = 0.02$) and preterm birth (yes versus no; HR 2.50, 95% CI 1.29–4.87, $P = 0.007$) were associated with increased incidence of hip arthroplasty independent of age, sex, body mass index, education level, hypertension, diabetes mellitus, smoking, and physical activity. No significant association was observed for knee arthroplasty.

Conclusion.—Although these findings will need to be confirmed, they suggest that individuals born with LBW or at preterm are at increased risk of hip arthroplasty for OA in adult life. The underlying mechanisms warrant further investigation.

▶ If the findings in this study are corroborated by other investigators, it would appear that osteoarthritis (OA) of the hip severe enough to require replacement can be added to the growing list of adverse adult outcomes associated with preterm birth and/or low birth weight (LBW).

The population in this study is a subset of the Australian Diabetes, Obesity and Lifestyle study, a national population-based cohort study of 11 247 people > 24 years of age recruited during 1999-2000. Study subjects were restricted to those who were self-designated as preterm or LBW at enrollment and 40 years of age or older when the Australian Association National Joint Replacement Registry was initiated on January 1, 2002. The rationale for the latter was that in Australia hip and knee arthroplasty rarely occurs before 40 years of age.

In the discussion, the authors elaborate on the possible mechanisms for the relationship between LBW and preterm birth, and OA of the hip, including abnormal development of the hip after birth and reduced bone mass. The former may relate to not sustaining the in utero position of hip flexion and abduction after birth, factors that influence the development of the acetabulum. In addition, the decreased muscle tone prevalent in very preterm and critically ill infants may facilitate the "frog leg" position, which consists of wide hip abduction and external rotation. As to the latter, there is emerging evidence that preterm birth results in a decrease in bone formation and an increase in bone resorption, resulting in a net decrease in bone accretion.[1,2] Preliminary reports have demonstrated that physical activity improves bone mineralization in preterm infants.[3,4]

Although additional studies are needed to refute or support the findings in this report, placing preterm and LBW infants in an environment where hip flexion and abduction can be maintained, as well as providing physical barriers against which they can push, may be prudent.

L. A. Papile, MD

References

1. Miller ME. The bone disease of preterm birth: a biomechanical perspective. *Pediatr Res.* 2003;53:10-15.

2. Aly H, Moustafa MF, Amer HA, Hassanien S, Keeves C, Patel K. Gestational age, sex and maternal parity correlate with bone turnover in premature infants. *Pediatr Res.* 2005;57:708-711.
3. Aly H, Moustafa MF, Hassanien S, Massaro AN, Amer HA, Patel K. Physical activity combined with massage improves bone mineralization in premature infants: a randomized trial. *J Perinatol.* 2004;24:305-309.
4. Limanovitz I, Duffin T, Friedland O, et al. Early physical activity intervention prevents decrease of bone strength in very low birth weight infants. *Pediatrics.* 2003;112:15-19.

15 Ethics

Parents report positive experiences about enrolling babies in a cord-related clinical trial before birth
Ayers S, Sawyer A, Düring C, et al (City Univ London, UK; Univ of Sussex, Brighton, UK; et al)
Acta Paediatr 104:e164-e170, 2015

Aim.—The aim of this study was to evaluate parents' perceptions when they were asked to enrol their unborn preterm infant in a randomised trial involving delayed cord clamping or cord milking.

Methods.—The parents of 58 infants were asked to take part in a qualitative study using semi-structured interviews to provide feedback about how they felt about their infants being included in the research project. A total of 37 parents — 15 fathers and 22 mothers — agreed to take part.

Results.—Parents were generally positive about their experiences of their baby taking part in the trial, but the findings raised some concerns about the validity of the consent obtained before delivery, as it was given in a hurry, and some participants had difficulty remembering that they had agreed to take part. Four themes were identified from the interviews: implications of taking part, reasons for enrolling infants, experiences of recruitment and suggestions for improvement.

Conclusion.—Overall, the parents were positive about their baby taking part in the trial, but the consent process could be improved, by providing information about relevant trials earlier in the pregnancy or implementing continuous consent at key points in the trial.

▶ Medical research has played a key role in improving survival of critically ill newborns. Unfortunately, controversy over the SUPPORT trial[1] has generated a lot of negative press and attention on neonatal research. If there is a silver lining to the cloud surrounding the controversy, however, it is the increased focus on informed consent and parental perspectives for clinical trials involving their children. In this study, Ayers et al evaluate parental perceptions after enrolling their children in a randomized trial involving delayed cord clamping or cord milking. Overall, parents were very positive about the experience, and their motivations were altruistic. They wanted to help, contribute to research, and possibly benefit their baby. The study also found, as have other studies, that there is still work to be done to optimize the consent process in both timing and content. Additionally, parents want to know what happened and are interested in the study results. Research about optimizing research may seem superfluous at times, but it is an ethical imperative and the only way to ensure progress in the field. Fortunately many parents recognize this. As one parent of a preemie born more than 2 decades ago noted about the SUPPORT controversy: "My daughters treatment was so much guessing. Should they do this—or not? I'm sure treatment has advanced greatly since then. But how can the medical community determine which are the best practices? The doctors NEED to do studies to learn how to treat these little babies correctly."[2]

J. M. Fanaroff, MD, JD

References

1. Fanaroff JM. Ethical support for surfactant, positive pressure, and oxygenation randomized trial (SUPPORT). *J Pediatrics*. 2013;163:1498-1499.
2. Comment by a2pam from The Diane Rehm Show—Clinical Trials and Premature Babies. Aired April 17, 2013. http://thedianerehmshow.org/shows/2013–04-17/clinical-trials-and-premature-babies. Access date is June 1, 2015.

Ethics and Etiquette in Neonatal Intensive Care
Janvier A, for the POST Investigators (Hôpital Sainte-Justine, Montréal, Québec, Canada; et al)
JAMA Pediatr 168:857-858, 2014

When parents voice their dissatisfaction with the neonatal intensive care unit (NICU), it is often not because they think their baby has not received good medical care. Instead, it is often because their needs have not been addressed. Policy statements and pedagogy alike urge professionals to be empathetic, compassionate, honest, and caring. However, these theoretical concepts are generally endorsed without practical suggestions on how to achieve these goals. Negative encounters for parents are generally not about the caregivers' technical expertise or knowledge and often reflect a failure in a different domain. Simple rules of etiquette are not always applied in a busy NICU or in the hospital at large. The investigators of the POST (Parents from the Other Side of Treatment) group are health care professionals who regularly communicate with parents of sick children and who were also "NICU parents". We have developed an etiquette-based systematic approach to communication with families in the NICU. These specific and practical recommendations may help parents feel well treated and respected as they go through a challenging NICU stay.

▶ This short article by Janvier and Lantos is poignant in its simplicity. The 10 essentials of etiquette they present are in some ways so obvious, but as I read them, I could think of at least 1 incident in which I had failed to uphold each of these minimal standards of human and decent communication. Sometimes it's hard to be a neonatologist, but this article reminds us that it is even harder to be the parent of a child who needs a neonatologist. We should all be willing to get this message from parents who do not have the education or clout of doctors (or world-famous bioethicists), but the authors here do a great job of bringing together their personal and professional experiences. This article forces us to step back from science and even philosophy and ask ourselves if we are doing right by our patients' families. When I teach residents about ethics in the neonatal intensive care unit (NICU), I often surprise them by starting with the premise that it is not so hard—there are a few basic principles, yes, but really talking about the ethics of real patients in real time is about communication, and hurt feelings and moral distress can often be avoided if we share a common language. In my view, Janvier and Lantos have a similar message: respectfully and empathetically engaging the parents of babies in the NICU is not a bonus skill for those with God-given talent, it is a basic requirement of being a doctor, and we can all do it.

S. M. Donn, MD

Should Life Insurers Have Access to Genetic Test Results?
Klitzman R, Appelbaum PS, Chung WK (Columbia Univ Med Ctr, NY; Columbia Univ, NY)
JAMA 312:1855-1856, 2014

Background.—Insurers consider applicants' risk factors, but should genetic information be available to them or excluded from consideration?. With the rapid lowering of costs for genetic testing and their increasing use by the public, the question has become more salient. The concerns and several proposals were outlined.

Insurance Concerns.—Life insurance is designed to help people share the financial risks of premature death. The larger the pool of policy holders who share the risk, the more fairly premiums can be set. However, the pool should reflect the population risk or specify the ways it differs. Expanding predictive genetic testing may complicate risk calculations. If individuals learn they have a higher risk of death, disability, or both, they may be more likely to purchase insurance without sharing test results. This leads to an "adverse selection" of persons at higher risk.

Access to genetic information can be gained through family history, review of medical records, asking applicants if they have undergone genetic testing, or requesting that they undergo such tests. Having electronic health records (EHRs) makes the data more accessible, with most insurance applications routinely including the release of medical records.

Insurance companies are debating how to approach the issue. Legally, there are no set rules in many countries, such as the United States, although others have set moratoria on sharing or will allow sharing to some degree.

Insurers should be encouraged to avoid unfair discrimination, but the definition of fairness rests on a balance of stakeholders' interests. Although having applicants' genetic test results could stratify risks more accurately, conservative approaches to insurance are likely to lead to risk overestimation. Adjustments based on these estimates could price applicants out of life insurance coverage.

Patient and Health Care Concerns.—If the results of genetic testing will ultimately help in diagnosing, preventing, or treating disease, tests could actually lower the individual's risk. Often genetic tendencies can be modified by lifestyle changes and medical interventions. In addition, persons who lack the familial mutation for a potentially lethal disorder are at lower risk for that disease, a side of the issue that is not generally considered by insurers.

Patients may also avoid seeking genetic testing for fear that the results could be used to increase their premiums. In this way, they are depriving themselves of possible interventions to lower their risk or even eliminate the influence of genetic factors.

Courses of Action.—Solutions include changing government policy to ban the use of genetic tests by insurers. Such an approach may be countered by insurers amortizing possible losses by raising rates for all customers.

If insurers' access is limited to certain defined sets of well-characterized, high-risk, high-penetrance genes and variants, the number of persons denied coverage would be limited and insurers' strongest interests addressed. However, an accompanying measure should be to have modified rates for persons who take medically effective measures to reduce their risks.

The pattern in the United Kingdom could be adopted. In this model, a certain amount of insurance is available to everyone, with companies allowed to use genetic information only if people want to purchase additional insurance. Alternatively, insurers could be permitted unlimited access to genetic test results. The latter approach would deny certain applicants access to insurance coverage.

Conclusions.—Genetic data should be treated differently from other data with predictive value used by life insurers because of the complications that are likely to arise. Public policy should seek to maintain the general availability of coverage, with insurers allowed to access only the information related to clinically well-characterized, high-risk, high-penetrance genes and variants–and only when these individuals desire to purchase additional coverage. Further input from genetic and policy experts and public transparency should be sought.

> ▶ "The problem [with genetic research] is, we're just starting down this path, feeling our way in the dark. We have a small lantern in the form of a gene, but the lantern doesn't penetrate more than a couple of hundred feet. We don't know whether we're going to encounter chasms, rock walls or mountain ranges along the way. We don't even know how long the path is."
> — Francis S. Collins MD, PhD

Since DNA was first discovered by Swiss physician Friedrich Miescher in 1869,[1] there have been incredible advances in our understanding of the genetic basis of disease. It has also become clear that in determining clinical course or prognosis, genetics often is just one part of a complex interplay of environmental factors such as nutrition, sleep, exercise, and several other exposures. Insurance companies often take these environmental factors into account when providing insurance. An obese motorcycle-riding smoker, for example, will pay a higher premium for insurance than a thin nonsmoker who does not drive. But what about genetic testing? Can that same insurance company demand testing for Huntington's disease before agreeing to provide insurance? In the United States, the Genetic Information Nondiscrimination Act (GINA)[2] makes it illegal for health insurers to use genetic information to determine eligibility for health insurance or to determine premiums, contribution amounts, or the length of coverage. As the authors of this article point out, however, GINA only includes health insurance, and thus excludes life, long-term care, or disability insurance. This means that, unless prohibited by state law, a life insurance company could possibly demand genetic testing, and the authors address the issue of whether they should incorporate genetic testing. In neonatology and pediatrics, these issues are even more complex, and the American Academy of Pediatrics Committee on Bioethics states that "[p]redictive genetic testing for adult-onset conditions generally should be deferred unless an intervention initiated in childhood may reduce morbidity or mortality."[3] The authors of the opinion piece have done a nice job of summarizing the current debate, and to date insurance companies have been cautious in their approach to these issues. As one executive quoted in the article noted, "his company would request genetic information but does not want to be the first to do so." Insurance companies will not wait forever. National Institutes of Health Director, Francis S. Collins has recognized that there are more questions than answers, and the rapid increase in the use of genetic testing adds to the urgency with which society must consider and approach these issues.

J. M. Fanaroff, MD, JD

References

1. Dahm R. Discovering DNA: Friedrich Miescher and the early years of nucleic acid research. *Hum Genet.* 2008;122:565-581.
2. 42 U.S. Code Chapter 21F - Prohibiting Employment Discrimination on the Basis of Genetic Information. American Academy of Pediatrics
3. Committee on Bioethics, Committee on Genetics, American College of Medical Genetics and Genomics Social, Ethical, Legal Issues Committee. Ethical and policy issues in genetic testing and screening of children. *Pediatrics.* 2013;131:620-622.

Scientific, Economic, Regulatory, and Ethical Challenges of Bringing Science-Based Pediatric Nutrition Products to the U.S. Market and Ensuring Their Availability for Patients
Merritt RJ, Goldsmith AH (Univ of Southern California, Los Angeles, CA; Washington and Lee Univ, Lexington, VA)
JPEN J Parenter Enteral Nutr 38:17S-34S, 2014

Many nutrition products and related drugs are unavailable or not consistently available to clinicians despite a body of clinical data and experience supporting their use. Many of these can be related to drug shortages that have increased since 2009. In addition, there are potentially useful products that are not approved for a specific use or are no longer being manufactured. This review broadly examines the product availability gap from the perspectives of a clinician/former nutrition industry medical director and an economist. The process of pediatric nutrition product and related drug innovation, as well as its drivers and the steps involved in bringing a product to market, is first described. This is followed by an assessment of factors influencing product availability beyond the innovation process, including regulatory issues, manufacturing compliance, purchasing practices, and other factors related to drug and nutrition product pricing and reimbursement. Three pediatric case examples are reviewed and placed in the context of the prior review. Last, recent and future possible steps toward closing the product availability gap are discussed.

▶ This is a must-read review for neonatologists. It is written by a highly experienced nutritionist who has worked with several companies and an economist. The review aptly describes several aspects of why certain products are so difficult to bring from research or even manufacturing to the bedside. It also describes the cause of some of the recent product shortages, such as vitamin A and certain minerals, that unquestionably have threatened the well-being of neonates in our intensive care units. In addition to addressing certain shortages, there is an apt discussion of why certain products are so difficult to bring to the bedside of neonatal patients. Examples are provided. One includes the difficulty of bringing certain fish oil-containing intravenous preparations to the US patient while it is being used in many other countries, where there are strong data to suggest safety and where it is known that the currently used soy-based products are far from optimal. It discusses the fact that US neonatologist are able to use probiotics that are poorly controlled for their patients, whereas an Investigational New Drug (IND) approval (which is not easy to obtain) is needed to do the badly needed probiotic trials.

J. Neu, MD

16 Behavior Pain

Single-Family Room Care and Neurobehavioral and Medical Outcomes in Preterm Infants

Lester BM, Hawes K, Abar B, et al (Warren Alpert Med School of Brown Univ, Providence, RI; et al)
Pediatrics 134:754-760, 2014

Objective.—To determine whether a single-family room (SFR) NICU, including factors associated with the change to a SFR NICU, is associated with improved medical and neurobehavioral outcomes.

Methods.—Longitudinal, prospective, quasi-experimental cohort study conducted between 2008 and 2012 comparing medical and neurobehavioral outcomes at discharge in infants born <1500 g. Participants included 151 infants in an open-bay NICU and 252 infants after transition to a SFR NICU. Structural equation modeling was used to determine the role of mediators of relations between type of NICU and medical and neurobehavioral outcomes.

Results.—Statistically significant results (all $Ps \leq .05$) showed that infants in the SFR NICU weighed more at discharge, had a greater rate of weight gain, required fewer medical procedures, had a lower gestational age at full enteral feed and less sepsis, showed better attention, less physiologic stress, less hypertonicity, less lethargy, and less pain. NICU differences in weight at discharge, and rate of weight gain were mediated by increased developmental support; differences in number of medical procedures were mediated by increased maternal involvement. NICU differences in attention were mediated by increased developmental support. Differences in stress and pain were mediated by maternal involvement. Nurses reported a more positive work environment and attitudes in the SFR NICU.

Conclusions.—The SFR is associated with improved neurobehavioral and medical outcomes. These improvements are related to increased developmental support and maternal involvement

▶ There has been widespread adoption of the single-family room (SFR) model of care in the neonatal intensive care unit in lieu of the traditional open-bay model. The rationale for this change has been that minimizing stimulation by limiting noise, sound exposure, and sleep interruptions will reduce stress and optimize the neurodevelopment of preterm infants. In practice, this has resulted in single rooms that are very quiet, have continuous low light, and are often accompanied by a blanket draped over the isolette to further suppress light and sound exposure. In addition, contact with staff is minimized so as not to disturb the infant. What is not known is whether being cared for in an SFR truly results in improved medical and developmental outcomes.

The beneficial results of the SFR model of care reported above is in contrast to a previously published US study by Pineda et al[1] that suggested the model may not be beneficial, particularly when studied in an underprivileged population. In the above study, the SFR model of care was associated with increases in developmental support and maternal involvement, whereas the previous study noted no changes in maternal involvement. In addition, Pineda et al noted less brain maturation at term gestation for the SFR cohort.

Most likely the contrasting outcomes relate, not to the SFR model of care but rather to the amount of stimuli infants received. In both studies infants cared for in SFRs were not exposed to white noise and bright lights. However, in the Pineda study, the elimination of these stimuli was not replaced by appropriate physical stimulation and may have resulted in neurosensory deprivation. Thus, the SFR model of care alone may not be optimal for all acutely ill newborn infants unless it is supplemented by the provision of the appropriate amount and type of stimuli.

L. A. Papile, MD

Reference

1. Pineda RG, Neil J, Dierker D, et al. Alterations in brain structure and neurodevelopmental outcome in preterm infants hospitalized in different neonatal intensive care environment. *J Pediatr.* 2014;164:52-60.e52.

Maternal Sensitivity in Parenting Preterm Children: A Meta-analysis
Bilgin A, Wolke D (Univ of Warwick, Coventry, UK)
Pediatrics 136:e177-e193, 2015

Background and Objectives.—Preterm birth is a significant stressor for parents and may adversely impact maternal parenting behavior. However, findings have been inconsistent. The objective of this meta-analysis was to determine whether mothers of preterm children behave differently (eg, less responsive or sensitive) in their interactions with their children after they are discharged from the hospital than mothers of term children.

Methods.—Medline, PsychInfo, ERIC, PubMed, and Web of Science were searched from January 1980 through May 2014 with the following keywords: "premature", "preterm", "low birth weight" in conjunction with "maternal behavio*r", "mother-infant interaction", "maternal sensitivity", and "parenting". Both longitudinal and cross-sectional studies that used an observational measure of maternal parenting behavior were eligible. Study results relating to parenting behaviors defined as sensitivity, facilitation, and responsivity were extracted, and mean estimates were combined with random-effects meta-analysis.

Results.—Thirty-four studies were included in the meta-analysis. Mothers of preterm and full-term children did not differ significantly from each other in terms of their behavior toward their children (Hedges' $g = -0.07$; 95% confidence interval: -0.22 to 0.08; $z = -0.94$; $P = .35$). The heterogeneity between studies was significant and high ($Q = 156.42$; $I^2 = 78.9$, $P = .001$) and not explained by degree of prematurity, publication date, geographical area, infant age, or type of maternal behavior.

Conclusions.—Mothers of preterm children were not found to be less sensitive or responsive toward their children than mothers of full-term children.

▶ Despite the best efforts of well-intentioned, caring neonatal intensive care unit (NICU) caregivers, there are substantial barriers to parenting in the NICU, an experience that leads to parental trauma and is thought to disrupt infant–parent bonding. This meta-analysis performed by Bilgin and Wolke examines post-NICU maternal sensitivity in parenting. The strength of this analysis is that only studies in which assessments were based on direct observation of maternal–infant interaction were included. Although there was substantial heterogeneity among studies, the happy news is that, overall, mothers of (former) preterm children were not seen as being less sensitive or responsive to their children. This is not, however, to say that mothers (and fathers) are not traumatized by the experience of having a preterm baby in the NICU. The incidence of posttraumatic stress disorder is substantial among parents of former preemies; this is a condition about which I think we must be more cognizant and proactive in preventing and/or addressing. Furthermore, neuroscientists are gaining progressively greater insights regarding the ways in which neonatal care can foster or inhibit neonatal neurodevelopment. There is growing evidence that parents play important roles in enhancing their baby's neurodevelopment, and we must endeavor both to more effectively support and also to better engage parents in effective and meaningful parenting of their preterm infants, beginning in the NICU.

L. J. Van Marter, MD, MPH

Maternal Sensitivity in Parenting Preterm Children: A Meta-analysis
Bilgin A, Wolke D (Univ of Warwick, Coventry, UK)
Pediatrics 136:e177-e193, 2015

Background and Objectives.—Preterm birth is a significant stressor for parents and may abstract adversely impact maternal parenting behavior. However, findings have been inconsistent. The objective of this meta-analysis was to determine whether mothers of preterm children behave differently (eg, less responsive or sensitive) in their interactions with their children after they are discharged from the hospital than mothers of term children.

Methods.—Medline, PsychInfo, ERIC, PubMed, and Web of Science were searched from January 1980 through May 2014 with the following keywords: "premature", "preterm", "low birth weight" in conjunction with "maternal behavio*r", "mother-infant interaction", "maternal sensitivity", and "parenting". Both longitudinal and cross-sectional studies that used an observational measure of maternal parenting behavior were eligible. Study results relating to parenting behaviors defined as sensitivity, facilitation, and responsivity were extracted, and mean estimates were combined with random-effects meta-analysis.

Results.—Thirty-four studies were included in the meta-analysis. Mothers of preterm and full-term children did not differ significantly from each other in terms of their behavior toward their children (Hedges' $g = -0.07$; 95% confidence interval: -0.22 to 0.08; $z = -0.94$; $P = .35$). The heterogeneity between studies was significant and high ($Q = 156.42$; $I^2 = 78.9$, $P = .001$) and not explained by degree of prematurity, publication date, geographical area, infant age, or type of maternal behavior.

Conclusions.—Mothers of preterm children were not found to be less sensitive or responsive toward their children than mothers of full-term children.

▶ Maternal sensitivity has been reported to be a predictor of the development of secure infant-to-mother attachment, and in preterm infants maternal sensitivity has been associated with positive developmental outcomes.[1,2] However, there is considerable inconsistency in published studies as to whether mothers of preterm infants are as sensitive or responsive as mothers of full-term infants in their interactions with their infants. The authors of this study sought to answer this question by conducting a meta-analysis of cross-sectional and longitudinal studies of maternal behavior in preterm infant—mother dyads published between January 1980 and May 2014. Studies included in the analysis needed to use an observable instrument to measure maternal parenting behavior and had to include a full-term comparison group. The results of the meta-analysis indicate that mothers of preterm infants/children provide, on average, similar observed sensitive and responsive parenting for their preterm offspring as mothers of full-term infants. However, the authors' additional statement that the degree of prematurity did not influence this observation needs clarification. For study purposes, gestational age was truncated into 2 categories, very preterm (less than 32 weeks' gestation) and moderate-to-late preterm (32-36 weeks' gestation). In addition, in the 34 studies included in the analysis, the mean gestational age was 30.4 weeks (standard deviation [SD], = 2.2 weeks) and the mean birth weight was 1374 g (SD = 234). Thus, although the above observation is encouraging, it may not pertain to mothers of infants who are extremely low gestational age or extremely low birth weight.

L. A. Papile, MD

References

1. De Wolff MS, van Ijzendoorn MH. Sensitivity and attachment, a meta-analysis on parental antecedents of infant attachment. *Child Dev.* 1997;68:571-591.
2. Magill-Evans J, Harrison MJ. Parent-infant interactions, parenting stress, and developmental outcomes at 4 years. *Child Health Care.* 2001;30:135-150.

Maternal singing during kangaroo care led to autonomic stability in preterm infants and reduced maternal anxiety

Arnon S, Diamant C, Bauer S, et al (Meir Med Ctr, Kfar Saba, Israel)
Acta Paediatr 103:1039-1044, 2014

Aim.—Kangaroo care (KC) and maternal singing benefit preterm infants, and we investigated whether combining these benefitted infants and mothers.

Methods.—A prospective randomised, within-subject, crossover, repeated-measures study design was used, with participants acting as their own controls. We evaluated the heart rate variability (HRV) of stable preterm infants receiving KC, with and without maternal singing. This included low frequency (LF), high frequency (HF) and the LF/HF ratio during baseline (10 min), singing or quiet phases (20 min) and recovery (10 min). Physiological parameters, maternal anxiety and the infants' behavioural state were measured.

Results.—We included 86 stable preterm infants, with a postmenstrual age of 32—36 weeks. A significant change in LF and HF, and lower LF/HF ratio, was observed during KC with maternal singing during the intervention and recovery phases, compared with just KC and baseline (all p-values <0.05). Maternal anxiety was lower during singing than just KC ($p = 0.04$). No differences in the infants' behavioural states or physiological parameters were found, with or without singing.

Conclusion.—Maternal singing during KC reduces maternal anxiety and leads to autonomic stability in stable preterm infants. This effect is not detected in behavioural state or physiological parameters commonly used to monitor preterm infants.

▶ Mothers of preterm infants are increasingly interested in how they can contribute to their infant's growth and well-being during the neonatal intensive care unit (NICU) stay. This led to the adaptation of kangaroo care, a technique initially developed for indigent populations in South America, and more recently, music therapy, as part of developmental care in the NICU.

In this clinical study the investigators evaluated the effect of maternal singing during kangaroo care in the NICU and compared the results with the effects of kangaroo care alone. Two 40-minute sessions were performed over 2 days, starting with kangaroo care on its own for 10 minutes, followed by either maternal singing and kangaroo care or just kangaroo care for 20 minutes and subsequently followed by another 10 minutes of just kangaroo care. The mother was instructed to sing with a repetitive soothing tone, softly, simply and with slow tempo. She was asked to include lullabies, preferably those that she sang during pregnancy. The change in heart rate variability and a reduction in maternal anxiety associated with maternal singing are not unexpected; previous studies of ive music interventions applied by musical therapist have yielded similar results. Of note, one of the exclusion criteria was hyper-alertness to maternal voice, defined as crying when the mother started singing and relaxing when the singing stopped. Thus, it may be prudent to have a mother audition before she is encouraged to sing to her infant.

L. A. Papile, MD

Assessment of pain during application of nasal-continuous positive airway pressure and heated, humidified high-flow nasal cannulae in preterm infants
Osman M, Elsharkawy A, Abdel-Hady H (Mansoura Univ Children's Hosp, Egypt)
J Perinatol 35:263-267, 2015

Objective.—To assess pain and compare its severity in preterm infants during application of nasal-continuous positive airway pressure (nCPAP) and heated, humidified high-flow nasal cannulae (HHHFNC).

Study Design.—An observational cross-sectional study. Sixty preterm infants, categorized into nCPAP ($n = 37$) and HHHFNC groups ($n = 23$). Pain response was assessed using Premature Infant Pain Profile (PIPP), duration of first cry and salivary-cortisol concentrations.

Result.—The PIPP scores were significantly higher in the nCPAP compared with HHHFNC group (10 (7–12) vs 4 (2–6), $P < 0.01$). None of the infants in the HHHFNC group had severe pain defined as a PIPP score >12, compared with 5 (13.5%) infants in the nCPAP group. Salivary-cortisol concentrations were significantly higher in nCPAP group compared with the HHHFNC group (5.0 (3.6–5.9) vs 1.6 (1.0–2.3) nmol l^{-1}, $P < 0.01$). A lower incidence of cry was observed for infants in the HHHFNC group compared with the nCPAP group (11 (47.8%) vs 30 (81.1%), $P < 0.001$), however, the duration of first cry was not significantly different between groups. The respiratory rate was significantly lower after application of HHHFNC compared with nCPAP ($P < 0.001$). There were no significant differences between groups with regard to fraction of inspired oxygen (FiO_2), oxygen saturation by pulse oximeter (SpO_2) and heart rate.

Conclusion.—The application of HHHFNC in preterm infants is associated with less pain compared with nCPAP, as it is associated with less PIPP scores and lower salivary-cortisol concentrations.

▶ Neonatal intensive care is by necessity associated with patient discomfort. Some procedures are clearly painful (eg, heel sticks, venipuncture, and mechanical ventilation), whereas others (eg, chest physiotherapy or noninvasive respiratory support) are generally used without analgesia or comforting interventions. In an observational cross-sectional study, Osman et al compared pain scores, cortisol levels, and crying in 60 infants receiving nasal continuous positive airway pressure (nCPAP) or heated humidified high flow nasal cannula (HHHFNC). Pain was assessed using the Premature Infant Pain Profile (PIPP) directly after administration of the nasal support device and salivary cortisol 30 minutes after the application of HHHFNC or nCPAP. The PIPP scores and salivary cortisol levels were significantly higher in infants receiving nCPAP. The authors acknowledge the limitations of the study: small sample size, lack of blinding or randomization, and no baseline cortisol values.

There have been 3 large randomized clinical trials comparing HHHFNC with nCPAP either as a primary mode of respiratory support or preventing postextubation failure.[1-4] In none of the trials was HHHFNC superior to nCPAP, and in the largest study of infants < 30 weeks' gestation, there was a trend for the superiority nCPAP especially for infants < 26 weeks' gestation.[1] Nasal trauma scores were less in the HHHFNC group in 2 of the studies.[2,3] In the only other study evaluating infant pain, Klingenberg et al found no differences in pain scores between the 2 modes of noninvasive support.[5]

There is no question that application of noninvasive respiratory support can be associated with patient discomfort. The skill of bedside nurses is critical to ensure that pain is minimized by correct application of the devices and assessment of pain after the infant has been repositioned and stabilized. Infants with continued discomfort should receive nonpharmacologic interventions.

R. A. Polin, MD

References

1. Osman M, Elsharkawy A, Abdel-Hady H. Assessment of pain during application of nasal-continuous positive airway pressure and heated, humidified high-flow nasal cannulae in preterm infants. *J Perinatol.* 2015;35:263-267.
2. Manley BJ, Owen LS, Doyle LW, et al. High flow nasal cannulae in very preterm infants after extubation. *N Engl J Med.* 2013;369:1425-1433.
3. Yoder BA, Stoddard RA, Li M, King J, Dirnberger DR, Abbasi S. Heated humidified high-flow nasal cannula versus nasal CPAP for respiratory support in neonates. *Pediatrics.* 2013;131:e1482-e1490.
4. Collins CL, Barfield C, Horne RS, Davis PG. A randomized controlled trial to compare heated humidified high-flow nasal cannulae with nasal continuous positive airway pressure post extubation in premature infants. *J Pediatr.* 2013;162: 949-954.
5. Klingenberg C. Patient comfort during treatment with heated humidified high-flow treatment versus nasal continuous positive airway pressure: a randomized crossover trial. *Arch Dis Child Fetal Neonatal Ed.* 2014;99:F134-F137.

The utility of pain scores obtained during 'regular reassessment process' in premature infants in the NICU
Rohan AJ (State Univ of New York at Stony Brook)
J Perinatol 34:532-537, 2014

Objective.—To examine the association of pain assessment scores achieved through regular reassessment practice, as required by the Joint Commission (JC), with painful events and the use of analgesics in premature, ventilated infants.

Study Design.—A cross-sectional study was performed in two tertiary level neonatal intensive care units. Pain was assessed at regular intervals at each center using validated multidimensional instruments in accordance with the JC standards.

Result.—Sample comprised 196 ventilated premature infant patient-days. Overall, 2% of scores suggested the presence of pain, and 0.1% of pain scores were associated with analgesia. Ventilated infants who were exposed to multiple pain-associated procedures in a day never demonstrated pain score elevations despite infrequent preemptive or continuous analgesic administration.

Conclusion.—Pain assessment scores achieved using regular reassessment processes were poorly correlated with exposure to pain-associated procedures or conditions. Low pain scores achieved through regular reassessment may not correlate to low pain exposure. Resources that are expended on regular reassessment processes may need to be reconsidered in light of the low yield for clinical alterations in care in this setting.

▶ Several years ago, the assertion that pain should be considered to be "the fifth vital sign" led to a Joint Commission mandate for pain assessment with each vital sign assessment for all hospital inpatients. Despite universal adoption of this practice, there remains a paucity of evidence for improvement in pain control as a result. That seems to be particularly problematic for preverbal patients, including newborn infants, who cannot report the subjective experience of pain. This report provides empiric evidence that 2 well-validated pain assessment tools fail to identify pain episodes in ventilated preterm infants, given that pain scores were rarely significantly elevated despite frequent exposures to presumably painful procedures. Although regression analysis demonstrated a modest association between painful events and pain scores, that association disappeared when gestational age adjustments were eliminated, suggesting that the observed correlation simply reflected greater frequency of both slight score increases and frequency of painful procedures in less mature infants. These discrepancies could result from either poor sensitivity of the assessment tools or from excellent anticipatory pain relief. The latter does not seem to be plausible, however, because only 10% of the procedures performed were associated with administration of analgesic medications. It therefore appears that this may be another instance in which the performance of a diagnostic procedure was much better in validation trials than turns out to be the case in actual practice. Accordingly, the author courageously points out that the Joint Commission mandate for these regularly scheduled pain assessments may require reconsideration, at least as applied to patients in the neonatal intensive care unit (NICU). On the other hand, the study data demonstrate a substantial difference between the 2 study centers in the daily number of documented pain exposures, implying that differences in practice patterns (avoidance of intubation and early extubation, in particular) may offer a more effective strategy for pain reduction in these patients. In addition, the author wisely suggests that "dynamic provider perceptions of the infant pain experience may be a more important factor than pain scores in driving pain management in the NICU." In other words, provider empathy coupled with anticipatory and compassionate use of analgesic medications appears to be our current best option for pain prevention and control in our neonatal patients.

W. E. Benitz, MD

Article Index

Chapter 1: The Fetus

Fetal Surgery: Principles, Indications, and Evidence	1
Risk of selected structural abnormalities in infants after increased nuchal translucency measurement	2
Accuracy of prenatal ultrasound in detecting jejunal and ileal atresia: systematic review and meta-analysis	4
Thoracoamniotic shunts for the management of fetal lung lesions and pleural effusions: a single-institution review and predictors of survival in 75 cases	5

Chapter 2: Epidemiology and Pregnancy Complications

A population-based, multifaceted strategy to implement antenatal corticosteroid treatment versus standard care for the reduction of neonatal mortality due to preterm birth in low-income and middle-income countries: the ACT cluster-randomised trial	7
A Universal Transvaginal Cervical Length Screening Program for Preterm Birth Prevention	9
Urinary Bisphenol A Levels during Pregnancy and Risk of Preterm Birth	12
Climate change is associated with male:female ratios of fetal deaths and newborn infants in Japan	13
Prescription Opioid Epidemic and Infant Outcomes	15
Etiologies of NICU Deaths	16
Etiologies of NICU Deaths	17
Impact of Late Preterm and Early Term Infants on Canadian Neonatal Intensive Care Units	19
Measuring Gestational Age in Vital Statistics Data: Transitioning to the Obstetric Estimate	21
Survival and Morbidity of Preterm Children Born at 22 Through 34 weeks' Gestation in France in 2011: Results of the EPIPAGE-2 Cohort Study	22
Using Satellite-Based Spatiotemporal Resolved Air Temperature Exposure to Study the Association between Ambient Air Temperature and Birth Outcomes in Massachusetts	24
Neonatal and early childhood outcomes following early vs later preterm premature rupture of membranes	25

Chapter 3: Genetics and Teratology

Severity of Birth Defects After Propylthiouracil Exposure in Early Pregnancy	27
Hypermethylation of *SHH* in the pathogenesis of congenital anorectal malformations	29
FUT 2 polymorphism and outcome in very-low-birth-weight infants	31

Dexamethasone but not the equivalent doses of hydrocortisone induces
neurotoxicity in neonatal rat brain   32

Chapter 4: Labor and Delivery

Endotracheal Suction for Nonvigorous Neonates Born through Meconium Stained
Amniotic Fluid: A Randomized Controlled Trial   35

Endotracheal Suction for Nonvigorous Neonates Born through Meconium Stained
Amniotic Fluid: A Randomized Controlled Trial   37

Diagnostic Accuracy of Fetal Heart Rate Monitoring in the Identification of
Neonatal Encephalopathy   38

Delivery of Breech Presentation at Term Gestation in Canada, 2003–2011   40

Delayed cord clamping with and without cord stripping: a prospective randomized
trial of preterm neonates   42

Effect of umbilical cord milking on morbidity and survival in extremely low
gestational age neonates   44

Effect of gravity on volume of placental transfusion: a multicentre, randomised,
non-inferiority trial   46

Randomized Trial of Occlusive Wrap for Heat Loss Prevention in Preterm Infants   47

Low Apgar score, neonatal encephalopathy and epidural analgesia during labour: a
Swedish registry-based study   50

Extreme macrosomia – Obstetric outcomes and complications in birthweights
>5000 g   51

Between-Hospital Variation in Treatment and Outcomes in Extremely Preterm
Infants   52

Chapter 5: Infectious Disease and Immunology

Late-Onset Group B Streptococcal Meningitis Has Cerebrovascular Complications   55

The microbiota regulates neutrophil homeostasis and host resistance to *Escherichia
coli* K1 sepsis in neonatal mice   56

Effect of Fluconazole Prophylaxis on Candidiasis and Mortality in Premature
Infants: A Randomized Clinical Trial   57

Blood Transfusion and Breast Milk Transmission of Cytomegalovirus in Very
Low-Birth-Weight Infants: A Prospective Cohort Study   59

Blood Transfusion and Breast Milk Transmission of Cytomegalovirus in Very
Low-Birth-Weight Infants: A Prospective Cohort Study   61

Blood Transfusion and Breast Milk Transmission of Cytomegalovirus in Very
Low-Birth-Weight Infants: A Prospective Cohort Study   64

Oropharyngeal Colostrum Administration in Extremely Premature Infants: An
RCT   66

Oropharyngeal Colostrum Administration in Extremely Premature Infants: An
RCT   67

Effect of emollient therapy on clinical outcomes in preterm neonates in Pakistan: a
randomised controlled trial   69

Presepsin for the Detection of Late-Onset Sepsis in Preterm Newborns	71
Timely empiric antimicrobials are associated with faster microbiologic clearance in preterm neonates with late-onset bloodstream infections	73
The Role of Coagulase-Negative Staphylococci in Early Onset Sepsis in a Large European Cohort of Very Low Birth Weight Infants	74
Incidence, Etiology, and Outcome of Bacterial Meningitis in Infants Aged <90 Days in the United Kingdom and Republic of Ireland: Prospective, Enhanced, National Population-Based Surveillance	76
Clinical and laboratory characteristics of central nervous system herpes simplex virus infection in neonates and young infants	78
Valganciclovir for Symptomatic Congenital Cytomegalovirus Disease	79
Valganciclovir for Symptomatic Congenital Cytomegalovirus Disease	81
Anaerobic Antimicrobial Therapy After Necrotizing Enterocolitis in VLBW Infants	82
Mortality Due to Bloodstream Infections and Necrotizing Enterocolitis in Very Low Birth Weight Infants	84
Role of Guidelines on Length of Therapy in Chorioamnionitis and Neonatal Sepsis	86
Newborn Screening for Severe Combined Immunodeficiency in 11 Screening Programs in the United States	88
First Pertussis Vaccine Dose and Prevention of Infant Mortality	90

Chapter 6: Cardiovascular System

Natural evolution of patent ductus arteriosus in the extremely preterm infant	93
Use of ultrasound in the haemodynamic assessment of the sick neonate	95
Vasopressin versus Dopamine for Treatment of Hypotension in Extremely Low Birth Weight Infants: A Randomized, Blinded Pilot Study	97
Do small doses of atropine (<0.1 mg) cause bradycardia in young children?	98
Antidepressant Use Late in Pregnancy and Risk of Persistent Pulmonary Hypertension of the Newborn	99
Fetal Thrombotic Vasculopathy and Perinatal Thrombosis: Should all Placentas be Examined?	101
Transplantation-Free Survival and Interventions at 3 Years in the Single Ventricle Reconstruction Trial	103

Chapter 7: Respiratory Disorders

Spontaneously Breathing Preterm Infants Change in Tidal Volume to Improve Lung Aeration Immediately after Birth	105
Sustained Lung Inflation at Birth for Preterm Infants: A Randomized Clinical Trial	106
Safe oxygen saturation targeting and monitoring in preterm infants: can we avoid hypoxia and hyperoxia?	108
Oxygen Saturation Target Range for Extremely Preterm Infants: A Systemic Review and Meta-analysis	108

PaCO$_2$ in Surfactant, Positive Pressure, and Oxygenation Randomised Trial (SUPPORT)	110
A randomised controlled trial of an automated oxygen delivery algorithm for preterm neonates receiving supplemental oxygen without mechanical ventilation	112
Unbound Unconjugated Hyperbilirubinemia Is Associated with Central Apnea in Premature Infants	114
Very long apnea events in preterm infants	115
Less invasive surfactant administration is associated with improved pulmonary outcomes in spontaneously breathing preterm infants	116
Neurodevelopmental Outcomes of Very Low Birth Weight Preterm Infants Treated With Poractant Alfa versus Beractant for Respiratory Distress Syndrome	117
Bi-level CPAP does not improve gas exchange when compared with conventional CPAP for the treatment of neonates recovering from respiratory distress syndrome	119
Changes in ventilator strategies and outcomes in preterm infants	120
Congenital chylothorax: a prospective nationwide epidemiological study in Germany	122
Hospital Variation and Risk Factors for Bronchopulmonary Dysplasia in a Population-Based Cohort	123
Pulmonary Hypertension in Preterm Infants: Prevalence and Association with Bronchopulmonary Dysplasia	125
Noninvasive Inhaled Nitric Oxide Does Not Prevent Bronchopulmonary Dysplasia in Premature Newborns	126
Inhaled nitric oxide in preterm infants with prolonged preterm rupture of the membranes: a case series	128
An Update on the Impact of Postnatal Systemic Corticosteroids on Mortality and Cerebral Palsy in Preterm Infants: Effect Modification by Risk of Bronchopulmonary Dysplasia	129
Detection of Bloodstream Infections and Prediction of Bronchopulmonary Dysplasia in Preterm Neonates with an Electronic Nose	130
The Effect of the National Shortage of Vitamin A on Death or Chronic Lung Disease in Extremely Low-Birth-Weight Infants	131
Cardiovascular function in children who had chronic lung disease of prematurity	133

Chapter 8: Central Nervous System and Special Senses

Neonatal encephalopathy and the association to asphyxia in labor	137
Diagnostic Accuracy of Fetal Heart Rate Monitoring in the Identification of Neonatal Encephalopathy	138
Heart rate variability in hypoxic ischemic encephalopathy: correlation with EEG grade and 2-y neurodevelopmental outcome	139
Brain Temperature in Neonates with Hypoxic-Ischemic Encephalopathy during Therapeutic Hypothermia	141
Cognitive Outcomes After Neonatal Encephalopathy	142

Cognitive Outcomes of Preterm Infants Randomized to Darbepoetin, Erythropoietin, or Placebo — 143

Effects of Hypothermia for Perinatal Asphyxia on Childhood Outcomes — 146

Maternal allopurinol administration during suspected fetal hypoxia: a novel neuroprotective intervention? A multicentre randomised placebo controlled trial — 147

Melatonin use for neuroprotection in perinatal asphyxia: a randomized controlled pilot study — 148

Effect of Depth and Duration of Cooling on Deaths in the NICU Among Neonates With Hypoxic Ischemic Encephalopathy: A Randomized Clinical Trial — 149

Effect of Depth and Duration of Cooling on Deaths in the NICU Among Neonates With Hypoxic Ischemic Encephalopathy: A Randomized Clinical Trial — 151

Association Between Early Administration of High-Dose Erythropoietin in Preterm Infants and Brain MRI Abnormality at Term-Equivalent Age — 153

Association Between Early Administration of High-Dose Erythropoietin in Preterm Infants and Brain MRI Abnormality at Term-Equivalent Age — 155

Brain Magnetic Resonance Imaging in Infants with Surgical Necrotizing Enterocolitis or Spontaneous Intestinal Perforation versus Medical Necrotizing Enterocolitis — 157

Prenatal unilateral cerebellar hypoplasia in a series of 26 cases: significance and implications for prenatal diagnosis — 158

Eye disorders in newborn infants (excluding retinopathy of prematurity) — 159

The Pediatric Cataract Register (PECARE): analysis of age at detection of congenital cataract — 160

Late Reconstruction of Brachial Plexus Birth Palsy — 162

Chapter 9: Gastrointestinal Health and Nutrition

Intestinal Microbiota Development in Preterm Neonates and Effect of Perinatal Antibiotics — 167

Bacteriological, Biochemical, and Immunological Properties of Colostrum and Mature Milk From Mothers of Extremely Preterm Infants — 169

Breast milk, microbiota, and intestinal immune homeostasis — 170

Bioactive peptides released from *in vitro* digestion of human milk with or without pasteurization — 171

Human milk microRNA and total RNA differ depending on milk fractionation — 172

Enteral Granulocyte-Colony Stimulating Factor and Erythropoietin Early in Life Improves Feeding Tolerance in Preterm Infants: A Randomized Controlled Trial — 173

Enteral Granulocyte-Colony Stimulating Factor and Erythropoietin Early in Life Improves Feeding Tolerance in Preterm Infants: A Randomized Controlled Trial — 175

Influences of Breast Milk Composition on Gastric Emptying in Preterm Infants — 177

Influences of Breast Milk Composition on Gastric Emptying in Preterm Infants — 178

A randomised trial of re-feeding gastric residuals in preterm infants — 179

Abdominal Circumference or Gastric Residual Volume as Measure of Feed Intolerance in VLBW Infants	181
Breast-Feeding Improves Gut Maturation Compared With Formula Feeding in Preterm Babies	183
Randomized Trial of Human Milk Cream as a Supplement to Standard Fortification of an Exclusive Human Milk-Based Diet in Infants 750-1250 g Birth Weight	184
Glycerin Enemas and Suppositories in Premature Infants: A Meta-analysis	187
Guidelines for Feeding Very Low Birth Weight Infants	188
Balancing the risks and benefits of parenteral nutrition for preterm infants: can we define the optimal composition?	189
Cow's Milk Contamination of Human Milk Purchased via the Internet	190
Cow's Milk Contamination of Human Milk Purchased via the Internet	191
Network analysis suggests a potentially 'evil' alliance of opportunistic pathogens inhibited by a cooperative network in human milk bacterial communities	193
Utility of Gastrointestinal Fluoroscopic Studies in Detecting Stricture After Neonatal Necrotizing Enterocolitis	194
Fecal Short-Chain Fatty Acids of Very-Low-Birth-Weight Preterm Infants Fed Expressed Breast Milk or Formula	195
Long-Chain Polyunsaturated Fatty Acids and Cognition in VLBW Infants at 8 years: an RCT	197
Hirschsprung disease in the premature newborn: A population based study and 40-year single center experience	198
Nutritional outcomes in survivors of congenital diaphragmatic hernia (CDH)—Factors associated with growth at one year	200

Chapter 10: Hematology and Bilirubin

Why do four NICUs using identical RBC transfusion guidelines have different gestational age-adjusted RBC transfusion rates?	203
Early Discharge of Infants and Risk of Readmission for Jaundice	204
Early Discharge of Infants and Risk of Readmission for Jaundice	206
Discrepancies Between Transcutaneous and Serum Bilirubin Measurements	207
Peanut, milk, and wheat intake during pregnancy is associated with reduced allergy and asthma in children	209
Thrombocytopenia in late preterm and term neonates after perinatal asphyxia	211
Thrombocytopenia in late preterm and term neonates after perinatal asphyxia	213

Chapter 11: Renal, Metabolism, and Endocrine Disorders

Clinically stable very low birthweight infants are at risk for recurrent tissue glucose fluctuations even after fully established enteral nutrition	215
Preterm Birth Is Associated with Higher Uric Acid Levels in Adolescents	217

Neonatal Citrullinemia: Novel, Reversible Neuroimaging Findings Correlated
With Ammonia Level Changes	218

Chapter 12: Miscellaneous

Comparison of four near-infrared spectroscopy devices shows that they are only
suitable for monitoring cerebral oxygenation trends in preterm infants	221

Comparison of four near-infrared spectroscopy devices shows that they are only
suitable for monitoring cerebral oxygenation trends in preterm infants	222

Refractive Outcomes Following Bevacizumab Monotherapy Compared With
Conventional Laser Treatment: A Randomized Clinical Trial	223

Between-Hospital Variation in Treatment and Outcomes in Extremely Preterm
Infants	225

Pigmentary Lines of the Newborn: A Case Report and Review of the Literature	227

Origins of the breast milk-derived cells; an endeavor to find the cell sources	228

Diagnostic Yield of Sonography in Infants With Suspected Hip Dysplasia:
Diagnostic Thinking Efficiency and Therapeutic Efficiency	229

A comparison of the direct cost of care in an open-bay and single-family room
NICU	231

Evacuation of a Neonatal Intensive Care Unit in a Disaster: Lessons From
Hurricane Sandy	232

Chapter 13: Pharmacology

Antenatal magnesium sulfate and spontaneous intestinal perforation in infants less
than 25 weeks gestation	235

Diuretic Exposure in Premature Infants from 1997 to 2011	236

Azithromycin in Early Infancy and Pyloric Stenosis	238

A Randomized, Controlled Trial of Oral Propranolol in Infantile Hemangioma	239

Phthalates and critically ill neonates: device-related exposures and non-endocrine
toxic risks	241

Reduction in Developmental Coordination Disorder with Neonatal Caffeine
Therapy	242

Morphine Versus Clonidine for Neonatal Abstinence Syndrome	243

Chapter 14: Postnatal Growth and Development/Follow-up

Between-Hospital Variation in Treatment and Outcomes in Extremely Preterm
Infants	245

Bayley-III Cognitive and Language Scales in Preterm Children	247

International standards for newborn weight, length, and head circumference by
gestational age and sex: the Newborn Cross-Sectional Study of the
INTERGROWTH-21st Project	249

Nature and origins of mathematics difficulties in very preterm children: a different
etiology than developmental dyscalculia	251

Referral of Very Low Birth Weight Infants to High-Risk Follow-Up at Neonatal Intensive Care Unit Discharge Varies Widely across California	252
Cardiorespiratory events in extremely low birth weight infants: neurodevelopmental outcome at 1 and 2 years	253
Developmental outcomes at 3 years of age following major non-cardiac and cardiac surgery in term infants: A population-based study	255
In Utero and Childhood Polybrominated Diphenyl Ether Exposures and Body Mass at Age 7 Years: The CHAMACOS Study	256
Neurodevelopmental outcomes of preterm singletons, twins and higher-order gestations: a population-based cohort study	257
An Update on the Impact of Postnatal Systemic Corticosteroids on Mortality and Cerebral Palsy in Preterm Infants: Effect Modification by Risk of Bronchopulmonary Dysplasia	259
Effects of Hypothermia for Perinatal Asphyxia on Childhood Outcomes	260
Association of Low Birth Weight and Preterm Birth With the Incidence of Knee and Hip Arthroplasty for Osteoarthritis	261

Chapter 15: Ethics

Parents report positive experiences about enrolling babies in a cord-related clinical trial before birth	265
Ethics and Etiquette in Neonatal Intensive Care	266
Should Life Insurers Have Access to Genetic Test Results?	267
Scientific, Economic, Regulatory, and Ethical Challenges of Bringing Science-Based Pediatric Nutrition Products to the U.S. Market and Ensuring Their Availability for Patients	269

Chapter 16: Behavior Pain

Single-Family Room Care and Neurobehavioral and Medical Outcomes in Preterm Infants	271
Maternal Sensitivity in Parenting Preterm Children: A Meta-analysis	272
Maternal Sensitivity in Parenting Preterm Children: A Meta-analysis	273
Maternal singing during kangaroo care led to autonomic stability in preterm infants and reduced maternal anxiety	275
Assessment of pain during application of nasal-continuous positive airway pressure and heated, humidified high-flow nasal cannulae in preterm infants	276
The utility of pain scores obtained during 'regular reassessment process' in premature infants in the NICU	277

Author Index

A

Abar B, 271
Abdel-Hady H, 276
Abraham RS, 88
Adami RR, 38, 138
Adhisivam B, 35, 37
Adzick NS, 5
Ågren J, 137
Aliaga S, 236
Almaas AN, 197
Alsaweed M, 172
Althabe F, 7
Aly H, 148
Ambalavanan N, 110
Amin SB, 114
Ancel P-Y, 22
Andersen SL, 27
Andresen D, 78
Appelbaum PS, 267
Araque Campo R, 112
Arboleya S, 167
Arnon S, 275
Ashby E, 229
Autmizguine J, 82
Awad HA, 173, 175
Ayers S, 265
Azpeitia A, 74
Azzopardi D, 146, 260

B

Bada HS, 243
Baer RJ, 2
Baer VL, 211, 213
Bagna R, 101
Bairdain S, 200
Bassil KL, 19
Bateman BT, 99
Bauer AS, 162
Bauer S, 275
Baughman AL, 90
Baxter JK, 9
Belizán JM, 7
Benders MJNL, 147
Benjamin DK Jr, 57
Bennett MV, 252
Bhat BV, 35, 37
Bhat R, 179
Bhutta ZA, 69
Bialkowski A, 122
Bianconi T, 71

Bilgin A, 272, 273
Blanco CL, 184
Boelig MM, 5
Boelig RC, 9
Botta G, 101
Bowen JR, 204, 206
Bunyavanich S, 209

C

Cagneaux M, 158
Caliendo AM, 59, 61, 64
Cantonwine DE, 12
Carr SR, 1
Chantala K, 236
Chessell L, 188
Chettri S, 35, 37
Cheung P-Y, 105
Chevrier J, 256
Christensen RD, 143, 203, 211, 213
Chuang AZ, 223
Chung WK, 267
Clark EAS, 44
Clark RH, 16, 17
Clark TA, 90
Clark WL, 223
Cook DJ, 108
Coull BA, 24
Cragg L, 251
Cruz H, 232
Cuna A, 179
Currier R, 88
Cutter GR, 126

D

D'antonio F, 4
Darmstadt GL, 69
de Vaan L, 183
Demmert M, 31
Deshmukh HS, 56
Diamant C, 275
Diomandé D, 93
Dizdar EA, 117
Doelling N, 78
Downey EC, 198
Doyle LW, 129, 242, 259
Drinker LR, 235
Dudley J, 15
Düring C, 265
Dutta S, 188

E

Easley KA, 59, 61, 64
Eberly MD, 238
Ehrenkranz RA, 129, 259
Eide MB, 238
Eisa L, 98
Ekéus C, 50
El-Dib M, 148
El-Farrash RA, 173, 175
El-Ganzoury MM, 173, 175
Elmahdy H, 148
Elsharkawy A, 276
Embleton ND, 189
Eras Z, 117
Erkin-Cakmak A, 256
Espiritu M, 232
Eyal FG, 42

F

Feng Y, 32
Ferguson KK, 12
Fernández L, 169
Fisher J, 200
Clark EAS, 44
Ford S, 125
Fosse N, 227
Fox MA, 241
Franta J, 128
Friedlich P, 141
Fukuda K, 13
Fukuda M, 13

G

Gage SC, 123
Garel C, 158
Geloneck MM, 223
Gibson J, 243
Gilmore C, 251
Gnanendran L, 257
Goldsmith AH, 269
Golombek SG, 108
Gómez JJ, 112
Goodwin A, 195
Göpel W, 116
Gorenstein AN, 46
Gould JB, 252
Goulding RM, 139
Gozzini E, 71
Graham EM, 38, 138
Greene MM, 253

H

Guan Q, 193
Gui L, 153, 155

Haargaard B, 160
Hair AB, 184
Halliday HL, 129, 259
Halliday R, 255
Harley KG, 256
Hawes K, 271
Hehir MP, 51
Helseth CC, 231
Henry E, 203
Hepworth AR, 172, 177, 178
Herrmann N, 130
Hintz SR, 252
Hoeger P, 239
Hofstätter E, 221, 222
Hosseini SM, 228
Huang Y, 29
Hughes E, 198
Hultin M, 50
Hussain SM, 261
Huybrechts KF, 99

I

Itin P, 227
Iyengar RS, 170

J

Jacob J, 16, 17
James MA, 162
Janvier A, 266
Jonsson M, 137
Josephson CD, 59, 61, 64
Joshi S, 133
Jung YH, 66-67

K

Kaandorp JJ, 147
Kaiser JR, 97
Kamath-Rayne BD, 143
Kamitsuka M, 16, 17
Kan P, 123
Kanmaz G, 117
Kaur A, 181
Keim SA, 190, 191
Khalil A, 4
Khan FA, 200
Khan S, 253
Kim H-S, 66, 67
Kimberlin DW, 79, 81
King C, 189
Kinsella JP, 126
Kirmeyer SE, 21
Kiser C, 86
Klemme M, 215
Kler N, 181
Klitzman R, 267
Kloog I, 24
Kluckow M, 95
Kotecha S, 133
Kotzbauer D, 78
Kramer BW, 183
Kraus DM, 235
Kraus SJ, 194
Krueger MS, 42
Kulkarni MM, 190, 191
Kumar P, 32
Kwan A, 88

L

Lain SJ, 204, 206
Lakshminrusimha S, 108
Lampland AL, 119
Lapcharoensap W, 123
Laughon MM, 236
Léauté-Labrèze C, 239
Lee H, 115
Lee J, 66, 67
Lee KJ, 247
Lefèvre C, 172
Legacy J, 218
Lerman J, 98
Lester BM, 271
Leuchter RH-V, 153, 155
Lista G, 106
Liu Y, 56
Livingston MH, 187
Lönnerdal B, 171
Loughran-Fowlds A, 255
Lyons J, 40

M

(Sam) Ma Z, 193
Madrid M, 74
Magnetti F, 101
Maguire PJ, 51
Maier RF, 130
Mallow EB, 241
Manja V, 108
Manuck TA, 25
Manzano S, 169
Martin JA, 21
Martin PR, 15
Massoud M, 158
Mazereeuw-Hautier J, 239
McClure EM, 7
Mchugh AF, 51
McKenna K, 86
McKenney SL, 38, 138
McKinley PS, 131
McLean C, 141
McNamara K, 190, 191
Meinzen-Derr J, 157
Melly SJ, 24
Menkiti OR, 56
Merhar SL, 157
Merritt RJ, 269
Mian Q, 105
Milani C, 167
Minnich B, 221, 222
Mirza H, 125
Mohr MA, 115
Mola-Schenzle E, 215
Moles L, 169
Monday L, 73
Montes Bueno MT, 108
Moreira AG, 184
Morgan C, 189
Mukherjee B, 12
Mularoni A, 74
Murray DM, 139
Murthy K, 131

N

Nakstad B, 197
Natarajan G, 73
Nawab U, 86
Newburger JW, 103
Nixon PA, 217
Nolan VG, 195
Nordén-Lindeberg S, 137
Norton ME, 2
Nyström A, 160

O

O'Donnell SM, 128
Ohls RK, 143
Okike IO, 76
Olsen J, 27

O'Reilly M, 105
Orzechowski KM, 9
Osman M, 276
Osterman MJK, 21

P

Palmsten K, 99
Pappas A, 142
Passi Y, 98
Patel S, 44
Patil U, 232
Patra K, 253
Patrick SW, 15
Peevy KJ, 42
Peranteau WH, 5
Perrella SL, 177, 178
Piening B, 84
Platts-Mills TA, 209
Plumm B, 119
Poggi C, 71
Poncet A, 153, 155
Pourcyrous M, 195
Putnam AR, 198

R

Ramos Y, 157
Rattray BN, 235
Reilly MC, 47
Reisinger KW, 183
Rifas-Shiman SL, 209
Rios DR, 97
Roberts CL, 204, 206
Rodriguez CE, 44
Rogosch T, 130
Rohan AJ, 277
Rolland A, 93
Roposch A, 229
Rosenbaum PL, 187
Rosensvärd A, 160
Ruder J, 218
Russell GB, 217
Russo G, 218
Rysavy MA, 52, 225, 245

S

Salam RA, 69
Salas AA, 179
Salmannejad M, 228
Saluja S, 181
Sánchez B, 167
Sani M, 228
Satragno DS, 46
Sawyer A, 265
Scheer T, 73
Schneider A, 221, 222
Schuit E, 147
Schwab F, 84
Semberova J, 128
Shankar-Aguilera S, 93
Shankaran S, 149, 151
Shaw GM, 2
Shawyer AC, 187
Sheffield MJ, 203
Shimizu T, 13
Sibbel SE, 162
Simmer KN, 177, 178
Simms V, 251
Sinclair A, 55
Singh B, 188
Sithisarn T, 243
Sola A, 108
South AP, 194
Spencer-Smith MM, 247
Spittle AJ, 247
Staffler A, 215
Steinhorn RH, 126
Stevens DC, 231
Stevenson NJ, 139

T

Tamnes CK, 197
Taylor JA, 207
Thompson JL, 238
Thompson PA, 231
Tibussek D, 55
Tiwari TSP, 90
Tolia VN, 131
Törnell S, 50

V

Vain NE, 46
VanderVeen DK, 159
Varner MW, 25
Vendettuoli V, 120
Vergales BD, 115
Villar J, 249
Virgone C, 4

W

Wada Y, 171
Walker K, 255
Walker WA, 170
Wan MJ, 159
Wang H, 114
Wang J, 32
Wang Y, 261
Washburn LK, 217
Wenstrom KD, 1
Wiland EL, 194
Wilson DG, 133
Wluka AE, 261
Wolke D, 272, 273
Worwa C, 119
Wu CS, 27
Wu T-W, 141

Y

Yaish HM, 211, 213
Yau I, 55
Ye C, 193

Z

Zapata J, 112
Zhang P, 29
Zheng S, 29
Zibell R, 84
Ziegler J, 125

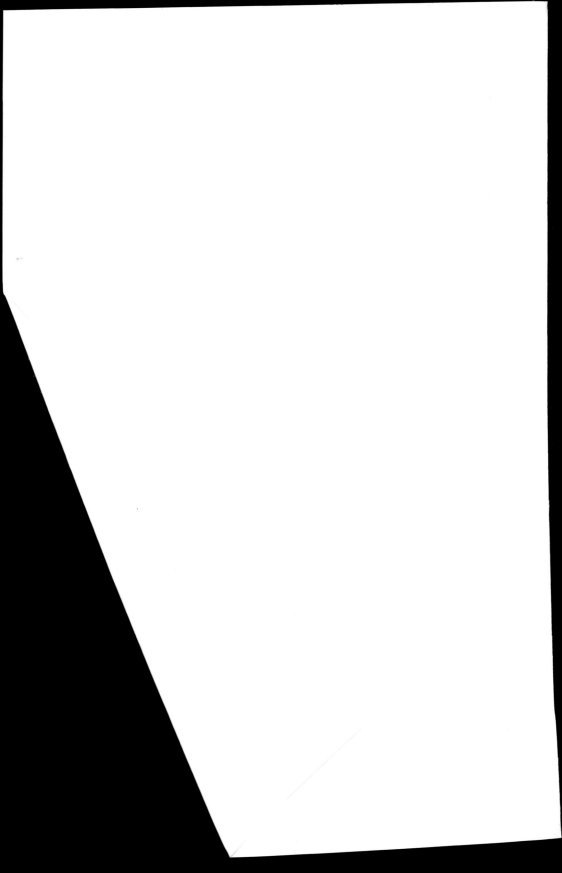

O'Reilly M, 105
Orzechowski KM, 9
Osman M, 276
Osterman MJK, 21

P

Palmsten K, 99
Pappas A, 142
Passi Y, 98
Patel S, 44
Patil U, 232
Patra K, 253
Patrick SW, 15
Peevy KJ, 42
Peranteau WH, 5
Perrella SL, 177, 178
Piening B, 84
Platts-Mills TA, 209
Plumm B, 119
Poggi C, 71
Poncet A, 153, 155
Pourcyrous M, 195
Putnam AR, 198

R

Ramos Y, 157
Rattray BN, 235
Reilly MC, 47
Reisinger KW, 183
Rifas-Shiman SL, 209
Rios DR, 97
Roberts CL, 204, 206
Rodriguez CE, 44
Rogosch T, 130
Rohan AJ, 277
Rolland A, 93
Roposch A, 229
Rosenbaum PL, 187
Rosensvärd A, 160
Ruder J, 218
Russell GB, 217
Russo G, 218
Rysavy MA, 52, 225, 245

S

Salam RA, 69
Salas AA, 179
Salmannejad M, 228
Saluja S, 181
Sánchez B, 167
Sani M, 228
Satragno DS, 46
Sawyer A, 265
Scheer T, 73
Schneider A, 221, 222
Schuit E, 147
Schwab F, 84
Semberova J, 128
Shankar-Aguilera S, 93
Shankaran S, 149, 151
Shaw GM, 2
Shawyer AC, 187
Sheffield MJ, 203
Shimizu T, 13
Sibbel SE, 162
Simmer KN, 177, 178
Simms V, 251
Sinclair A, 55
Singh B, 188
Sithisarn T, 243
Sola A, 108
South AP, 194
Spencer-Smith MM, 247
Spittle AJ, 247
Staffler A, 215
Steinhorn RH, 126
Stevens DC, 231
Stevenson NJ, 139

T

Tamnes CK, 197
Taylor JA, 207
Thompson JL, 238
Thompson PA, 231
Tibussek D, 55
Tiwari TSP, 90
Tolia VN, 131
Törnell S, 50

V

Vain NE, 46
VanderVeen DK, 159
Varner MW, 25
Vendettuoli V, 120
Vergales BD, 115
Villar J, 249
Virgone C, 4

W

Wada Y, 171
Walker K, 255
Walker WA, 170
Wan MJ, 159
Wang H, 114
Wang J, 32
Wang Y, 261
Washburn LK, 217
Wenstrom KD, 1
Wilard EL, 194
Wilson DG, 133
Wluka AE, 261
Wolke D, 272, 273
Worwa C, 119
Wu CS, 27
Wu T-W, 141

Y

Yaish HM, 211, 213
Yau I, 55
Ye C, 193

Z

Zapata J, 112
Zhang P, 29
Zheng S, 29
Zibell R, 84
Ziegler J, 125